TRENDS IN CERVICAL CANCER RESEARCH

TRENDS IN CERVICAL CANCER RESEARCH

HECTOR T. VARAJ
EDITOR

Nova Biomedical Books
New York

NOTICE TO THE READER

The Publisher has taken reasonable care in the preparation of this book, but makes no expressed or implied warranty of any kind and assumes no responsibility for any errors or omissions. No liability is assumed for incidental or consequential damages in connection with or arising out of information contained in this book. The Publisher shall not be liable for any special, consequential, or exemplary damages resulting, in whole or in part, from the readers' use of, or reliance upon, this material.

Independent verification should be sought for any data, advice or recommendations contained in this book. In addition, no responsibility is assumed by the publisher for any injury and/or damage to persons or property arising from any methods, products, instructions, ideas or otherwise contained in this publication.

This publication is designed to provide accurate and authoritative information with regard to the subject matter covered herein. It is sold with the clear understanding that the Publisher is not engaged in rendering legal or any other professional services. If legal or any other expert assistance is required, the services of a competent person should be sought. FROM A DECLARATION OF PARTICIPANTS JOINTLY ADOPTED BY A COMMITTEE OF THE AMERICAN BAR ASSOCIATION AND A COMMITTEE OF PUBLISHERS.

LIBRARY OF CONGRESS CATALOGING-IN-PUBLICATION DATA

New research on cervical cancer / Hector T. Varaj (editor).
    p. ; cm.
Includes bibliographical references and index.
ISBN 13: 978-1-60021-299-4
ISBN 10: 1-60021-299-9
1. Cervix uteri--Cancer--Research. 2. Papillomavirus diseases. I. Varaj, Hector T.
[DNLM: 1. Uterine Cervical Neoplasms--etiology. 2. Uterine Cervical Neoplasms--genetics. 3. Mass Screening. 4. Papillomavirus Infections--complications. WP 480 N5313 2006]
RC280.U8N49   2006
616.99'466--dc22   2006018918

Published by Nova Science Publishers, Inc. ✦ New York

CONTENTS

PREFACE

Cervical cancer is a malignancy of the cervix. Worldwide, it is the second most common cancer of women. It may present with vaginal bleeding but symptoms may be absent until the cancer is in advanced stages, which has made cervical cancer the focus of intense screening efforts utilizing the Pap smear. Most scientific studies point to human papillomavirus (HPV) infection is responsible for 90% of the cases of cervical cancer. There are 7 most common types of HPV - 16, 18, 31, 33, 42, 52 and 58. Types 16 and 18 being the most common cause of the cancer. Treatment is with surgery (including local exicision) in early stages and chemotherapy and radiotherapy in advanced stages of the disease. This book presents cutting edge research in this study of cervical cancer. This involves, new perspectives in pharmacological treatments, antihormonal agents, therapeutic trends for patients, nerve sparing treatments, antibodies in single chain formats, predictors of radiation response, lymphatic mapping and docetaxel labeling with radionuclides.

Chapter I - Cervical cancer, known to be a common female gynacologic cancer and a common cause of death in women, can nowadays be easily detected and prevented by appropriate measures. Recently, it has been estimated that approximately 420 women out of the 1400 women diagnosed with cervical cancer will die during 5 years from diagnosis. It is therefore been classified as the second most common cancer in women worldwide. Current understanding of apoptosis and regulators of apoptosis as well as their implication in carcinogenesis is considered critical to closely understand the molecular biology of cervical cancer. This, in turn, will enhance the development of treatment strategies that will modulate, transform and regulate essential factors involved in the pathogenesis of cervical cancer. This review addresses the pathogenesis of cervical cancer in humans with a special emphasis on the human papilloma virus as a predominant cause of cervical cancer in humans. Apoptosis, apoptotic and anti-apoptotic factors will be discussed. A special focus will be given to the role of Rel/NF-kappaB family of genes in the growth and chemotherapeutic treatment of the malignant HeLa cervical cells. Emphasis will be on Xrel3, being a cRel homologue. Finally, the importance of genetic testing and the currently available genetic testing tools will be further highlighted and described.

Chapter II - Cisplatin [CDDP]-based concomitant chemotherapy and irradiation is the standard treatment for advanced cervical cancer. A randomised Gynecologic Oncologic Group [GOG] study found no difference in pelvic failures between weekly CDDP or continuous infusion of 5- fluorouracil [5-FU] in combination with pelvic irradiation and brachytherapy, whereas there was an increase in distant failures in the 5- FU arm. CDDP-based neoadjuvant chemotherapy followed by radical hysterectomy with pelvic lymphadenectomy appears to be an effective therapeutic option for patients with stage Ib2-IIb disease. The combination of paclitaxel [TAX] + ifosfamide + CDDP is associated with a higher pathological optimal response rate than the combination of ifosfamide + CDDP, without any statistically significant benefit on overall survival. Neoadjuvant chemotherapy followed by conization and laparoscopic pelvic lymphadenectomy can represent an interesting therapeutic option, alternative to radical treachelectomy, to preserve fertility in accurately selected patients with early-stage cervical cancer. As for metastatic or recurrent disease, single-agent CDDP achieves an overall response rate of 18 to 31 % approximately, and recent phase III trials have shown response rates of 27% or 39% when CDDP has been combined with either TAX or topotecan, respectively. In particular, the combination of CDDP + topotecan has obtained a significantly better response rate, median progression-free survival, and median overall survival when compared with single- agent CDDP. However most of the responses to chemotherapy are partial and short-lived, thus encouraging the research of novel drugs and new combinations also including molecularly targeted agents (i.e. antiangiogenic agents, apoptosis inducers, and telomerase inhibitors).

Chapter III - Cervical cancer continues to be the major cause of cancer mortality in women in developing countries. Although detection routine screening programs have been implemented since 1975, an increased rate of new cases has also been detected. Some studies have demonstrated a relationship between HPV, cervical intraepithelial neoplasia, and invasive carcinoma of cervix. Additionally, it has been predicted that within 10 years, 66% of all dysplasia -without medical intervention- would progress to carcinoma in situ. It is important to bear these data in mind in order to be able to search new alternatives for cervical cancer treatment.

Cisplatin and its derivatives are important drugs in cervical cancer therapy. However, the administration of cisplatin is associated with serious side effects, including nephrotoxic and neurotoxic events. This issue has motivated the search for new agents or new regimens for cisplatin combinations with the purpose of increasing antitumoral activity and decreasing secondary events.

Among the chemosensitizer drugs, antihormonal agents have been used to modulate the cytotoxic activity of antineoplastic agents, principally in hormone-dependent cancers such as breast and prostate cancers. Although the normal cervix is known to respond to steroid sex hormones, hormonal treatments are not frequently employed in cervical carcinoma therapy. In fact, this carcinoma is traditionally considered not to respond to antihormonal therapy. We hypothesize that exposure to antihormonal agents for sensitizer cervical cancer cells to the antineoplastic treatment can be independent of steroid-receptors. The importance of antihormonal agents used to modulate the cytotoxic activity of anticancer drugs in cervical cancer will be explored in this article.

Chapter IV - In uterine cervical cancers, lymph node metastasis, recognized as a common form of metastasis, and recurrence after curative resection are critical to patient prognosis. The growth of secondarily spreading and initial recurrent lesions must be suppressed to improve patient prognosis. Chemotherapy and radiation are often not very specific to cancer cells, and it produces severe effects on even normal cells, especially bone marrow and renal cells. On the other hand, anti-angiogenic therapy is specific to the rapidly growing vascular endothelial cells in tumors, without any effect on slow growing vascular endothelial cells and other normal cells. Therefore, anti-angiogenic therapy should be an excellent strategy to suppress the growth of secondarily spreading and initial recurrent lesions. However, if an angiogenic factor is suppressed by anti-angiogenic therapy for a long period, another angiogenic factor might be induced by an alternately linked angiogenic pathway, which is recognized as tolerance. Therefore, we have studied the expression manner of angiogenic factors and one angiogenic transcription factor in uterine cervical cancers, and herein introduce novel gentle therapeutic trends for patients of uterine cervical cancers.

Chapter V - Five-year survival rates of over 90% have been reported after radical surgery for early cervical cancer. An increasing number of technical modifications have been suggested since this procedure was first described by Wertheim. Changes in the way radical surgery is viewed have led to the idea that benefits from oncological surgery must not be evaluated simply in terms of disease control but also by the functional end-results that may affect the quality of life.

Major causes of radical hysterectomy (RH) morbidity are disturbances in bladder, sexual and rectal functions. These negative sequelaes could derive from damage to the sympathetic and parasympathetic nervous systems.

Yabuki pioneered a nerve-sparing radical hysterectomy (NSRH) technique for cervical cancer to reduce morbidity. In Europe, some investigators have also begun practicing NS surgery, based on studies of the anatomy of the autonomic nervous system of the pelvis. Results have been encouraging.

Raspagliesi et al. reported on 23 cervical cancer patients treated by NSRH. The endpoints were the assessment of the feasibility of the NS technique and the rate of early bladder dysfunctions. Two (9%) patients were discharged with self-catheterization and one of them recovered the ability to void her bladder. They concluded that the NSRH technique was feasible, with promising results in terms of preventing early bladder dysfunction.

Recently, the same group of investigators decided to retrospectively compare the safety of the procedure with that of other types of RH. Accordingly class III NSRH was compared with other classes of RH in terms of incidence of early bladder dysfunctions and complications. One hundred and ten patients with cervical cancer were submitted to class II RH (group 1), class III NSRH (group 2) and class III RH (group 3). The groups did not differ significantly in terms of GIII/IV morbidity. Group 1 and 2 presented a prompt recover of bladder function, significantly different from that of the group 3. The class III NSRH is comparable to class II RH and superior to class III RH in terms of early bladder dysfunctions.

There is a deep gap between the information contained in anatomic textbooks and the reality of operating theatre. Despite the growing number of papers addressing the issue of NSRH, with the emergence of several techniques, no consensus has been reached. In this chapter we are going to discuss some landmarks of the neuroanatomy and neurophysiology, highlighting the most significant elements which support the performance of a NS technique in RH.

Chapter VI - The recognized causal relation between the "high risk" human papillomavirus (HPV) genotypes and the cervical neoplasia has allowed exploring new ways for prevention and treatment of the HPV-associated tumors. One challenge of the non-invasive cancer therapy is to generate tumor-specific strategies in order to achieve targeted efficacy and to limit side effects. Most of the cervical carcinomas are caused by the HPV genotype 16 (HPV16). The viral oncoproteins E6 and E7 are tumor-antigens that play a crucial role in the virus-associated tumorigenicity by inhibiting apoptosis and promoting cellular proliferation. They are considered as molecular targets for the development of therapeutic strategies against the HPV-associated tumors. A main goal of therapy is to impair the E6 and E7 oncogenic activity. Among the different strategies of protein "knock out" used in gene-therapy, intracellular antibodies have emerged as powerful tools. They offer the chance to interfere with the antigen function in a precise intracellular compartment by a restricted and targeted expression. Recently, the phage display technology has been used to select antibodies in single-chain format (scFv) against the E7 oncoprotein of the high-risk HPV16. One of these scFvs has been expressed in different compartments of HPV16-positive cells, showing a specific effect of proliferation inhibition when expressed in the nucleus and in the secretory compartment. The antiproliferative efficacy is, with high confidence, related to the antigen localization and to the scFv stability. The results obtained *in vitro* are encouraging and open the way to wide applications in gene therapy.

Chapter VII - Radiotherapy is the treatment of choice for locally advanced carcinoma of the cervix. Clinical trials have shown that the addition of concurrent platinum-based chemotherapy improves 3-year survival by 8-19%. Whilst the survival gains are impressive, the risk of serious late toxicity and its effect on long-term quality of life is a major concern. This is particularly important as a significant proportion of patients with advanced stage disease can be cured by radiotherapy alone. If techniques that have the potential to predict the response to radiotherapy could be identified, it may be possible to individualise treatment strategy in order to improve the therapeutic index of treatment. This could minimise morbidity in good prognosis patients (e.g. by omitting chemotherapy) whilst local control in poor prognosis patients could be maximised by intensification of treatment (e.g. by increasing the total dose, utilising alternative fractionation regimes, implementing novel sequencing of treatments, or by including additional modalities of treatment such as hypoxic cell sensitisers). For these predictive assays to be clinically useful, they would have to be reliable, reproducible and practical.

Several studies have attempted to identify potential predictive assays of radiation response in cervical cancer. Initial studies have investigated radiobiological predictors including cell proliferation kinetics, intrinsic tumour radiosensitivity and hypoxia. These assays assess the characteristics of the tumour and its microenvironment at the cellular level. Other studies have explored the potential of imaging techniques such as dynamic contrast enhanced magnetic resonance imaging, magnetic resonance spectroscopy and positron emission tomography, to predict radiation response. The early emphasis is on techniques for evaluating tumour vascular physiology and its effect on tumour oxygenation. More recently, new techniques and probes for studying other processes at the cellular and molecular levels have been developed, so-called molecular imaging. These techniques include immunohistochemistry assays as well as genomic and tissue microarray technology, and proteomics analyses.

This article reviews the published studies on predictive assays for cervix cancer and discusses their clinical relevance.

Chapter VIII - The concept for sentinel lymph node is one of the most significant and interesting achievements in surgical oncology in the last 10 years. The sentinel lymph node (SLN) is defined as the first draining lymph node of an anatomical region, so that a histologically negative SLN would predict the absence of tumor metastases in the other non-sentinel lymph nodes. The detection of SLN is currently a standard component of the surgical treatment of malignant melanoma, breast cancer and is a promising staging technique for patients with vulvar cancer. In cervical cancer SLN mapping is more recent and only a few studies have been published so far, those preliminary studies indicated that is a feasible technique. SLN are currently detected by the application of two techniques, blue dye and radioactive tracer technetium-99-m. The combination of the two techniques increases its sensitivity.

Lymph node status is a major prognostic factor for patients with cervical carcinoma and is a decision criterion for adjuvant therapy. Radical hysterectomy with pelvic and with or without paraaortic lymphadenectomy is the most commonly performed definitive surgical procedure for patients with early cervical cancer. In patients with early stage cervical cancer, pelvic node metastases are expected in 10-15% of the cases. This means that in the most favorable group of patients, the majority who undergo lymphadenectomy derive no benefit from the procedure yet must endure the associated increase in the risk of lymphocyst and lymphedema. Furthermore, in case of lymph node metastases, patients with cervical cancer could be treated with primary chemoradiotherapy without radical surgery.

SLN identification in early stage cervical cancer is feasible, and extends our knowledge on the pathways of lymphatic spread of cervical cancer. The use combination technique with of technetium-99-m-labeled nanocolloid and blue dye achieved in the majority of trials near than 100% detection rate, and a predictive negative value of 100%. This method currently allows a more precise examination of the most critical nodes through serial sections and immunohistochemistry. The results obtained at this moment with the use of lymphatic mapping and SLN biopsy in cervical cancer must be confirmed in multicentric and controlled trials before it could be considered a standard of care.

Chapter IX - Advanced carcinoma of the uterine cervix is conventionally treated with radiotherapy. Moreover, several lines of evidence show that chemotherapy administered concurrently with radiotherapy often overcomes developed resistance of cancer cells, thereby improving therapeutical efficiency of this treatment modality. Besides traditionally used cytostatics such as cisplatin or fluorouracil, taxanes represent a relatively new group of agents in this field, showing cytostatic activity against some advanced forms of cervical carcinoma. In addition, recently, it has been experimentally demonstrated that paclitaxel and docetaxel act as radiosensitizing agents, promisingly enhancing the cytotoxic effect of radiation in the treatment of cervical cancer. In this study, we present a new treatment modality in which chemotherapeutic agent (docetaxel) was labeled with radionuclide iodine 131 which is an emittor of β- and γ-radiation and its cytotoxic potential was evaluated and compared with non-labeled docetaxel on the HeLa Hep2 cell lines (chemosensitive and resistant) during 48 hours. Unlike non-labeled docetaxel which induced apoptosis in sensitive HeLa Hep-2 cell line only, the radiolabeled docetaxel was significantly more toxic in both cell lines, inducing cell cycle arrest, DNA damage and subsequent p53-dependent apoptosis as early as 12 hours after the beginning of the treatment. Our results thus show that ^{131}I-docetaxel holds a promising therapeutic potential whose mechanism as well as efficacy might be worth of further investigation both *in vitro* as well as *in vivo*.

In: Trends in Cervical Cancer
Editor: Hector T. Varaj, pp. 1-30
ISBN: 1-60021-299-9
© 2007 Nova Science Publishers, Inc.

Chapter I

CERVICAL CANCER RESEARCH: A CURRENT AND COMPREHENSIVE UPDATE

Marlene Shehata[*]

Department of Cellular and Molecular Medicine, Faculty of Medicine, University of Ottawa Heart Institute, Ottawa, Canada.

ABSTRACT

Cervical cancer, known to be a common female gynacologic cancer and a common cause of death in women, can nowadays be easily detected and prevented by appropriate measures. Recently, it has been estimated that approximately 420 women out of the 1400 women diagnosed with cervical cancer will die during 5 years from diagnosis. It is therefore been classified as the second most common cancer in women worldwide. Current understanding of apoptosis and regulators of apoptosis as well as their implication in carcinogenesis is considered critical to closely understand the molecular biology of cervical cancer. This, in turn, will enhance the development of treatment strategies that will modulate, transform and regulate essential factors involved in the pathogenesis of cervical cancer. This review addresses the pathogenesis of cervical cancer in humans with a special emphasis on the human papilloma virus as a predominant cause of cervical cancer in humans. Apoptosis, apoptotic and anti-apoptotic factors will be discussed. A special focus will be given to the role of Rel/NF-kappaB family of genes in the growth and chemotherapeutic treatment of the malignant HeLa cervical cells. Emphasis will be on Xrel3, being a cRel homologue. Finally, the importance of genetic testing and the currently available genetic testing tools will be further highlighted and described.

---

[*] Correspondence concerning this article should be addressed to Marlene Shehata Department of Cellular and Molecular Medicine, Faculty of Medicine, University of Ottawa Heart Institute, 40 Ruskin Street, K1Y-4W7, Ottawa, Canada. mshehata@ottawaheart.ca.

Keywords: Cervical cancer, NF-κB, HeLa cells, Xrel3, Human Papilloma Virus, apoptosis

INTRODUCTION

1.1. Carcinogenesis

1.1.1. Etiology of Cancer: Focus on Cervical Cancer

The process of oncogenesis or carcinogenesis presents itself as a mass of tissue whose growth is uncoordinated with that of adjacent normal tissue. Before the formation of that mass of tissue, some morphologic changes have to take place in the cell nucleus. These morphologic achanges cause the nuclei of affected cells to be crowded, overlapping, and with high mitotic activity. This forms the pre-malignant stage known as dysplasia. Dysplasia then progresses to neoplasia when cell growth disorders occur and abnormal masses of tissues are formed, known as neoplasms. Neoplasms can be benign or malignant. Neoplasms can also be classified as primary or metastatic depending on whether the tumor will remain localized to a particular organ, tissue space (primary neoplasm) or whether it will spread to adjacent tissues, lymph nodes, cavities and organs (metastatic). At the molecular level, carcinogenesis fundamentally arises from defects in the balance between the activity of proto-oncogenes, which promote cell survival, differentiation and proliferation, and tumor suppressor genes, which regulate the cell cycle. DNA damage and repair occurs normally in every living cell. DNA damage occurs at a rate of 50,000 to 500,000 molecular lesions per cell per day. DNA damage occurs due to normal metabolic processes inside the cell, and it compromises the integrity and accessibility of essential information in the genome. Depending on the type of damage inflicted on the DNA's double helical structure, the appropriate repair strategy has evolved to restore lost information. Once damage is identified, and further localized, specific DNA repair molecules are summoned to, and bind at or near the site of damage, inducing other molecules to bind and form a complex that enables actual repair to occur. When the rate of DNA damage exceeds that of repair, accumulation of DNA damage and defects might trigger the initiation of cancer (Furomoto and Irahara, 2002, Munoz *et al.*, 2003, Garland, 2002).A single unrepaired lesion to a critical cancer-related gene (such as tumor suppressor gene) can have catastrophic consequences for an individual.

Uterine cervical cancer is a serious gynecologic malignancy in women. It affects that part of the uterus attached to the top of the vagina.There are two main types of cervical cancer, squamous cell carcinoma and adenocarcinoma, based on the type of cells that become cancerous. It is known that almost 90% of cervical cancer cases reported arises from squamous cells covering the cervix (squamous cell carcinoma). The remaining 10% of cases arise from the glandular cells that lead to the uterus (adenocarcinoma). Like other types of cancer, the development of cervical cancer is gradual and manifests itself at the cellular level as dysplasia. In other words, when the combined actions of a group of carcinogens cause the normal, physiological events to go awry, the pre-malignant dysplasia state will be the expected outcome (Josefson, 1999). Dysplasia can ultimately resolve without treatment. This usually occurs in young women. It might also progress to cervical carcinoma in situ (CIS), when the cancer does not spread to adjacent tissues and is only localized to a specific area.

Microinvasive cervical carcinoma occurs when the cancer spreads few millimeters around the affected area, without lymph node involvement or further spreading to blood vessels. It might take years for the dysplasia to progress to carcinoma in situ or microinvasive carcinoma. However, once progression to any of the above mentioned conditions occur, then further spreading to neighbouring tissues, organs, lymph nodes and blood vessels becomes faster. Poor prognosis is usually associated with positive pelvic lymph nodes, indicating that the tumor cells have become metastatic (Kim *et al.,* 2003). High morbidity of the disease is highly related to the conservative attitude towards Pap smear (Walboomers et al., 1999). Furthermore, the high infection rate with human papillomavirus among affected women has greatly contributed to the poor prognosis of the disease (Walboomers et al., 1999).

Recent studies have demonstrated that estrogen, which is the female sex hormone, might have a contributory role in increasing vaginal epithelium proliferation and thus promoting the malignant transformation of the squamous and columnar cells at the junction of the cervical and vaginal epithelium (Park *et al.,* 2003). In a recent report by Nair and other co-workers, it has been estimated that 35% of the 19 cases of cervical carcinoma tested showed a positive expression of aromatase enzyme (Nair et al., 2005). This enzyme is responsible for converting androgen to estrogen. On the other hand, aromatase was neither detected in normal cervical tissue (n = 17) nor precancerous tissues (n = 42). Increased aromatase was associated with increased estrogen receptor (ER) levels suggesting that estrogen signaling via the ER might play a role in tumor growth (Nair et al., 2005). Levels of estrogen are significantly higher in a dose-dependant fashion in cervical cancer patients as compared to controls (Wang et al., 2005). Furthermore, the degree of proliferation of SiHa cervical cancer cells was directly proportional to the duration of estrogen therapy (Brewer et al., 2005). The previously mentioned results support the proposed theory of estrogen contribution in cervical mailgnancy. Besides estrogen involvement, infection by the Human Papilloma Virus, HPV, is a necessary requirement for cervical cancer, but not all women infected by this virus develop cervical cancer (Castellsague *et al.,* 2002). Some HPV infections, for instance are associated with benign proliferation or wart formation. Recent studies by Ueda and other co-workers, demonstrated the ability of HPV to provoke local inflammation that can ultimately lead to drug resistance encountered in uterine cervical cancer (Ueda et al., 2006). In the next section, we will look in depth on the involvement of HPV in carcinogenesis and its role in the pathogenesis of cervical cancer.

1.1.2. Human Papilloma Virus (HPV)

HPVs are small DNA viruses. HPVs are implicated in the mucosal and epithelial infections that may range from a benign lesion to a malignant carcinoma (Garland, 2002). HPV has also been reported to be associated with anal, genital cancers as well as some head and neck cancers (Heilmann and Kreienberg, 2002, Sisk and Robertson, 2002). There are more than 100 different types of HPVs, most of them are harmless. About 30 of these 100 different kinds of HPV are known to be transmitted sexually by sexual contact. Some types of HPVs are associated with genital warts (Sisk and Robertson, 2002). Genital warts are small bumps localized in the genital areas of men and women including the vagina, cervix, vulva (area outside of the vagina), penis, and rectum. Among the many different kinds of HPVs reported, only 15 kinds cause virtually all kinds of cervical cancer (Castle et al., 2006).

Recent studies have shown 13 to 15 different types of HPV to be associated with carcinogenesis (Munoz *et al.,* 2003, Castle et al., 2006). Many patients with HPV infection remain symptom free. However, infection with high-risk HPV is known to be the most common cause of cervical cancer (Ghim *et al.,* 2002). That's why HPVs are classified into high and low risk viruses based on their virulence and potential for inducing diseases. The most widely known factors associated with HPV are the E6 and E7 oncoproteins known to interact with p53 and Rb tumor suppressors respectively (Furumoto and Irahara, 2002). The interaction of E6 and E7 with these cellular proteins results in their suppression (Ghim *et al.,* 2002), thus disrupting the normal physiological process of programmed cell death in response to DNA damage (See Figure 1) (Finzer *et al.,* 2002). The net result will be cell growth disorders leading to overproliferation and mass formation. HPV type 38 E6 and E7 oncogenes stabilize wild type p53, which in turn activates the transcription of DeltaNp73, an isoform of the p53-related protein p73. This isoform then inhibits the ability of p53 to transcribe genes involved in apoptosis (Accardi et al., 2006) resulting in immortal cells. The high risk HPV 16 and HPV 18 are associated with malignant transformation and carcinogenesis in 85% of the diagnosed cervical cancer cases (Garland, 2002). HPV-16 E6 and not E7 promotes the transactivation of survivin promotor (Borbely et al., 2006). Survivin not only serves as a significant inhibitor of apoptosis, but also it controls the cell division (Borbely et al., 2006). In the presence of carcinogens, therefore, the accumulation of DNA damage without apoptosis is presumed to lead to cancer.

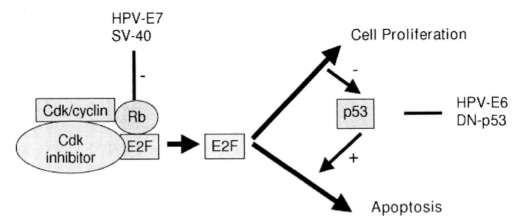

Figure 1: A schematic illustration of RB/p53 interactions to regulate cell cycle and apoptosis Cell cycle transition from G_1-S phase is mediated by RB interactions with the E2F transcription factor family, which is considered an important regulator of the cell cycle. Growth factors lead to the phosphorylation of RB in late G_1 phase by cdk/cyclin. This is followed by the release of E2F, allowing transcriptional activation of E2F target genes, which promotes S-phase entry and cell proliferation. HPV E7 and Simian Virus 40 (SV40) promote the release of E2F from RB, whereas HPV E6 and the dominant negative, DN-p53 inhibit p53 activity leading to cell proliferation (Reproduced with permission from Cancer Cell International Copyright (Shehata et al., 2005).

Prevalence of carcinogenic HPV increased among young middle aged women as compared to old women who harboured the non carcinogenic types of HPV (Castle et al., 2006). The mechanism of action of HPV in the pathogenesis of cervical cancer is proposed to be via suppressing the dendritic cells. Dendritic cells are present in tissues with high antigenic exposure like the skin and mucous membranes. HPVs suppress dendritic cells significantly and thus interfere with antigen handling of the immune system (Jimenez-Flores et al., 2006).

It should be made clear that viral infection by itself does not cause cancer. It is the interaction of the viral genome with host genes that disrupts the normal cell cycle and transforms the cell into a pre-malignant state. For instance, some viruses might interact with specific genes (like tumor suppressor genes mentioned above) in the host cells, switching some systems on or off, thus leaving the cell free to divide in an uncontrolled way and raising the risk of cancer (Zur Hausen *et al.,* 2003).

Other cellular proteins may be affected by HPV infection as well. For instance, cervical cancer cell lines showed overexpression of the anti-apoptotic protein BAG-1, which might contribute to its malignant proliferation (Yang *et al.,* 1998, Shehata et al., 2004, 2005). Recent studies have assessed the potential for developping prophylactic and therapeutic vaccines by delivering the E6 and E7 oncogenes in nucleic acid form by utilizing viral or bacterial vectors (Govan, 2005). This approach was further investigated by Shillitoe who encouraged targetting HPVs for cancer gene therapy (Shillitoe, 2005). Therefore, understanding the molecular mechanisms leading to this disease will be of importance for generating means for its early detection and possible prevention and treatment.

1.2. Apoptosis: Definition and Regulators

1.2.1. Definition

The term apoptosis is derived from the Greek word that signifies the dropping of leaves from the trees. Apoptosis, or programmed cell death, is the process by which the organism can protect its integrity by destroying threatening cells. Apoptosis was first described in 1972 by John Kerr, Andrew Wyllie and Alistair Currie as a curious form of cell death (Kerr et al., 1972). It now became the most intensively studied topic in modern biology. It is clearly different from necrosis which usually occurs as a result of acute cell injury when inflammatory cells rush in to clear away the debris. Apoptosis is a clean, quick and predictable sequence of structural changes causing a cell to shrink and be rapidely digested by neighbouring cells. It is orchestrated by a highly organized group of signaling pathway proteins (for review see Miller and Marx, 1998; Fiers *et al.,* 1999). Although, long ago biologists predicted that cell suicide plays an important role in tissue sculpture within developping embryos, Kerr et al in 1972 were the first to report that apoptosis also occurred in mature cells. Over the last 15 years, scientists have shown that apoptosis plays an integral part in organism development by molding neural and immune systems and shaping tissue specificity. They also demonstrated that apoptosis maintains the balance between cell death and renewal by getting rid of excess, damaged and abnormal cells. In 1988, the first link between apoptosis and cancer was established when David Vaux and colleagues demonstrated the blockade of death of B cells in follicular lymphoma by the effect of *bcl-2* gene (Vaux et al., 1988). Since then, scientists gathered considerable information about *bcl-2* gene, being a suicide "brake" gene. Bcl-2 protein production has been identified in several cancers including lymphomas, B-cell leukemias, colon, prostate, neuroblastoma and cervical cancers.

Apoptosis can be triggered by internal or external factors (for review, see Miller and Marx, 1998). When a cell is triggered by an internal stimulus like reactive oxygen species, the Bcl-2 protein displayed on the outer surface of the mitochondria will activate a related protein known as Bax (See figure 2). Bax will then form holes on the outer membrane of the mitochondria causing a leak of cytochrome c from the mitochondria (for review, see Green and Reed, 1998). The released cytochrome c binds to the protein Apaf-1 ("apoptotic protease activating factor-1"). This process utilizes the energy provided by ATP. These complexes then aggregate forming apoptosomes which then bind and activate caspase-9. Caspase-9 belongs to a class of protein-splitting enzymes called caspases, which are activated upon detection of DNA damage and eventually cause cell death (for review, see Thornberry and. Lazebnik, 1998). Caspase-9 activates caspases-3 and 7 creating a cascade of proteolytic activity. This will ultimately lead to digestion of structural cellular proteins and degradation of chromosomal DNA and finally phagocytosis of cells (for review, see Green and Reed, 1998). The control of programmed or physiological cell death acts as a protective mechanism for the organism because accumulation of DNA damage without concomitant repair could lead to the development of cancer, while unregulated apoptosis can cause autoimmune diseases.

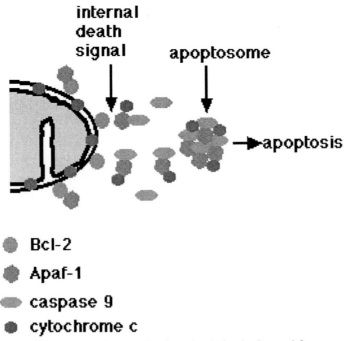

Figure 2: Illustration of the process of apoptosis after stimulation by internal factor.

On the other hand, when a cell is triggered by an external factor (eg. Xray, UV light), the pathway leading to apoptosis is different from that mentioned above. Fas and TNF receptor are integral proteins in the membrane with their receptor domains exposed at the surface of the cell (for review, see Ashkenazi and Dixit, 1998). Upon stimulation, binding of the complementary death activator (FasL and TNF respectively) transmits a signal to the cytoplasm that finally leads to activation of caspase 8 (See figure 3). Caspase 8 (like caspase 9) initiates a cascade of caspase activation leading to phagocytosis of the cell.

A third and final mechanism by which the cell can undergo apoptosis usually involve a different pathway than those previously mentioned. It involves apoptosis-inducing factor (AIF) and it is the mechanism by which neurons and perhaps other cells undergo self-destruction. AIF is present in the intermembrane space of the mitochondria. When a death stimulus is perceived by the cell, AIF is released from the mitochondria in a manner similar to that of cytochrome release. After its release, it translocates to the nucleus, and binds to the DNA triggering DNA damage and ultimately cell death.

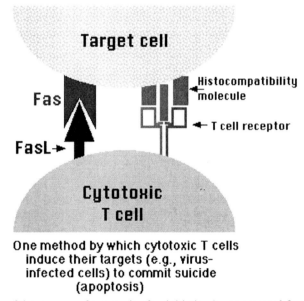

One method by which cytotoxic T cells induce their targets (e.g., virus-infected cells) to commit suicide (apoptosis)

Figure 3: Illustration of the process of apoptosis after initiation by an external factor.

The process of apoptosis is essential in stopping the uncontrolled proliferation of cells (for review, see Nicholson, 2000). Any defects in this dynamic process may eventually lead to the development of benign proliferative lesions or even malignant tumors (for review, see Nicholson, 2000).

As mentioned above, David Vaux and co-workers in 1988 established the first link between apoptosis and cancer. Since then, apoptosis has been associated with the topic of cancer. For example, HPVs that are known to cause cervical cancer presumably act by inhibiting apoptosis. This is mainly through the E6 oncoprotein that binds to and inactivate the apoptosis promotor protein p53. Epstein Barr Virus (EBV) implicated in mononucleosis and some kinds of lymphomas has a mechanism of action involving the apoptosis pathway. EBV is proposed to work by producing a protein similar to Bcl-2. This protein enhances the cell's own expression of Bcl-2. Bcl-2 promotes further cell proliferation by hindering apoptosis. Even without viral involvement, the process of carcinogenesis has been significantly dependant on inhibiting the apoptosis pathway. For example, Lymphomas and B-cell leukemias are know to express high levels of Bcl-2. Bcl-2 gene then translocate to the enhancer region for more antibody production. Melanoma, which is considered a serious skin cancer, inhibits the expression of the gene encoding Apaf-1 thus it avoids apoptosis.

Apoptosis acts as a double-edged sword. Despite its importance in restricting cell proliferation and maintaining constant cell number, excessive apoptosis is associated with stroke, Alzheimer's disease and other neurodegenerative disorders (for review, see Yuan and Yankner, 2000). Damaged neurons in these disorders commit suicide inappropriately. Alzheimer's disease, for instance, was found to be associated with a genetic component that involves mutations in the chromosomes (1, 14, 21) as well as the tau gene on chromosome 17 and results in unscheduled or unregulated death of brain cells (Rich *et al.*, 2000).

Understanding the details and the signaling pathways of this phenomenon might be helpful in manipulating and intervening in the process of apoptosis. Apoptosis is required to restrict cell proliferation and to maintain a constant cell number. Attempts to suppress apoptosis, however, may be useful to treat neurodegenerative disorders, while attempts to activate apoptosis may be useful in disorders involving overproliferation.

1.2.2. Regulators of Apoptosis

Signaling for apoptosis occurs through a variety of mechanisms that involve multiple independent pathways (Strasser et al., 2000). The triggering events can be from outside or inside the cell as highlighed in the previous subsection. The apoptosis signaling pathways converge on a common machinary aiming at destroying the cell, and this is activated by caspases. Dismantling and removal of dead cells by proteolysis is followed by phagocytosis by neighbouring cells (Strasser et al., 2000). Four of the most important factors that regulate apoptosis are p53, the caspases, the Bcl-2 family of proteins and PARP (Reed, 1997; Packham *et al.*, 1997; for review, see Green, 2000).

Caspases are the executioners of cell death. They receive the signals that enable them to initiate apoptosis (for review, see Thornberry and Lazebnik, 1998; Savill and Fadok, 2000). All caspases share a similar structure that consists of three domains: an NH_2-terminal peptide (prodomain), a large subunit (approximately 20 kD) and a small subunit (approximately 10 kD) (for review, see Hengartner, 2000). Caspases are expressed as procaspases, which undergo cleavage to the 2 subunits mentioned above (for review, see Meier *et al.*, 2000). Cleavage of caspases is a sign of active apoptosis. The large and small subunits then associate to form a heterodimer (Boise *et al.*, 1995; Reed, 1997).

The exact mechanism of action of caspases is still unknown. However, several studies have shown that caspases exert both direct and indirect actions on the cell (for review, see Evan et *al.*, 1998). Direct action of caspases can be exemplified by their ability to act on cell structural integrity by destroying the nuclear lamina (Evan *et al.*, 1998) and cleaving the proteins responsible for regulating the cytoskeleton (Boyd *et al.*, 1995; Evan *et al.*, 1998). Indirect action of caspases is via their ability to inhibit the proteins that promote cell survival and growth (for review, see Hengartner, 2000). Among these proteins is the Bcl-2 family of proteins, which are cleaved by caspases resulting in inactivation of the Bcl-2 proteins and the release of a fragment that has a direct apoptotic effect (for review, see Evan *et al.*, 1998).

Initiator caspases are the first to be activated and include caspase-2, 8, 9 and 10. These cleave and activate the effector caspases (3, 6, 7), which cleave, degrade or activate other cellular proteins. Some caspases (1, 4, 5, 11, 12, 13, 14) have a specialized role in inflammation and their activation leads to the processing of pro-inflammatory cytokines (for review, see Hengartner, 2000). Caspase activation can be mediated by intrinsic factors such as Bcl-2 on the mitochondrial membrane.The Bcl-2 family of proteins has several members with various functions (for review, see Nicholson, 2000). The Bcl-2 gene family comprises pro-apoptotic and anti-apoptotic proteins sharing one or more Bcl-2 homology (BH) domains (Reed, 1997). For example, bcl-2 and bcl-XL are anti-apoptotic, while others such as Bad or Bax are pro-apoptotic. The sensitivity of cells to apoptotic stimuli can depend on the balance of pro- and anti-apoptotic bcl-2 proteins (Christensen *et al.,* 1999; Stuart *et al.,* 1998; Yang *et al.,* 1998). When there is an excess of pro-apoptotic proteins the cells are more sensitive to apoptosis, when there is an excess of anti-apoptotic proteins the cells will tend to be less sensitive (for review, see Hengartner, 2000). However, Bax, which promotes apoptosis (Christensen *et al.,* 1999) translocates to the mitochondrial membrane and releases cytochrome c, which can initiate the apoptotic cascade (for review, see Ferrer and Planas, 2003). It also competes for binding with Bcl-2 and with other members of the Bcl-2 superfamily of proteins (for review, see Ferrer and Planas, 2003). Such heterodimerization between anti-apoptotic and pro-apoptotic members of this family is very common and is considered a regulatory mechanism for the decision to undergo apoptosis (Reed, 1997). Thus, the balance between Bcl-2 and Bax is essential for the determination of the apoptotic potential of the cells, in which high apoptotic activity is often associated with a low Bcl-2/Bax level ratio (Reed, 1997). BAG-1 has been shown to provide an anti-apoptotic effect. Its overexpression in cervical cancer suppressed apoptosis both independently and by increasing Bcl-2 protective activity, which further increased the resistance of cervical carcinoma to the effect of DNA-damaging agents (Yang *et al.,* 1998; Naishiro, 1999).

The tumor suppressor protein p53 has numerous functions (Rosenthal *et al.,* 1998). Its principle role, however, is as a transcriptional regulator required for the expression of a number of genes involved in cell cycle regulation and apoptosis. The gene encoding p53 can be mutated in many forms of cancer including cervical, uterine, adenocarcinoma, adrenal and colorectal cancers. In cervical cancer, mutation patterns of p53 may vary from point mutation to deletion to base-pair alteration, however 30% of the cases showed a higher percentage of Guanine-Cytosine complementary base pairs compared to the Adenine-Thymine complementary base pairs suggesting that alteration in the base-pairing sequence is the major mutation pattern recognized in p53 (Rosenthal *et al.,* 1998). A recent clinical study showed that the overexpression of p53 in cisplatin-treated tumors might be associated with resistance of the tumor to further cell death and apoptosis (Nakayama *et al.,* 2003).

MDM2 is a p53-regulated protein that has a role in the translocation of p53 from the nucleus and enhances its proteosomal degradation (Rich, Allen and Wyllie, 2000). Therefore, increased levels of MDM-2 and subsequent low levels of p53 are associated with increased cell growth and proliferation. The p53 tumor suppressor protein can also be targeted for degradation by the E6 oncogene of the Human Papilloma virus (HPV), thus promoting neoplastic proliferations (refer to Figure 1.1) (Rosenthal *et al.,* 1998).

Poly (ADP-ribose) polymerase, PARP, has recently been found to promote cell death, but the exact mechanism of action of PARP remains largely obscure. Many cellular enzymes were found to contain the PARP catalytic subunit, but they have different cellular localizations (Nicoletti and Stella, 2003). Because PARP activation consumes much cellular energy, detection of abnormally high levels of PARP in cells might indicate excessive energy consumption and cellular exhaustion (for review, see Rich *et al.*, 2000). PARP is also known as an apoptosis-inducing factor and high levels of PARP are detected following DNA damage. Thus, this group of enzymes might also be involved in DNA repair, as well as apoptotic responses of the cells (for review, see Rich *et al.*, 2000).

1.3. Rel/NF-κB family

1.3.1. Introduction

Various studies have allowed the characterisation of a family of eukaryotic transcription factors with basic impact on oncogenesis, embryonic development and differentiation including immune response and acute phase reaction. NF kappa B is induced in response to many different noxious agents. It is activated by a myriad of agents including cytokines like IL-1 and TNF-alpha, bacterial LPS, viral infection and certain viral proteins such as HTLV-1 Tax, LMP1 of EBV, antigen receptor cross linking on T and B lymphocytes, calcium ionophores, phorbol esters, UV radiation and others. The genes regulated by NF kappa B family of transcription factors are just as diverse as the activators and include those involved in immune function, inflammatory response, cell adhesion, cell growth, and cell death. First characterized in mature B and plasma cells as a nuclear protein that binds specifically to a 10-bp sequence in the kappa intronic enhancer, NF kappa B has now been demonstrated in virtually all cells. In most cells with the exception of mature B cells, macrophages and some neurons, NF kappa B remains dormant in the cytoplasm bound to its inhibitor, I kappa B. Treatment with various agents leads to the dissociation of the inhibitor and the translocation of the free NF kappa B to the nucleus.

NF kappa B was originally identified as a B lymphocyte nuclear factor binding to a site in the immunoglobulin kappa light chain enhancer. It is now recognized as a pleiotropic transcription factor binding to many cellular and viral gene promoters. NF kappa B is recognized for its central role in immunological processes via the expression of a wide variety of immune response genes. Recent studies have provided evidence for the involvement of NF kappa B in growth control of certain tumors. NF kappa B is maintained in the cytoplasm of the cell by the inhibitor kappa B (I kappa B) which tightly regulates the nuclear expression and biological function of NF kappa B. The speed of induction and its ubiquitous expression makes NF kappa B an ideal regulator of rapid-response genes. NF kappa B family of transcription factors are homo- and heterodimeric complexes formed from combinations of members of the Rel family of proteins. The Rel family of proteins belong to the v-rel oncogene found in the Reticuloendotheliosis Virus Strain T (RevT) and are characterized by having a common Rel homology domain (RHD) which consists of 300 amino acids in length. Specific sites within the RHD are responsible for DNA binding to kappa B sites, dimerization with other Rel family proteins, and interaction with I kappa B. The C-terminal portion of the RHD contains a group of positively charged amino acids that function as the nuclear localization signal (NLS). There are five mammalian members of the Rel family of proteins. These include c-Rel, NF kappa B1 (p105/p50), NF kappa B2 (p100/p52), RelA (p65), and RelB. NFATp(nuclear factor of activated T cells) is considered to be related to the Rel family of proteins as it has a region of 430 amino acids that shares 17% amino acid identity to RelA (p65). There also appears to be some functional similarities between p65 and NFATp since both these proteins can interact with c-fos and c-jun.

Theoretically, five members of the Rel family proteins can form almost any possible combination of homo or heterodimers although only certain combinations have been detected in vivo. The classic and most well studied NF kappa B molecule is a heterodimer of p50/p65 subunits. This heterodimer is the most abundant complex and is found in virtually all cell types. Heterodimers of p50/p65 are rapidly translocated to the nucleus following cellular activation and bind the consensus sequence 5'GGGRNNYYCC3'. The transactivation function in vivo is mediated by RelA (p65), RelB, and c-Rel which contain transactivation domains in their C-terminal domains, while the p50 and p52 subunits primarily serve as DNA binding subunits. Transcriptionally active complexes are usually heterodimers consisting of p50 or p52 in combination with one of the transactivating subunits (p65, c-Rel, or RelB), while homodimers of p50 correlate with transcriptional repression. Each of the heterodimers exhibit unique properties including cell type specificity, DNA binding site preference, differential interactions with I kappa B isoforms, differential activation requirements, and kinetics of activation, thus being capable of regulating gene expression in a uniquely specific manner. For example, in pre-B cells the active NF kappa B complexes are primarily dimers of p50/p65 while the constitutive form of NF kappa B in mature B cells are c-Rel/p50 dimers. While p50/p65 dimers rapidly appear in the nucleus following stimulation, dimers of p50/c-Rel exhibit a more delayed response and accumulate in the nucleus more slowly.

The Rel/NF-kappa B family is a group of structurally-related, tightly-regulated transcription factors that control the expression of a multitude of genes involved in key cellular and organismal processes. The Rel/NF-kappa B signal transduction pathway is misregulated in a variety of human cancers, especially ones of lymphoid cell origin, due either to genetic changes (such as chromosomal rearrangements, amplifications, and mutations) or to chronic activation of the pathway by epigenetic mechanisms. Constitutive activation of the Rel/NF-kappa B pathway can contribute to the oncogenic state in several ways, for example, by driving proliferation, by enhancing cell survival, or by promoting angiogenesis or metastasis. In many cases, inhibition of Rel/NF-kappa B activity reverses all or part of the malignant state. Thus, the Rel/NF-kappa B pathway has received much attention as a focal point for clinical intervention. NF-kappa B is a transcription factor that consists of 2 subunits: a 50 kilodalton subunit (p50) and a 65 kilodalton subunit (p65, also known as RelA). The generation of knockouts of members of the NF-kappa B/I kappa B family has allowed the study of the roles of these proteins in normal development and physiology. The first identified member of the nuclear factor-kappa (κ) B (Rel/NF-κB) family was a protein found to be associated with a decameric oligonucleotide sequence in the enhancer element of the immunoglobulin kappa light chain in B-lymphocytes (Verma et al., 1995; Baeuerle and Baltimore, 1988; Govind, 1999). The Rel/NF-κB family is now known to be made up of a plethora of transcriptional regulators which share a 300 amino acid terminal domain called the Rel homology domain (RHD) (Castranova et al., 1998; Gerondakis et al., 1999). This RHD in turn comprises the DNA binding domain, nuclear localization signal (NLS), dimerization domains and the IκB binding domain (See Figure 4) (Liou and Baltimore, 1993; May and Ghosh, 1998). Members of this family include p50, p52, p65, c-

Rel, v-Rrel, RelB, and the Drosophila proteins, Dorsal and Dif. Most of these transcription factors bind as homo- and heterodimers to the consensus a DNA sequence motif termed kappa-B according the first described factor-binding sequence motif located in the immunoglobulin kappa light chain enhancer region (Verma et al., 1995). Mice devoid of *p65* generated by targeted "knock-out" gene disruption resulted in defects in fetal development localized to the spleen and liver. However, knock-out mice devoid of *p105/p50* expression showed no defects during their development. Lyt-10 (p100), including p100 and p52, are required in spleen development. c-rel knock-out mice showed defects in the proliferation of B and T cells. relB knock-out mice showed defects in thymus development. Dorsal, which is involved in the formation of the dorsal-ventral axis of the fruit fly Drosophila (Liou and Baltimore, 1993).

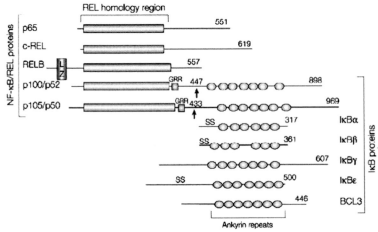

Figure 4: NF-κB and IκB proteins (Adapted from Karin *et al.*, 2002). A schematic representation of various domains in (Rel)/nuclear factor of kappa B (NF-κB) proteins including the Rel Homology Domain, RHD, which comprises the DNA binding domain, nuclear localization signal (NLS), dimerization domains and the IκB binding domain. (Rel)/nuclear factor of κB (NF-κB) proteins include those that do not require proteolytic processing and those that do require proteolytic processing. The first group consists of: RelA (known as p65), c-Rel and RelB and the second group includes NF-κB1 (known as p105) and NF-κB2 (known as p100), which further produce p50 and p52 proteins, respectively. These two groups dimerize, the most commonly detected NF-κB dimer is p50–RelA. RelA is responsible for most of NF-κB transcriptional activity due to the presence of a strong transcriptional activation domain. p50–c-Rel dimers are less abundant. Both p50–RelA and p50–c-Rel dimers are regulated by interactions with the inhibitor of κB (IκB) proteins, which cause their cytoplasmic localization. RelB, however, mostly associates with p100 and the p100–RelB dimers are exclusively cytoplasmic. Proteolytic processing of p100 results in the release of p52–RelB dimers, which translocate to the nucleus. RelB, unlike RelA and c-Rel, can function as an activator or repressor (May and Ghosh, 1998, Verma *et al.,* 1998).

Rel/nuclear factor of kappa B (NF-κB) proteins include those that do not require proteolytic processing and those that do require proteolytic processing. The first group consists of: RelA (known as p65), c-Rel and RelB. The second group includes NF-κB1 (known as p105) and NF-κB2 (known as p100), which further produce p50 and p52 proteins, respectively (See Figure 4). Members of these two groups pair with each other with the most commonly detected NF-κB being a heterodimer of p50 and RelA. RelA is responsible for most of NF-κB's transcriptional activity due to the presence of a strong transcriptional activation domain at its C-terminus. p50–c-Rel dimers are less abundant.

Both p50–RelA and p50–c-Rel dimers are regulated by interactions with the inhibitor of κB (IκB) proteins, which cause their cytoplasmic localization. RelB, however, mostly associates with p100 and the p100–RelB dimers are exclusively cytoplasmic. Proteolytic processing of p100 results in the release of p52–RelB dimers, which then translocate to the nucleus. RelB, unlike RelA and c-Rel, can function as an activator or repressor (May and Ghosh, 1998, Verma *et al.*, 1998). Of the above-mentioned proteins, only p50 and p52 are produced from the cytoplasmic precursors p105 and p100, in the presence of ATP as an energy source (May and Ghosh, 1998). However, the other members contain trans-activation domains and can act as activators or inhibitors of transcription based on dimers containing or lacking trans-activation domains (See Figure 1.3) (for review, see Beg and Baldwin 1993).

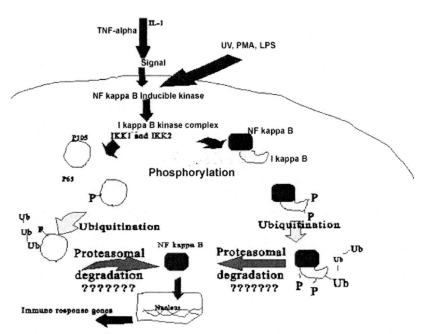

Figure 5: The steps involved in the activation of NF-κB family of transcription factors. Activators of NF-κB like TNF-alpha, PMA, UV or LPS activate the NF-κB inducible kinase, which in turn phosphorylates at least IKK1 (I kappa B kinase-alpha) and sometimes IKK2 (I kappa B kinase-beta) in the I kappa B-kinase complex. Activators of NF-κB may directly activate the kinase complex as well. This may be followed by phosphorylation of the p105/p65 complex by the kinase complex, which is in turn followed by ubiquitination, proteasomal degradation and the nuclear translocation of NF kappa B. Inside the nucleus; NF kappa B promotes the transcription of immune response genes. The "??????" indicates the possibility of lowered translocation and consequent activation of NF-κB, which occurs in various diseases (Adapted from Ponnappan, 1998).

The functions of the Rel/NF-κB family of proteins are strongly related to the target genes that contain the response elements for the protein (Grilli *et al.*, 1993; Collins *et al.*, 1995; for review, see Verma *et al.*, 1995; Wang *et al.*, 1999). For example, κB response elements are localized in *IL-2, IL-2R, Ig κ* and *MHC Classes (I) and (II) genes*, and here the Rel/NF-κB family of proteins function in modulating the immune system responses by binding to these target sequences and recruiting other immune system and inflammatory reaction mediators (See Figure 5 and Table 2). However, the Rel/NF-κB family of proteins is also directly involved in inflammatory reactions and acute phase responses when the κB binding sites are found in the regulatory sequences for the *IL-1, IL-6, TNF-α, TNF-β* and *serum amyloid A protein* genes. Also, the Rel/NF-κB family of proteins is involved in viral infections when the κB sites are found in the HIV-LTR, SV 40, CMV and adenovirus. Other functions of Rel/NF-κB proteins include growth regulation, immune system responses and cell adhesion molecules (see Table 2).

Table 2: Localization of κB binding motifs in the body suggests the functions of Rel/NF-κB (for review, see Verma *et al.,* 1995; Wang *et al,* 1999).

κB sites	Related functions
IL-2, IL-2R, Igκ, MHC Classes I and II	Immune system reaction and responses.
IL-1, IL-6, TNF-α, TNF-β, serum amyloid A protein	Inflammatory reactions and acute phase responses.
HIV-LTR, SV 40, CMV, adenovirus	Viral infections
Rel/NF-κB family (NF-κB1, NF-κB2, c-rel, RelB)	Immune system responses.
p53, c-Myc, Ras, pRB1	Growth regulation.
IκB-α, IκB-γ, p105, p100 and Bcl-3	IκB family members
I-CAM, V-CAM, E-selectin, ELAM1	Cell adhesion molecules

Table 3: The factors associated with activation of NF-κB transcription factor (Schottelius *et al.,* 1999; Sun and Ballard, 1999; McFarland *et al.,* 1999; Liou and Baltimore, 1993; Verma *et al.,* 1995; Kawakami *et al.,* 1999; Meyskens *et al.,* 1999; Haddad, 2002).

- Cytokines (TNF-α, IL-1, IL-2, IL-6)
- Bacterial lipopolysaccharides
- Phytohemagglutinin (PHA)
- Cross-linking surface CD2, CD3, CD28 and T-cell receptors.
- Proteins secreted by viruses, for example, tax, X, E1A
- Viral infections, for example, HIV-1, Hepatitis B, HSV, HTLV-1
- Antigenic stimulants for the T and B-cells receptors
- Ultraviolet light exposure
- X-irradiation
- Nitric oxide
- Hydrogen peroxide and other oxidizing agents
- Calcium ionophores

Activation of NF-κB transcription involves the translocation of NF-κB proteins to the nucleus as illustrated in Figure 1.4 (Liou and Baltimore, 1993; May and Ghosh, 1998; Verma *et al.,* 1995; Shain *et al,* 1998). The factors involved in the transcriptional activation of different members of the Rel/NF-κB family are mentioned in Table 3 (for review, see Verma *et al.,* 1995; Liou and Baltimore, 1993; May and Ghosh, 1998).

1.3.2. IκB Inhibitor System

The rapid inducibility of NF kappa B can be attributed to the fact that it preexists in the cytoplasm of cells in an inactive form complexed to I kappa B, thus requiring no new protein synthesis. I kappa B proteins regulate the cellular location, DNA binding, and transcriptional properties of NF kappa B/Rel family of proteins. The current mammalian I kappa B family of proteins includes I kappa B-alpha, I kappa B-beta, I kappa B-gamma, I kappa B-delta, (generated from alternative splicing of the NF kappa B1 gene, NF kappa B1, NF kappa B2), I kappa B-epsilon and the predominantly nuclear protein Bcl-3. All I kappa B proteins have in common a conserved domain containing six to eight repeats of the erythrocyte protein ankyrin. I kappa B binds to the NF kappa B dimer and masks its nuclear localization signal thereby sequestering NF kappa B in the cytoplasm of the cell. The NF kappa B/I kappa B complex itself cannot bind to DNA, however disassociation of I- kappa B from NF kappa B which can be achieved in vivo with various activating agents or in vitro with agents such as deoxycholate will produce an NF kappa B dimer which is capable of translocating to the nucleus and binding DNA.

I kappa B-alpha is the most extensively studied and most abundant I kappa B family member and unlike I kappa B-beta, is primarily involved in regulating the rapid and transient activation of NF kappa B. I kappa B-alpha is a 37 kd protein which can be structurally divided into a 70 amino acid N terminus, a central section of 205 amino acids composed of 6 ankyrin repeats, and an acidic 42 amino acid C- terminus that contains a PEST (pro-glu-ser-thr) sequence, a motif correlated with rapid protein turnover. I kappa B-alpha performs several critical functions including cytoplasmic retention of NF kappa B in resting cells, release of NF kappa B in response to activating signals, and inhibition of DNA binding by NF-kappa B. I kappa B-alpha binds to specific Rel subunits and masks the NLS of all dimers containing any of the transactivating subunits (RelA, c-Rel, RelB), especially those containing RelA, thereby retaining these complexes in the cytoplasm. Studies of stoichiometry have shown that one dimer of NF kappa B is bound to one I kappa B-alpha molecule. Thus the classic cytoplasmic NF KAPPA B complex contains a p50/p65 dimer bound to one I kappa B-alpha. I kappa B-alpha can have differential affinity for the various NF kappa B dimers. For example, I kappa B-alpha binds a RelB/p50 heterodimer more efficiently than a RelB/p52 heterodimer. Complexes with the highest affinity for I kappa B-alpha are thought to be mainly cytoplasmic and represent the inducible pool, while those complexes with low affinity for I kappa B-alpha are nuclear and provide constitutive activity.

Removing DNA bound dimers in the absence of an activating signal may also be a role of I kappa B-alpha since I kappa B-alpha not only prevents DNA binding of strongly activating complexes but can also dissociate bound complexes from DNA. The underlying mechanism for the inhibition of DNA binding mediated via I kappa B-alpha is not clearly understood, however, it has been shown to require the C-terminal region of I kappa B-alpha.

Recent studies have shown that exogenously introduced, over expressed, or newly synthesized I kappa B-alpha can be found not only in the cytoplasm, but in the nucleus as well. In addition, recent studies of I kappa B-alpha knockout mice have demonstrated that TNF-alpha treatment of embryonic fibroblasts from these mice results in a prolonged and sustained nuclear induction of NF kappa B indicating that I-kappa B-alpha plays a role in the termination of an NF kappa B response. Thus, it is likely that newly synthesized I kappa B-alpha may enter the nucleus and regulate NF kappa B activity, resulting in a transient response.

The multiple targets of Rel/NF-κB proteins and their multiple modes of regulation indicate that this family possesses diversity in function. Interestingly, their major mode of regulation appears to be well conserved through the IκB inhibitor system. IκB is a protein of 60-70 kDa (Baeuverle and Baltimore, 1988; May and Ghosh, 1998). The IκB inhibitor system comprises seven molecules IκB-α, IκB-β, IκB-γ, Bcl-3, p105, p100 and I κB R (Garcia et al., 1999). The inhibitor of κB (IκB) kinase (IKK) complex is composed of two catalytic subunits, IKKα and IKKβ, and one regulatory subunit, IKKγ.

The IκB inhibitor system regulates NF-κB (p50, p65) by retaining it as a complex in the cytoplasm (Henkel et al., 1993). As a result, the NF-κB family members remain in the cytoplasm in an inactive form. In response to stimuli such as tumour-necrosis factor-α (TNF-α), CD40 ligand (CD40L), interleukin-1 (IL-1) or lipopolysaccharide (LPS), the IKKβ subunit is activated, and phosphorylates the IκB proteins (bound to the NF-κB heterodimers) at two conserved serines. This phosphorylation event triggers the ubiquitin-dependent degradation of IκB by the 26S proteasome, resulting in the nuclear translocation of RelA–p50 (or c-Rel–p50) heterodimers and transcriptional activation of target genes (See Figure 1.5). In response to other stimuli, such as the TNF family members lymphotoxin B (LTβ) and BAFF, IKKα is activated to induce the phosphorylation of p100 (bound to RelB) at two serine residues at its carboxyl terminus. This phosphorylation event triggers the ubiquitin-dependent degradation of the carboxy-terminal half of p100, releasing its amino-terminal half, the p52 polypeptide, which together with its heterodimer partner, RelB, translocates to the nucleus to activate transcription (Garcia et al., 1999, Baeuverle and Baltimore, 1988; May and Ghosh, 1998, McKenzie et al., 2000) (See Figure 6 and Table 4).

Rel/NF-κB family members also cooperate with other transcriptional regulators such as the non-Rel/NF-κB protein Ets-1. Recent data has provided evidence that physical interaction between Ets and NF-kappaB proteins is required for the transcriptional activity of the HIV-1 and HIV-2 enhancers (Bassuk et al., 1997). These interactions represent a potential target for the development of novel immunosuppressive and antiviral therapies.

1.3.3. Role of NF-κB in Apoptosis and Cell Survival

The dual role of NF-κB in enhancing or inhibiting apoptosis and cell death has attracted much attention in regard to its role in carcinogenesis (Mercurio and Manning, 1999; Tickle, 1998; Sonenshein, 1997; Muller et al., 2003; Bushdid et al., 1998; Huang et al., 2000; Romano et al., 2000; Bukowski et al., 1998; Bash et al., 1999).

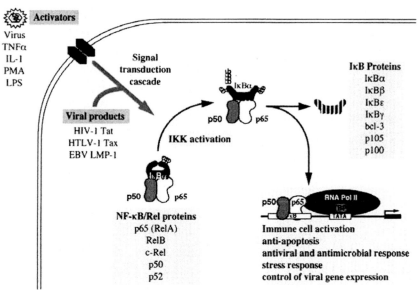

Figure 6: Illustration of the Rel/NF-κB pathway. In response to stimuli such as tumour-necrosis factor-α (TNF-α), CD40 ligand (CD40L), interleukin-1 (IL-1) or lipopolysaccharide (LPS), the IKKβ subunit is activated, and phosphorylates the IκB proteins (bound to the NF-κB heterodimers) at two conserved serines. This phosphorylation event triggers the ubiquitin-dependent degradation of IκB by the 26S proteasome, resulting in the nuclear translocation of RelA–p50 (or c-Rel–p50) heterodimers and transcriptional activation of target genes (Adapted from Hiscott *et al.*, 2001).

Table 4: Steps involved in Rel/NF-κB activation (Shain *et al.*, 1998).

1. Exposure to a stimulus that activates NF-κB such as UV light.
2. Degradation of IκB or its inactivation by phosphorylation by means of protein kinases (McKenzie et al., 2000).
3. Dissociation of the complex between NF-κB family members and IκB inhibitor system.
4. Translocation of NF-κB proteins to the nucleus.
5. DNA binding of NF-κB proteins.
6. Transcriptional induction by NF-κB proteins.

1.3.3.1. NF-κB Involvement in Apoptosis

The role of Rel/NF-κB proteins in apoptosis has been well studied (Hogerlinden *et al.*, 1999; Manna *et al.*, 2000). NF-κB, for instance, was found to be activated following TNF-α-induced apoptosis in several cell lines (Miyamoto *et al.*, 1994). Treatment of cell lines derived from acute B-cell leukemia and human thymocytes with etoposide was found to activate NF-κB and this activation occurred prior to the initiation of apoptosis (Beg and Baldwin, 1993). Further evidence supporting the involvement of NF-κB in apoptosis is the presence of NF-κB binding sites in the genes encoding *IL-1β converting enzyme protease, c-myc,* and *TNFα,* which are all involved in apoptosis and cell death (Collins *et al.*, 1995; Beg and Baldwin, 1993). Also, several studies showed that p65 is involved in apoptosis. This was based on an original observation whereby inhibition of apoptosis was achieved by overexpression of a dominant-negative p65 protein (Higgins *et al.*, 1993).

1.3.3.2. Rel/NF-κB Role in Cell Protection and Survival

The role of Rel/NF-κB proteins in cell survival is generally associated with their ability to upregulate the expression of myc (for review, see Foo and Nolan, 1999; Chen *et al.*, 1998). Myc is a protein that mediates the transcriptional activation of cyclin A and cyclin D3, which are cell cycle regulators. A decrease in the myc protein concentration in the cell has been associated with apoptosis. Another pathway that leads to high myc levels is through the stimulation of CD40, a member of TNF receptor family, which results in NF-κB activation (Madrid *et al.*, 1999; Furman *et al.*, 2000) and whose stimulation has been implicated in cell survival and protection (Madrid *et al.*, 1999).

The role of Rel/NF-κB as a factor in both cancerous and normal cell survival is well documented. Recent results, for instance, have shown NF-κB to be activated in the early malignant transformation of mammary cells of the breast (Kim *et al.*, 2000). Furthermore, NF-κB is constitutively active in pancreatic adenocarcinoma in humans (Wang *et al.*, 1999), in T-cell leukemia cells (Mori *et al.*, 1999), in human breast cancer (Cogswell *et al.*, 2000) and in head and neck squamous cell carcinoma cell lines (Ondrey *et al.*, 1999).

In non-cancer cells, NF-κB was reported to be essential for the growth and survival of sympathetic nerve cells independently of the *de novo* protein synthesis (Maggirwar *et al.*, 1998). Further evidence of severe liver degeneration was associated with lack of NF-κB activation (Rudolph *et al.*, 2000). This was based on the death of murine embryonic fibroblasts that lack detectable NF-κB DNA binding activity in response to TNF-α, LPS, IL-1 and do not show IκB kinase activity required for NF-κB activation (Rudolph *et al.*, 2000).

The anti-apoptotic activity of Rel/NF-κB can be regulated by other proteins. For instance, the X chromosome-linked inhibitor of apoptosis (XIAP) induces NF-κB activation by increasing the nuclear translocation of its p65 subunit (Hofer-Warbinek *et al.*, 2000; Stehlik *et al.*, 1998). In addition, CD95, which is known as Fas and possesses an apoptotic effect, was found to stimulate NF-κB degradation by caspases (Ravi *et al.*, 1998), but when an antibody against CD95 was used, caspases were inhibited and the inducibility of NF-κB was restored (Ravi *et al.*, 1998).

1.3.4. Xrel3

Xrel3 encodes an embryonic protein found to be related to the rel family of proteins. The *Xrel3* gene is present in the genome of the amphibian, <u>Xenopus laevis</u> and is expressed in and is essential for the normal development of the head of <u>Xenopus laevis</u> embryos (Lake *et al.*, 2001). *Xrel3* is also normally expressed in the otocysts and notochord of the embryonic larval stages (Lake *et al.*, 2001). Interestingly, Xrel3 overexpression has been implicated in the development of epidermal tumors in embryos (Yang *et al.*, 1998; Lake *et al.*, 2001), but little is known about how these tumors form, or whether they have similar properties to human tumors. Therefore, I was interested in investigating whether the Xrel3 protein had properties that could contribute to human cancer. By applying what is known about the role of Xrel3 in embryos to human cell lines, it may be possible to uncover new knowledge about the mechanism of Rel/NF-κB activity in general. I considered this to be a novel approach to the study of this important family of oncogenes.

In addition to its ability to cause embryonic tumor formation, the rationale for studying the effects of Xrel3 in human cervical cancer cells has basis in practicality. When a DNA vector encoding tagged-Xrel3 was transiently transfected into HeLa cells, Xrel3 protein constitutively localized in the nuclei, suggesting its ability to be active constantly in mammalian cells (Green, 2003). In addition, HeLa cells do not normally express Rel/NF-☐B, so the transfection of Xrel3 into these cells gave me the opportunity to study the activity of an interesting Rel/NF-κB protein in a negative background. Therefore, even though Xrel3 is not a mammalian gene, its homology to the mammalian Rel/NF-κB family indicates that it may serve as a good model for gene regulation by this family enabling us to understand the mechanism of action of the Rel/NF-κB family of transcriptional regulators in cancer cells.

1.4. Cancer Chemotherapy

1.4.1. Introduction

Many chemical agents are used in the treatment of cancer. Some can be used alone in single therapy and others have to be combined or added to other regimens for an effective outcome. The five groups of single chemotherapeutic agents are: alkylating agents, antimetabolites, plant derivatives, antitumor antibiotics and the miscellaneous group which contains the platinums, procarbazine, mitotane and gallium nitrate (British Medical Association, 2002).

1.4.2. Platinums

The platinum-containing compounds are carboplatin, cisplatin and oxaliplatin. This group of chemotherapeutic drugs is very effective in monotherapy regimens (Gadducci et al., 1997). They are the most active agents in the treatment of ovarian and cervical cancers. However, they are associated with three major drawbacks (Reedijk, 2003):

1. Severe toxicity in the form of nephrotoxicity, ototoxicity, myelosuppression and peripheral neuropathy.
2. Narrow range of tumors upon which they are effective.
3. The development of resistance after a short period of treatment.

New approaches are now designed in an attempt to expand the mechanism of action of platinums. This is done by developing a new generation of platinum-containing compounds that exhibited a broader spectrum of activity on different tumors, lower toxicity potential as well as delayed resistance to treatment (Fuertes et al., 2002; for review, see Jakupec, 2003).

1.4.3. Cisplatin

Cis DiamminedichloroplatinII (cisplatin) is one of the platinum-containing anti-cancer agents. It can be recognized from its chemical name that the cis form is the active form of the drug. The trans form was found to possess no biologic activity (Reedijk, 2003). The mechanism of action of cisplatin is similar to the alkylating agents, but it is not identical. Cisplatin works by promoting DNA cross-linking and chelation (United States Pharmacopeia, 2003). Recent clinical studies have shown that improved cytotoxicity of cisplatin can be attained by increasing the exposure time of the tumor to the drug (Markman, 2003).

1.4.4. Rel/NF-κB and Chemoresistance

Many researches have attempted to investigate the role that NF-κB family might have in chemotherapeutic resistance (Shehata et al., 2004, 2005). Activation of the Rel/NF-κB was found to be associated with chemotherapeutic resistance by suppressing the apoptotic potential of the chemotherapeutic drug. Recent data demonstrate that the protection from apoptosis induced in response to carbonyloxycamptothecin (CPT-11) treatment is effectively inhibited by the transient inhibition of NF-κB in a variety of human colon cancer cell lines (Cusack *et al.*, 2000). This might be due to the cell survival effects associated with the upregulation of Rel/NF-κB family as previously mentioned. In addition, genetic manipulation aimed at inhibiting Rel/NF-κB, was found to cause sensitization of different tumor cells, like lung cancer cells, to the effect of chemotherapeutic drugs (Jones *et al.*, 2000). This makes the Rel/NF-κB family an attractive set of proteins to study in chemoresistant tumors.

1.5. Genetics of Cervical Cancer

Family history often identifies people with a moderately increased risk of cancer, and in some cases may be an indicator of the presence of polymorphisms that influence cancer susceptibility, through such mechanisms as changes in the rate of metabolism of agents that predispose to cancer or catabolism of carcinogens, or effects on DNA repair or regulation of cell division. Less often, family history indicates the presence of an inherited cancer predisposition conferring a relatively high lifetime risk of cancer. In some cases, DNA-based testing can be used to confirm a specific mutation as the cause of the inherited risk, and to determine whether family members have inherited the mutation.

Identifying a person with an increased risk of cancer can reduce the occurrence of cancer through clinical management strategies (e.g., tamoxifen for breast cancer, colonoscopy for colon cancer) or improve that person's health outcome or quality of life through intrinsic benefits of the information itself (e.g., no genetic predisposition). Intrinsic benefits may include better ability to plan for the future (having children, career, retirement or other decisions) with improved knowledge about cancer risk. Methods of genetic risk assessment include assessment of personal and family history of disease and genetic testing; the latter is generally undertaken only when family history of disease or other clinical characteristics, such as early onset of cancer, indicate a substantial likelihood of an inherited predisposition to cancer.

Genetic testing may also be sought by people affected with cancer, both newly diagnosed individuals and survivors of earlier cancers. Testing may be desired to define personal cancer etiology, to clarify risk to offspring, to define the appropriateness of particular surveillance approaches, or to aid in decision-making about risk-reducing prophylactic surgery. While there are effective interventions specific for some cancer genetic syndromes (e.g., multiple endocrine neoplasia type 2A [MEN 2A], familial adenomatous polyposis [FAP], retinoblastoma [RB]), genetic testing is still being integrated into the management of patients with hereditary forms of common cancers (e.g., breast cancer). Some patients and physicians may wish to include genetic risk status as a factor in consideration of treatment options.

CONCLUSION

Clinical trials are on their way to test the efficacy and safety of multiple new apoptosis-inducing drugs. Among these drugs are Velcade developped by NCI and Millenium Pharmaceuticals, and Genasense developped by Genta Company (Spano et al., 2005). Velcade targets the proteosome, that machinary which serves as a cellular "garbage disposal", removing damaged, aged and abnormal proteins. The net result will be a built up of proteins, among which is Bax protein that blocks bcl-2 promoting apoptosis. Bax levels increase in response to Velcade and Bax inhibition of bcl-2 also increases and the cell ultimately undergoes apoptosis. Genasense acts by blocking cellular production of bcl-2 protein leaving cancer cells more vulnerable to apoptosis-inducing chemotherapies (Cotter FE, 2004). These medications, as well as many others yet to be discovered, will be outstanding candidates for better controlling cervical cancer progression

REFERENCES

Abbadie, C., Kabrun, N., Bouali, F., Smardova, J., Stehelin, D., Vandenbunder, B., & Enrietto, P.J. (1993). High levels of c-rel expression are associated with programmed cell death in the developing avian embryo and in bone marrow cells in vitro. *Cell, 75(5)*, 899-912.

Accardi, R, Dong W, Smet, A, Cui, R, Hautefeuille, A, Gabet, AS, Sylla, BS, Gissmann L, Hainaut P, Tommasino M. Skin human papillomavirus type 38 alters p53 functions by accumulation of DeltaNp73. *EMBO Rep.* 2006 Jan 6; [Epub ahead of print]

Adams, J.M., & Cory, S. (1998). The Bcl-2 Protein Family: Arbiters of Cell Survival. *Science, 281*, 1322-1326.

Alarcon, C.M., Pedram, M., Donelson, D.E. (1999). Leaky transcription of variant surface glycoprotein gene expression sites in bloodstream african trypanosomes. *Journal of Biological Chemistry, 274(24)*, 16884-16893.

Anonymous. (2002). *Platinum compounds*. British Medical Association, The Royal Pharmaceutical Society of Great Britain.

Ashkenazi, A., & Dixit, V.M. (1998). Death receptors: Signalling and Modulation. *Science, 281*, 1305-1308.

Baeuerle, P.A., & Baltimore, D. (1988). IκB: A Specific Inhibitor of the NF-κB Transcription Factor. *Science, 242*, 540-546.

Baldwin, A.S. (2001). Control of angiogenesis and cancer therapy resistance by the transcription factor NF- κB. *The Journal of Clinical Investigation, 107*, 241-246.

Barkett, M., & Gilmore, T.D. (1999). Control of apoptosis by Rel/NF- κB transcription factors. *Oncogene, 18*, 6910-6924.

Bash, J., Zong, W.X., Banga, S., Rivera, A., Ballard, D.W., Ron, Y., & Gelinas, C. (1999). Rel/NF- κB can trigger the Notch signaling pthway by inducing the expression of Jagged1, a ligand for Notch receptors. *The EMBO Journal, 18*, 2803-2811.

Bassuk, A.G., Anandappa, R.T., Leiden, J.M. (1997). Physical interactions between Ets and NF-kappaB/NFAT proteins play an important role in their cooperative activation of the human immunodeficiency virus enhancer in T cells. *Journal of Virology, 71(5)*, 3563-3573.

Becton, D. (2003). The mechanism of action of the Tet-On system.

Beg, A.A., & Baldwin Jr.,A.S. (1993). The IκB proteins: multifunctional regulators of Rel/NF-κB trancription factors. *Genes and Development, 7*, 2064-2070.

Bennett, M.R., Macdonald, K., Chan, S.W., Boyle, J.J., Weissberg, P.L. (1998). Cooperative Interactions Between RB and p53 Regulate Cell Proliferation, Cell Senescence, and Apoptosis in Human Vascular Smooth Muscle Cells From Atherosclerotic Plaques. *Circulation Research.*;82:704-712.

Boise, L.H., Gottschalk, A.R., Quintans, J., & Thonpson, C.B. (1995). Bcl-2 and Bcl-2-related proteins in apoptosis regulation. *Curr Top Microbiol Immunol., 200*, 107-121.

Borbely, AA, Murvai, M, Konya, J, Beck, Z, Gergely, L, Li F, Veress, G. Effects of human papillomavirus type 16 oncoproteins on survivin gene expression. *J Gen Virol.* 2006 Feb;87(Pt 2):287-94.

Botti, G., Chiappetta, G., Aiuto, G., Angelis, E., Matteis, A., Montella, M., Picone, A., & Cascione, F. (1993). PCNA/cyclin and P-glycoprotein as prognostic factors in locally advanced breast cancer. An immunohistochemical, retrospective study. *Tumori, 79*, 214-218.

Boyd, J.M., Gallo, G.J., Elangovan, B., Houghton, A.B., Malstrom, S., Avery, B.J., Ebb, R.G., Subramanian, T., Chittenden, T., & Lutz, R.J. (1995). Bik, a novel death-inducing protein shares a distinct sequence motif with Bcl-2 family proteins and interacts with viral and cellular survival-promoting proteins. *Oncogene, 11(9)*, 1921-1928.

Brewer, J, Benghuzzi, H, Tucci, M. The role of route of estrogen adminstration on the proliferation of SiHa cells in culture. *Biomed Sci Instrum.* 2005;41:68-73.

Bukowski, R.M., Rayman, P., Uzzo, R., Bloom, Sandstrom, K., Peereboom, D., Olencki, T., Budd, T., McLain, D., Elson, P., Novick, A., & Finke, J.H. (1998). Signal Transduction Abnormalities in T Lymphocytes from Patients with Advanced Renal Carcinoma: Clinical Relevance and Effects of Cytokine Therapy. *Clinical Cancer Research, 4*, 2337-2347.

Bushdid, P.B., Brantley, D.M., Yull, F.E., Blaeuer, G.L., Hoffman, L.H., Niswander, L., & Kerr, L.D. (1998). Inhibition of NF-kappaB activity results in disruption of the apical ectodermal ridge and aberrant limb morphogenesis. *Nature, 392*, 615-618.

Castellsague, X., Bosch, F.X., & Munoz,N. (2002). Environmental co-factors in HPV carcinogenesis. *Virus Research, 89*, 191-199.

Castle, PE, Jeronimo, J, Schiffman, M, Herrero, R, Rodriguez, AC, Bratti, MC, Hildesheim, A, Wacholder, S, Long, LR, Neve, L, Pfeiffer, R, Burk, RD. Age-related changes of the cervix influence human papillomavirus type distribution. *Cancer Res.* 2006 Jan 15;66(2):1218-24.

Castranova, V., Chen, F., Shi, X., & Demers, L.M. (1998,1999). New Insights into the Role of Nuclear Factor- κB, a Ubiquitous Transcription Factor in the Initiation of Diseases. *Clinical Chemistry*, 45, 7-17.

Chen, F., Castranova, V. & Shi, X. (2001). New Insights into the Role of Nuclear Factor- κB in Cell Growth Regulation. *American Journal of Pathology*, 159, 387-397.

Chen, J., Willingham, T., Shuford, M., Bruce, D., Rushing, E., Smith, Y., & Nisen, P.D. (1996). Effects of ectopic overexpression of p21(WAF1/CIP1) on aneuploidy and the malignant phenotype of human brain tumor cells. *Oncogene, 13(7)*, 1395-1403.

Christensen, J.G., Romach, E.H., Healy, L.N., Gonzales, A.J., Anderson, S.P., Malarkey, D.E., Corton, J.C., Fox,T .R., Cattley, R.C., & Goldsworthy, T.L. (1999). Altered Bcl-2 family expression during non-genotoxic hepatocarcinogenesis in mice. *Carcinogenesis, 20*, 1583-1590.

Cotter, FE. Unraveling biologic therapy for Bcl-2-expressing malignancies. *Semin Oncol.* 2004 Dec;31(6 Suppl 16):18-21; discussion 33. Review.

Cogswell, P.C., Guttridge, D.C., Funkhouser, W.K., & Baldwin Jr.,A.S. (2000). Selective activation of NF- κB subunits in human breast cancer: potential roles for NF- κB2/p52 and for Bcl-3. *Oncogene, 19*, 1123-1131.

Cohen, C., Lohmann, C.M., Cotsonis, G., Lawson, D., & Santoianni, R. (2003). Survivin expression in ovarian carcinoma: correlation with apoptotic markers and prognosis. *Mod Pathol, 16*, 574-583.

Collins,T., Read,M.A., Neish,A.S., Whitley,M.Z., Thanos,D., & Maniatis,T. (1995). Transcriptional regulation of endothelial cell adhesion molecules: NF-kappa B and cytokine-inducible enhancers. *FASEB J., 9(10)*, 899-909.

Cusack, J.C., Jr., Liu R. & Baldwin, A.S., Jr. (2000). Inducible Chemoresistance to 7-Ethyl-10-[4-(1-piperidino)-1-piperidino]carbonyloxycamptothecin (CPT-11) in Colorectal Cancer Cells and a Xenograft Model Is Overcome by Inhibition of Nuclear Factor-κB Activation. *Cancer Research*, 60, 2323-2330.

Deligdisch, L., Miranda, C.R.R., Wu, H.S., & Gil, J. (2003). Human papillomavirus-related cervical lesions in adolescents: a histologic and morphometric study. *Gynecologic Oncology, 89*, 52-59.

Evan, G., & Littlewood, T. (1998). A Matter of Life and Cell Death. *Science, 281*, 1317-1322.

Famuboni, A.K., Graveling, A.J., Markey, A.L., Minns, F.C., Patel,A. (2002). Apoptosis. http://www.portfolio.mvm.ed.ac.uk/studentwebs/session2/group28/index.html

Ferrer, I., & Planas, A.M. (2003). Signaling of cell death and cell survival following focal cerebral ischemia: life and death struggle in the penumbra. *J Neuropathol Exp Neurol., 62(4)*, 329-339.

Fiers, W., Beyaert, R., Declercq, W., & Vandenabeele, P. (1999). More than one way to die: apoptosis, necrosis and reactive oxygen damage. *Oncogene, 18*, 7719-7730.

Finzer, P., Lemarroy, A.A., & Rosl, F. (2002). The role of human papillomavirus oncoproteins E6 and E7 in apoptosis. *Cancer Letters, 188*, 15-24.

Foo, S.Y., & Nolan, G.P. (1999). NF-κB to the rescue. *Trends Genet, 15*, 229-235.

Fuertes, M.A., Castilla, J., Alonso, C., & Perez, J.M. (2002). Novel concepts in the development of platinum antitumor drugs. *Curr Med Chem Anti-Canc Agents, 2*, 539-551.

Furman, R.R., Asgary, Z., Mascarenhas, J.O., Liou, H.C., & Schattner, E.J. (2000). Modulation of NF-κB Activity and Apoptosis in Chronic Lymphocytic Leukemia B Cells. *Journal of Immunology, 164*, 2200-2206.

Furomoto, H.IM., & Irahara. (2002). Human papilloma virus (HPV) and cervical cancer. *J Med Invest, 49*, 124-133.

Gadducci, A., Brunetti, I., Cisco, S., Giannessi, PG., Genazzani, AR., & Conte, P. (1997). Platinum compounds and paclitaxel in advanced epithelial ovarian cancer. *Anticancer Research, 17*, 4703-4708.

Garcia, G.E., Xia, Y., Chen, S., Wang, Y., Ye, R.D., Harrison, J.K., Bacon, K.B., Zerwes, H.G., & Feng, L. (2000). NF- κB -dependent fractalkine induction in rat aortic endothelial cells stimulated by IL-1beta, TNF-alpha, and LPS. *Journal of Leukocyte Biology, 67*, 577-584.

Garland, S.M. (2002). Human papillomavirus update with a particular focus on cervical disease. *Pathology, 34*, 213-224.

Gerondakis, S., Grossmann, M., Nakamura, Y., Pohl, T., & Grumont, R. (1999). Genetic approaches in mice to understand Rel/NF- κB and I κB function: transgenics and knockouts. *Oncogene, 18*, 6888-6895.

Ghim, S.J., Basu, P.S., & Jenson, A. (2002). Cervical Cancer: Etiology, Pathogenesis, Treatment, and Future Vaccines. *Asian Pac J Cancer, 3*, 207-214.

Govan, VA. Strategies for human papillomavirus therapeutic vaccines and other therapies based on the e6 and e7 oncogenes. *Ann N Y Acad Sci.* 2005 Nov;1056:328-43.

Govind, S. (1999). Control of development and immunity by Rel transcription factors in Drosophila. *Oncogene, 18*, 6875-6887.

Green, A. (2003). Effect of Xrel3 on TGF-β Signalling Pathway in Human Cervical Cancer cells. Memorial University of Newfoundland.

Green, D.R., & Reed, J.C. (1998). Mitochondria and Apoptosis. *Science, 281*, 1309-1312.

Green, D.R. (2000). Apoptotic Pathways: Paper Wraps Stone Blunts Scissors. *Cell, 102*, 1-4.

Greider, C., Chattopadhyay, A., Parkhurst, C., & Yang, E. (2002). BCL-x_L and Bcl-2 delay Myc-induced cell cycle entry through elevation of p27 and inhibition of G1 cyclin-dependent kinases. *Oncogene, 21(51)*, 7765-7775.

Grilli, M., Chen-Tran, A., & ,L.M.J. (1993). Tumor necrosis factor alpha mediates a T cell receptor-independent induction of the gene regulatory factor NF-kappa B in T lymphocytes. *Mol Immunol.*1993 Oct;30(14):1287-1294.

Haddad, J. (2002). Science review: Redox and oxygen-sensitive transcription factors in the regulation of oxidant-mediated lung injury: role for nuclear factor-kappaB. *Critical Care, 6*, 481-490.

Heckman, C.A., Mehew, J.W., & Boxer, L.M. (2002). NF- κB activates Bcl-2 expression in t(14;18) lymphoma cells. *Oncogene, 21*, 3898-3908.

Heilmann, V., & Kreienberg, R. (2002). Molecular biology of cervical cancer and its precursors. *Curr Womens Health Rep, 2*, 27-33.

Hengartner, M.O. (2000). The biochemistry of apoptosis. *Nature Insight, 407*, 770-776.

Henkel, T., Machleidt, T., Alkalay, I., Kronke, M., Ben-Neriah, Y., & Baeuerle, P.A. (1993). Rapid proteolysis of I kappa B-alpha is necessary for activation of transcription factor NF-kappa B. *Nature, 365*, 182-185.

Hida, A., Kawakami, A., Nakashima, T., Yamasaki, S., Sakai, H., & Urayama, H.I.S. (2000). Nuclear factor-κB and caspases co-operatively regulate the activation and apoptosis of human macrophages. *Immunology, 99*, 553-560.

Higgins, K.A., Coleman, T.A., McComas, W.A., Perez, J.R., Dorshkind, K., Sarmiento, U.M., Rosen, C.A., & Narayanan, R. (1993). Antisense inhibition of the p65 subunit of NF-kappa B blocks tumorigenicity and causes tumor regression. *Proc Natl Acad Sci U S A, 90(21)*, 9901-9905.

Hiscott, J., Kwon, H.& Genin, P. (2001). Hostile takeovers: viral appropriation of the NF-kB pathway. *J. Clin. Invest., 107(2)*, 143 - 151.

Hogerlinden, M.V., Rozell, B.L., Richter, L.A., & Toftgard, R. (1999). Squamous Cell Carcinomas and Increased Apoptosis in Skin with Inhibited Rel/Nuclear Factor- κB Signaling. *Cancer research, 59*, 3299-3303.

Huang, Y., Johnson, K.R., Norris, J.S., & Fan, W. (2000). Nuclear Factor- κB /I κB Signaling Pathway May Contribute to the Mediation of Paclitaxel-induced Apoptosis in Solid Tumor Cells. *Cancer research, 60*, 4426-4432.

Jakupec,M.A., Galanski,M., & Keppler,B.K. (2003). Tumour-inhibiting platinum complexes--state of the art and future perspectives. *Rev Physiol Biochem Pharmacol*, 146-154.

Jiang,M., & Milner,J. (2003). Bcl-2 constitutively suppresses p53-dependent apoptosis in colorectal cancer cells. *Genes Dev., 17*, 832-837.

Jimenez-Flores R, Mendez-Cruz R, Ojeda-Ortiz J, Munoz-Molina R, Balderas-Carrillo O, de la Luz Diaz-Soberanes M, Lebecque S, Saeland S, Daneri-Navarro A, Garcia-Carranca A, Ullrich SE, Flores-Romo L. High-risk human papilloma virus infection decreases the frequency of dendritic Langerhans' cells in the human female genital tract. *Immunology.* 2006 Feb;117(2):220-8.

Jones, D.R., Broad, M., Madrid, L.V., Baldwin, A.S., Jr.& Mayo, M.W. (2000). Inhibition of NF-κB sensitizes non-small cell lung cancer cells to chemotherapy-induced apoptosis. *Ann Thorac Surg* 70, 930-936

Josefson, D. (1999). Mild cervical dysplasia often reverts to normal. *British Medical Journal, Feb 13*, 1999.

Kaltschmidt, B., Kaltschmidt, C., Hofmann, T.G., Hehner, S.P., Droge, W., & Schmitz, M.L. (2000). The pro- or anti- apoptotic function of NF- κB is determined by the nature of the apoptotic stimulus. *European Journal of Biochemistry, 267*, 3828-3835.

Karin, M., Cao, Y., Greten, F.R.,Li, Z.W. (2002). NF-κB in cancer: From innocent bystander to major culprit. Nature Reviews, *Cancer 2*, 301 –310.

Kawakami, A., Nakashima, T., Sakai, H., Urayama, S., Yamasaki, S., Hida, A., Tsuboi, M., Nakamura, H., Ida, H., Migita, K., Kawabe, Y., & Eguchi, K. (1999). Inhibition of Caspase Cascade by HTLV-I Tax Through Induction of NF-κB Nuclear Translocation. Immunobiology, *Blood, 94*, 3847-3854.

Kerr, JF, Wyllie, AH, Currie, AR. Apoptosis: a basic biological phenomenon with wide-ranging implications in tissue kinetics. *Br J Cancer.* 1972 Aug; 26(4):239-57. Review.

Kim, C.J., Jeong, J.K., Park, M., Park, T.S., Park, T.C., Namkoong, S.E., & Park, J.S. (2003). HPV oligonucleotide microarray-based detection of HPV genotypes in cervical neoplastic lesions. *Gynecologic Oncology, 89*, 210-217.

Kim, D.W., Sovak, M.A., Zanieski, G., Nonet, G., Romieu-Mourez, R., Lau, A.W., Hafer, L.J., Yaswen, P., Stampfer, M., Rogers, A.E., Russo, J., & Sonenshein, G.E. (2000).

Activation of NF- κB /Rel occurs early during neoplastic transformation of mammary cells. *Carcinogenesis, 21*, 871-879.

Kim, J.-S., Kim, S.Y., Kim, K.H., & Cho, M.J. (2003). Hyperfractionated Radiotherapy with Concurrent Chemotherapy for Para-aortic Lymph Node Recurrence in Carcinoma of the Cervix. *Int.J.Radiation Oncology Biol.Phys., 55(1247)*, 1253

Koivusalo, R., Krausz, E., Ruotsalainen, P., Helenius, H., & Hietanen, S. (2002). Chemoradiation of Cervical Cancer Cells: Targeting Human Papillomavirus E6 and p53 Leads to Either Augmented or Attenuated Apoptosis Depending on the Platinum Carrier Ligand. *Cancer research, 62*, 7364-7371.

Krammer, P.H. (2000). CD95's deadly mission in the immune system. *Nature Insight, 407*, 789-795.

Lake, B.B., Ford, R., & Kao, K.R. (2001). Xrel3 is required for head development in Xenopus laevis. *Development, 128(2)*, 263-273.

Liou, H.C., & Baltimore, D. (1993). Regulation of the NF- κB /rel transcription factor and I κB inhibitor system. *Current Opinion in Cell biology, 5*, 477-487.

Mackenzie, F.R., Connelly, M.A., Balzarano, D., Muller, J.R., Geleziunas, R., & Marcu, K.B. (2000). Functional Isoforms of I κB Kinase alpha (IKK alpha) Lacking Leucine and Helix-Loop-Helix Domains Reveal that IKK alpha and IKK beta Have Different Activation Requirements. *Molecular and Cellular Biology, 20*, 2635-2649.

Madrid, L.V., Wang, C.Y., Guttridge, D.C., Schottelius, A.J.G., Baldwin Jr.,A.S., & Mayo, M.W. (2000). Akt Suppresses Apoptosis by Stimulating the Transactivation Potential of the RelA/p65 Subunit of NF- κB. *Molecular and Cellular Biology, 20*, 1626-1638.

Maggirwar, S.B., Sarmiere, P.D., Dewhurst, S., & Freeman, R.S. (1999). Nerve Growth Factor-Dependent Activation of NF- κB Contributes to Survival of Sympathetic Neurons. *The Journal of Neuroscience, 18*, 10356-10365.

Manna, S.K., Mukhopadhyay, A., & Aggarwal, B.B. (2000). Resveratrol Suppresses TNF-Induced Activation of Nuclear Transcription Factors NF- κB, Activator Protein-1, and Apoptosis: Potential Role of Reactive Oxygen Intermediates and Lipid Peroxidation. *The Journal of Immunology, 164*, 6509-6519.

Markman, M. (2003). Intraperitoneal antineoplastic drug delivery: rationale and results. *The Lancet Oncology, 4*, 277-283.

May, M.J., & Ghosh, S. (1998). Signal transduction through NF- κB. *Immunology Today, 19*, 80-88.

McFarland, E.D.C., Izumi, K.M., & Mosialos, G. (1999). Epstein-Barr virus transformation: involvement of latent membrane protein 1-mediated activation of NF- κB. *Oncogene, 18*, 6959-6964.

Meier, P., Finch, A., & Evan, G. (2000). Apoptosis in development. *Nature Insight, 407*, 796-801.

Mercurio, F., & Manning, A.M. (1999). Multiple signals concerging on NF-kappaB. *Curr Opin Cell Biol, 11*, 226-232.

Meyskens Jr.,F.L., Buckmeier, J.A., McNulty, S.E., & Tohidian, N.B. (1999). Activation of Nuclear Factor κB in Human Metastatic Melanoma Cells and the Effect of Oxidative Stress. *Clinical Cancer Research, 5*, 1197-1202.

Mikeaelsdottir, E.K., Benediktsdottir, K.R., Olafsdottir, K., Arnadottir, T., Ragnarsson, G.B., Olafsson, K., Sigurdsson, K., Kristjansdottir, G.S., Imsland, A.K., Ogmundsdottir, H.M., & Rafnar, T. (2003). HPV subtypes and immunological parameters of cervical cancer in Iceland during two time periods, 1958-1960 and 1995-1996. *Gynecologic Oncology, 89*, 22-30.

Miller, L.J., & Marx, J. (1998). Apoptosis. *Science, 281*, 1301-1304.

Miyamoto, S., Maki, M., Schmitt, M.J., Hatanaka, M., & Verma, I.M. (1994). Tumor necrosis factor alpha-induced phosphorylation of I kappa B alpha is a signal for its degradation but not dissociation from NF-kappa B. *Proc Natl Acad Sci U S A., 91(26)*, 12740-12744.

Mori, N., Fujii, M., Ikeda, S., Yamada, Y., Tomonaga, M., Ballard, D.W., & Yamamoto, N. (1999). Constitutive Activation of NF- κB in Primary Adult T-Cell Leukemia Cells. *Blood*, 2360-2368.

Mosialos, G. (1997). The role of Rel/NF-kappa B proteins in viral oncogenesis and the regulation of viral transcription. *Semin Cancer Biol, 8*, 121-129.

Muller, I., Pfister, S.M., Grohs, U., Zweigner, J., Handgretinger, R., Niethammer, D., & Bruchelt, G. (2003). Receptor Activator of Nuclear Factor κB Ligand Plays a Nonredundant Role in Doxorubicin-induced Apoptosis. *Cancer research, 63*, 1772-1775.

Munoz, N., Bosch, F.X., Sanjose, S., Herrero, R., Castellsague, X., Shah, K.V., Snijders, P.J., Meijer, C.J., & International Agency for Research on Cancer Multicenter Cervical Cancer Study Group. (2003). Epidemiologic classification of human papillomavirus types associated with cervical cancer. *N Engl J Med, 348*, 518-527.

Nair, HB, Luthra, R, Kirma, N, Liu, YG, Flowers, L, Evans, D, Tekmal, RR. Induction of aromatase expression in cervical carcinomas: effects of endogenous estrogen on cervical cancer cell proliferation. *Cancer Res.* 2005 Dec 1;65(23):11164-73.

Naishiro, Y., Adachi, M., Okuda, H., Yawata, A., Mitaka, T., Takayama, S., Reed, J.C., Hinoda, Y., & Imai, K. (1999). *BAG-1 accelerates cell motility of human gastric cancer cells*. Stockton Press, 3244-3251.

Nakayama, K., Takebayashi, Y., Nakayama, S., Hata, K., Fujiwaki, R., Fukumoto, M., & Miyazaki, K. (2003). Prognostic value of overexpression of p53 in human ovarian carcinoma patients receiving cisplatin. *Cancer Letters, 192*, 227-235.

National Cancer Institute of Canada. 2003 *Canadian Cancer Statistics*. (2003). Anonymous.

Nicholson, D.W. (2000). From bench to clinic with apoptosis-based therapeutic agents. *Nature Insight, 407*, 810-816.

Nicoletti, V.G., & Stella, A.M. (2003). Role of PARP under stress conditions: cell death or protection? *Neurochem Res., 28(2)*, 187-194.

Ondrey, F.G., Dong, G., Sunwoo, J., Chen, Z., Wolf, J.S., Crowl-Bancroft, C.V., Mukaida, N., & Waes, C.V. (1999). Constitutive Activation of Transcription Factors NF κB, AP-1, and NF-IL6 in Human Head and Neck Squamous Cell Carcinoma Cell Lines that Express Pro-inflammatory and Pro-angiogenic Cytokines. *Molecular Carcinogenesis, 26*, 119-129.

Packham, G., Brimmell, M., & Cleveland, J.L. (1997). Mammalian cells express two differently localized Bag-1 isoforms generated by alternative translation initiation. *Journal of Biochemistry, 328*, 807-813.

Park, J.S., Rhyu, J.W., Kim, C.J., Kim, H.S., Lee, S.Y., Kwon, Y.I., Namkoong, S.I., Sin, H.S., & Um, S.J. (2003). Neoplastic change of squamo-columnar junction in uterine cervix and vaginal epitheluim by exogenous estrogen in hpv-18 URR E6/E7 transgenic mice small star, filled. *Gynecologic Oncology, 89*, 360-368.

Ponnappan, U. (1998). Regulation of transcription factor NFkappa B in immune senescence. *Frontiers in Bioscience, 3*, D152-168.

Pratt, M.A.C., & Niu, M.Y. (2003). Bcl-2 Controls Caspase Activation Following a p53-dependent Cyclin D1-induced Death Signal. *Journal of Biological Chemistry, 278*, 14219-14229.

Ravi, R., Bedi, A., Fuchs, E.J., & Bedi, A. (1998). CD95 (Fas)-induced Caspase-mediated Proteolysis of NF- κB. *Cancer research, 58*, 882-886.

Reed, J.C. (1997). Double identity for proteins of the Bcl-2 family. *Nature, 387,* 776

Reedijk, J. (2003). New Clues for platinum antitumor chemistry: Kinetically controlled metal binding to DNA. *National Academy of Sciences, 100*, 3611-3616.

Reuning, U., Guerrini, L., Nishiguchi, T., Page, S., Seibold, H., Magdolen, V., Graeff, H., & Schmitt, M. (1999). Rel transcription factors contribute to elevated urokinase expression in human ovarian carcinoma cells. *European Journal of Biochemistry, 259*, 143-148.

Rich, T., & Allen, R.L.W.A.H. (2000). Defying death after DNA damage. Nature Insight, 407, 777-783.

Romano, M.F., Lamberti, A., Bisogni, R., Tassone, P., Pagnini, D., Storti, G., Vecchio, L.D., Turco, M.C., & Venuta, S. (2000). Enhancement of cytosine arabinoside-induced apoptosis in human myeloblastic leukemia cells by NF- κB /Rel- specific decoy oligodeoxynucleotides. *Gene Therapy, 7*, 1234-1237.

Rosenthal, A.N., Ryan, A., Al-Jejani, R.M., Storey,A., Harwood, C.A., & Jacobs, I.J. (1998). p53 codon 72 polymorphism and risk of cervical cancer in UK. *The Lancet, 352*, 871-874.

Rudolph, D., Yeh, W.C., Wakeham, A., Rudolph, B., Nallainathan, D., Potter, J., Elia, A.J., & Mak, T.W. (2000). Severe liver degeneration and lack of NF- κB activation in NEMO/IKKγ-deficient mice. *Genes and Development*, 854-862.

Savill, J., & Fadok, V. (2000). Corpse clearance defines the meaning of cell death. *Nature Insight, 407*, 784-788.

Schottelius, A.J.G., Mayo, M.W., Sartor, R.B., & Baldwin Jr.,A.S. (1999). Interleukin-10 Signaling Blocks Inhibitor of κB Kinase Activity and Nuclear Factor-κB DNA Binding. *The Journal of Biological Chemistry, 274*, 31868-31874.

Seitz, C.S., Deng, H., Hinata, K., Lin, Q., & Khavari, P.A. (2000). Nuclear Factor- κB Subunits Induce Epithelial Cell Growth Arrest. *Cancer research, 60*, 4085-4092.

Shain, K.H., Jove, R., & Olashaw, N.E. (1999). Constitutive RelB Activation in v-Src-Transformed Fibroblasts: Requirement for I κB Degradation. *Journal of Cellular Biochemistry, 73*, 237-247.

Shehata, M, Shehata, M, Shehata, F, Pater, A. Apoptosis effects of Xrel3 c-Rel/Nuclear Factor-kappa B homolog in human cervical cancer cells. *Cell Biol Int.* 2005 Jun;29(6):429-40. Epub 2005 Mar 25.

Shehata, MF. Rel/Nuclear factor-kappa B apoptosis pathways in human cervical cancer cells. *Cancer Cell Int.* 2005 Apr 27;5(1):10.

Shehata, M, Shehata, M, Shehata, F, Pater, A. Dual apoptotic effect of Xrel3 c-Rel/NF-kappaB homolog in human cervical cancer cells. *Cell Biol Int.* 2004;28(12):895-904.

Shillitoe, EJ. Papillomaviruses as targets for cancer gene therapy. *Cancer Gene Ther.* 2005 Dec 9; [Epub ahead of print]

Shinoura, N., Yoshida, Y., Nishimura, M., Muramatsu, Y., Asai, A., Kirino, T., & Hamada, H. (2000). Expression Level of Bcl-2 Determines Anti- or Proapoptotic Function. *Cancer research, 59,* 4119-4128.

Sisk, E.A., & Robertson, E.S. (2002). Clinical implications of human papillomavirus infection. *Front Biosci, 1,* e77-e84

Sonenshein, G.E. (1997). Rel/NF-kappaB transcription factors and the control of apoptosis. *Semin Cancer Biol, 8,* 113-119.

Spano, JP, Bay, JO, Blay, JY, Rix,e O. Proteasome inhibition: a new approach for the treatment of malignancies. *Bull Cancer.* 2005 Nov;92(11):E61-6, 945-52. Review.

Stehlik, C., Rainer de Martin, Kumabashiri, I., Schmid, J.A., Binder, B.R., & Lipp, J. (1998). Nuclear Factor (NF)- κB -regulated X-chromosome-linked iap Gene Expression Protects Endothelial Cells from Tumor Necrosis Factor α-induced Apoptosis. *J.Exp.Med,* 188, 211-216.

Strasser, A., O'Connor, L., and Dixit, V.M. APOPTOSIS SIGNALING. *Annual Review of Biochemistry. Vol. 69*: 217-245 (Volume publication date July 2000).

Stuart, J.K., Myszka, D.G., Joss, L., Mitchell, R.S., McDonald, S.M., Xie, Z., Takayama, S., Reed, J.C., & Ely, K.R. (1998). Characterization of Interactions between the Anti-apoptotic Protein BAG-1 and Hsc70 Molecular Chaperones. *The Journal of Biological Chemistry, 273,* 22506-22514.

Sun, S.C., & Ballard, D.W. (1999). Persistant activation of NF- κB by the Tax transforming protein of HTLV-1: hijacking cellular I κB kinases. *Oncogene, 18,* 6948-6958.

Thornberry, N.A., & Lazebnik, Y. (1998). Caspases: Enemies Within. *Science, 281,* 1312-1316.

Tickle, C. (1998). Worlds in common through NF-kappaB. *Nature, 392,* 547-549.

Ueda, M, Hung, YC, Chen, JT, Chiou, SH, Huang, HH, Lin, TY, Terai, Y, Chow, KC. Infection of human papillomavirus and overexpression of dihydrodiol dehydrogenase in uterine cervical cancer. *Gynecol Oncol.* 2006 Jan 19; [Epub ahead of print]

United States Pharmacopeia, USP. (2003). Chemotherapeutic Drugs. In Anonymous,

Vaux, DL, Cory, S, Adams, JM. Bcl-2 gene promotes haemopoietic cell survival and cooperates with c-myc to immortalize pre-B cells. *Nature.* 1988 Sep 29;335(6189):440-2.

Verma, I.M., Stevenson, J.K., Schwarz, E.M., & Antwerp, D.V. (1995). Rel/NF- κB /I κB family: intimate tales of association and dissociation. *Genes and Development, 9,* 2723-2735.

Villiers, E.M. (2003). Relationship between steroid hormone contraceptives and HPV, cervical intraepithelial neoplasia and cervical carcinoma. *Int.J.Cancer, 103,* 705-708.

Walboomers, J.M, Jacobs, M.V., Manos, M.M., Bosch, F.X., Kummer J.A. and ShahK.V. *et al.,* Human papillomavirus is a necessary cause of invasive cervical cancer worldwide, *J. Pathol. 189* (1999), pp. 12–19.

Wang, JT, Gao, ES, Cheng, YY, Yan, JW, Ding, L. [Analysis on synergistic action between estrogen, progesterone and human papillomaviruses in cervical cancer] *Zhonghua Liu Xing Bing Xue Za Zhi.* 2005 May;26(5):370-3.

Wang, W., Abbruzzese, J.L., Evans, D.B., & Chiao, P.J. (1999). Overexpression of urokinase-type plasminogen activator in pancreatic adenocarcinoma is regulated by constitutively activated RelA. *Oncogene, 18,* 4554-4563.

Wang, W., Abbruzzese, J.L., Evans, D.B., Larry, L., Cleary, K.R., & Chiao, P.J. (1999). The Nuclear Factor-κB RelA Transcription Factor is Constitutively Activated in Human Pancreatic Adenocarcinoma Cells. *Clinical Cancer Research, 5,* 119-127.

Warbinek, R.H., Schmid, J.A., Stehlik, C., Binder, B.R., Lipp, J., & Martin, R. (2000). Activation of NF- κB by XIAP, the X Chromosome-linked Inhibitor of Apoptosis, in Endothelial Cells Involves TAK1. *The Journal of Biological Chemistry, 275,* 22064-22068.

Yang, X., Hao, Y., Ferenczy, A., Tang, S.C., & Pater, A. (1999). Overexpression of Anti-apoptotic Gene BAG-1 in Human Cervical Cancer. *Experimental Cell Research, 247,* 200-207.

Yang, X., Ferenczy, A., Tang, S.C., & Pater, A. (2000). Overexpression of anti-apoptotic gene BAG-1 in human cervical cancer. *Experimental Cell Research,* 2562-2583.

Yu, Q., Geng, Y., & Sicinski, P. (2001). Specific protection against breast cancers by cyclin D1 ablation. *Nature, 411,* 1001-1002.

Yuan, J., & Yanker, B.A. (2000). Apoptosis in the nervous system. *Nature Insight, 407,* 802-809.

Zhang, H.G., Huang, N., Liu, D., Bilbao, L., Zhang, X., Yang, P., Zhou, T., Curiel, D.T., & Mountz, J.D. (2000). Gene Therapy That Inhibits Nuclear Translocation of Nuclear Factor κB Results in Tumor Necrosis Factor alpha-induced Apoptosis of Human Synovial Fibroblasts. *Arthritis and Rheumatism, 43,* 1094-1105.

Zigarelli, B., Sheehan, M., & Wong, H.R. (2003). Nuclear factor- κB as a therapeutic target in critical care medicine. *Critical Care Medicine, 31,* S105-S111

zur Hausen, A., van Beek, J., Bloemena, E., ten Kate, F.J., Meijer, C.J., & van den Brule, A.J. (2003). No role for Epstein-Barr virus in Dutch hepatocellular carcinoma: a study at the DNA, RNA and protein levels. *J Gen Virol, 84(7),* 1863-1869.

In: Trends in Cervical Cancer
Editor: Hector T. Varaj, pp. 31-59

ISBN: 1-60021-299-9
© 2007 Nova Science Publishers, Inc.

Chapter II

NEW PERSPECTIVES IN THE PHARMACOLOGICAL TREATMENT OF CERVICAL CANCER: EXPERIMENTAL AND CLINICAL RESEARCHES

Angiolo Gadducci[1],, Stefania Cosio[1], Luca Cionini[2],
Andrea Riccardo Genazzani[1]*

[1]Department of Procreative Medicine, Division of Gynecology and Obstetrics, and
[2]Department of Oncology, Division of Radiotherapy, University of Pisa Italy.

ABSTRACT

Cisplatin [CDDP]-based concomitant chemotherapy and irradiation is the standard treatment for advanced cervical cancer. A randomised Gynecologic Oncologic Group [GOG] study found no difference in pelvic failures between weekly CDDP or continuous infusion of 5- fluorouracil [5-FU] in combination with pelvic irradiation and brachytherapy, whereas there was an increase in distant failures in the 5- FU arm. CDDP-based neoadjuvant chemotherapy followed by radical hysterectomy with pelvic lymphadenectomy appears to be an effective therapeutic option for patients with stage Ib2- IIb disease. The combination of paclitaxel [TAX] + ifosfamide + CDDP is associated with a higher pathological optimal response rate than the combination of ifosfamide + CDDP, without any statistically significant benefit on overall survival. Neoadjuvant chemotherapy followed by conization and laparoscopic pelvic lymphadenectomy can represent an interesting therapeutic option, alternative to radical treachelectomy, to preserve fertility in accurately selected patients with early-stage cervical cancer. As for metastatic or recurrent disease, single-agent CDDP achieves an overall response rate of 18 to 31 % approximately, and recent phase III trials have shown

---

* Correspondence concerning this article should be addressed to Angiolo Gadducci, Department of Procreative Medicine, Division of Gynecology and Obstetrics, University of Pisa, Via Roma 56, Pisa, 56127, Italy. Telephone number: 39 50 992609; Fax number 39 50 553410; E-mail: a.gadducci@obgyn.med.unipi.it.

response rates of 27% or 39% when CDDP has been combined with either TAX or topotecan, respectively. In particular, the combination of CDDP + topotecan has obtained a significantly better response rate, median progression-free survival, and median overall survival when compared with single- agent CDDP. However most of the responses to chemotherapy are partial and short-lived, thus encouraging the research of novel drugs and new combinations also including molecularly targeted agents (i.e. antiangiogenic agents, apoptosis inducers, and telomerase inhibitors).

1. INTRODUCTION

Cervical cancer is still a relevant health issue with a yearly incidence of almost half a million of new cases in the world and a mortality rate of 50% approximately [1]. The average annual incidence of this malignancy ranges widely according to geographical areas, with highest rates being reported in developing countries in Latin America, Caribbeans and Africa [2,3]. Moreover in developed countries most patients present with stage I cervical cancer, whereas in the developing ones 80 to 90% of patients have stage III-IV disease at presentation IV [3,4]. However, cervical cancer is still a common malignancy even in western countries, with 10520 new cases diagnosed and 3900 expected deaths in 2004 in the US [5]. Table 1 reports the distribution and survival by stage of the cervical cancer patients assessed in the International Federation of Gynecology and Obstetrics [FIGO] Annual Report n. 25 [6].

Table 1. Five year-survival of patients with cervical cancer by FIGO stage.

Stage	patients	5-year survival
Ia1	860	98.7%
Ia2	227	95.9%
Ib1	2530	88.0%
Ib2	950	78.8%
IIa	881	68.8%
IIb	2375	64.7%
IIIa	160	40.4%
IIIb	1949	43.3%
IVa	245	19.5%
IVb	189	15.0%

(Modified from Benedet et al. [6] Annual Report. N. 25)

Radical hysterectomy with pelvic lymphadenectomy and radiotherapy are equally effective in the treatment of early stage cervical cancer, but differ significantly as for morbidity and type of complications [7,8]. An Italian randomised trial on 343 women with stage Ib - IIa cervical cancer showed that 5-year overall survival and 5-year disease-free survival were identical in the radical hysterectomy and in radiotherapy arm (83% and 74%, respectively, for both groups), with severe morbidity being more frequent in surgically treated patients (28% versus 12%, p= 0.0004) [7]. A prospective randomised trial of the same authors detected that Piver II radical hysterectomy and Piver III radical hysterectomy are equally effective in the surgical treatment of stage Ib-IIa disease, but the former is associated with fewer late complications, especially of urological type [9]. Adjuvant postoperative external pelvic irradiation is routinely given to surgically treated patients with lymph node involvement, and is usually offered to those with negative nodes but with additional high-risk pathological factors, such as parametrial involvement, positive or close resection margins, lymph-vascular space involvement, deep cervical stromal invasion and large tumour size [10-24]. A phase III Gynecologic Oncology Group [GOG] study found that postoperative external irradiation significantly reduced the risk of recurrence (hazard ratio [HR], 0.54; 90% confidence interval [CI], 0.35-0.81; p= 0.007) and death (HR, 0.58; 90% CI, 0.40-0.85; p= 0.009) when compared to no adjuvant treatment in 277 stage Ib cervical cancer with negative lymph nodes but with two or more poor prognostic features including lymph-vascular space involvement, deep (more than one third) cervical stromal invasion, and tumor diameter $\geq$4 cm [22]. However, the addition of adjuvant pelvic irradiation increases the long-term complications of radical surgery, and especially of Piver III radical hysterectomy, and most gynecologists and radiation oncologists agree that a single treatment modality treatment is preferable to a planned combination of major therapeutic interventions [9,23-25].

External pelvic irradiation followed by brachytherapy has long been considered as the standard treatment of advanced cervical cancer, and the overall treatment time and total doses represent the major critical parameters for radiotherapy outcome [26-32]. The loss of local control and overall survival was found to be approximately 1% per day when treatment length exceeded 52 days [30]. Perez et al. [32] reported that among patients with stage IIb and III disease pelvic recurrence were 66.7% and 72%, 23.4% and 39%, 13.5% and 35%, respectively, according to radiation doses to point were below 60 Gy, 60 to 90 Gy, or 90 Gy. However the long–term clinical outcome of advanced cervical cancer patients treated with irradiation is unsatisfactory and has remained substantially unchanged during the last two decades. For instance the FIGO Annual Report n. 25 showed the 5-year survival of irradiation-treated patients was 64.2% for stage IIb, 40.9% for stage IIIa, 43.7% for stage IIIb, and 16.7% for stage IVa disease [6].

Chemotherapy has been often used as palliative treatment of patients with disseminated disease at the time of presentation or with recurrent/persistent disease after surgery and/or irradiation [33-42]. However, objective responses are short-lived, the impact of chemotherapy on survival, symptom control and quality of life is still unclear, and there have not been any randomised studies comparing chemotherapy versus the best supportive care. The poor chemoresponsiveness of recurrent cervical cancer depends on several factors. Drugs often fail to reach therapeutic intratumour concentrations because of altered post-irradiation blood supply. Previous irradiation decreases bone marrow reserve and causes poor tolerance for dose-intensive chemotherapy. The frequent ureteral involvement by recurrent disease makes the administration of certain nephrotoxic drugs difficult to be performed. Conversely, chemotherapy achieves satisfactory response rates in patients with untreated cervical cancer and therefore in the last two decades it has been investigated in the primary treatment of advanced disease with the aim of both increasing local control and eradicating distant lesions.

Chemotherapy is currently given as either treatment concomitant with irradiation (concurrent chemoradiation) or primary treatment before radical surgery (neoadjuvant chemotherapy).

Table 2. Concurrent chemo-radiation in advanced cervical cancer: chemotherapy regimens.

Author	drug	dose	schedule
Whitney [47]	CDDP	50 mg/m^2	days 1 and 29
	5-FU	1000 mg/m^2 x 96 hours	days 2 and 30
Whitney [47]	HU	80 mg/kg	twice weekly
Morris [48]	CDDP	75 mg/m^2	days 1, 22 and 43
	5-FU	1000 mg/m^2 X 96 hours	days 1, 22 and 43
Rose [49]	CDDP	50 mg/m^2	days 1 and 29
	5-FU	1000mg/m^2 x 96 hours	days 1 and 29
	HU	2 g/m^2	twice weekly
Rose [49]	CDDP	40 mg/m^2	weekly
Rose [49]	HU	3 g/m^2	twice weekly
Keys [50]	CDDP	40 mg/m^2	weekly
Peters [51]	CDDP	70 mg/m^2	days 1, 22, 43, 64
	5-FU	1000mg/m^2 x 96 hours	days 1, 22, 43, 64

2. CONCURRENT CHEMORADIATION FOR ADVANCED CERVICAL CANCER

Chemotherapy given concurrent to radiatiotherapy enhances the radiation damage, and offers the chance of spatial cooperation since the local effect of radiation is complemented by the systemic effect of chemotherapy on microscopic distant lesions [43,44]. Concurrent hydroxyurea and irradiation appeared to improve progression-free survival and overall survival when compared to irradiation alone [45,46]. In 1999 five prospective randomised trials showed the superiority of concurrent CDDP-based chemotherapy and irradiation versus hydroxyurea plus irradiation or irradiation alone [47-51) (Table 2) (Table 3). Whitney et al. [47] reported that severe leukopenia was more common in patients who received hydroxyurea plus irradiation than in those who received CDDP+ 5-fluorouracil [5-FU] plus irradiation (24% versus 4%), whereas overall survival was significantly better for the latter. The total elapsed time for radiotherapy did not exceed 10 weeks. In the series of Morris et al. [48], control arm received extended field irradiation on the basis of previous observations showing an improved 10-year survival when prophylactic para-aortic irradiation was added to standard pelvic irradiation in women with stage Ib bulky-IIb disease. [52]. Patients treated with concurrent CDDP + 5-FU and pelvic irradiation had a better overall survival and higher reversible haematologic toxicity than patients enrolled to extended field irradiation arm [48]. The total duration of radiotherapy was <8 weeks. Rose et al. [49] found that both patients enrolled to concurrent CDDP + 5-FU + hydroxydroxurea and irradiation and patients enrolled to concurrent CDDP and irradiation had a better overall survival than those treated with hydroxyurea and irradiation, and that single-agent CDDP arm was less toxic than three-drug regimen arm. The duration of irradiation was 10 weeks. In the trial of Keys et al. [50] radiotherapy followed by adjuvant hysterectomy was used as control arm on the basis of a previous GOG randomised trial showing a lower pelvic recurrence rate for women who received this integrated treatment compared to those who underwent irradiation alone. The authors found that stage Ib_2 cervical cancer patients who underwent concurrent CDDP and irradiation followed by extrafascial hysterectomy experienced a significantly reduced risk of death when compared to those who underwent irradiation followed by extrafascial hysterectomy. There was an higher frequency of grade 3-4 haematological toxicities (21% versus 2%) and gastrointestinal toxicities (14% versus 5%) among the former. The median duration of radiotherapy was 50 days in both arms. The trial of Peters et al. [51] randomised patients with high-risk early-stage cervical cancer after radical hysterectomy to receive concurrent adiuvant CDDP + 5-FU and pelvic irradiation or adjuvant pelvic irradiation alone, and observed that concurrent chemoradiaiton arm had a better clinical outcome. In all these five trials CDDP-based chemoradiation was the more effective therapy, reducing the risk of death by 30% to 50%, and the US National Cancer Institute Alert in February 1999 stated that concomitant chemoradiotherapy should be considered for all patients with for high-risk early stage and locally advanced cervical cancer [53,54]. However, in a Canadian randomised, the overall survival was not significantly different between advanced squamous cell cervical cancer patients who received concurrent weekly CDDP (40 mg/m^2) external irradiation and brachytherapy and those who received the same radiotherapy without chemotherapy (HR, 1.10; 95% CI, 0.75-1.62) [55]. It is noteworthy that median overall duration of irradiation was 49 days for the chemoradiation arm and 51 days for the irradiation arm, thus being clearly lower than that of the other studies.

The meta-analysis of data from 4921 cervical cancer patients enrolled in 24 trials (21 published, 3 unpublished) strongly suggested that chemoradiation improved progression- free survival and overall survival when compared with irradiation alone, with absolute benefits of 13% and 10% respectively [56]. Chemoradiation showed a significant benefit for local recurrences and a suggestion of a benefit for distant recurrences, thus suggesting that concomitant chemotherapy might afford radiosensitisation and systemic cytotoxic effects. Acute haematological and gastrointestinal toxicity was significantly greater in chemoradiation group, whereas late effects of treatment were not well reported and treatment-related deaths were rare.

A further randomised GOG trial compared weekly CDDP (40 mg/m^2) versus continuous infusion of 5-FU (225 mg/m^2/day for 5 days/week) in combination with pelvic irradiation plus high- or low-dose rate brachytherapy in patients with stage IIb-IVa cervical cancer and clinically negative para-aortic nodes [57]. An interim analysis showed an increased risk of progression of 35% in the 5-FU arm, mainly due to an higher distant failure rate.

A triple-modality therapy combining weekly CDDP (40 mg/m^2), weekly locoregional hyperthermia and irradiation obtained a complete response in 90% out of 68 advanced cervical cancer patients, with a disease-free survival and an overall survival of 74% and 84%, respectively, after a median follow-up of 538 days [58]. A phase III study comparing this novel triplet therapy with standard chemoradiation has been launched.

Paclitaxel [TAX] arrests the cell cycle in the more radiosensitive G_2/M phase [59-61], and in vitro studies have demonstrated that this drug has potent radiosensitizing effects on different tumour cell lines, including squamous cell cervical cancer cell lines [62-65]. Concurrent TAX (40-60 mg/m^2/week) and irradiation achieved a complete response in 12 out of 19 patients with locally advanced or recurrent squamous cell carcinoma of the uterine cervix, of whom 10 remained disease-free after a median follow-up of 47 months [66]. Five patients experienced grade 3 bowel toxicity, 1 patient had grade 3 bladder toxicity, and 1 patient had grade 4 mucositis.

Table 3. Concurrent chemoradiation in advanced cervical cancer: clinical outcome.

Authors	stage	patients		treatment	Clinical outcome	p
		R	E			
Whitney [47]	IIb-IVa[o+]	388	368	CDDP+5-FU+pelvic RT+ BCT	5y-OS: 64%	0.018
				HU + pelvic RT+ BCT	5y-OS : 48%	
Morris [48]	High-risk Ib-IIa or IIb-IVa[o++]	403	388	CDDP+ 5-FU+ pelvic RT+ BCT	5y-OS: 73%	0.004
				extended RT+ BCT	5y-OS: 58%	
Rose (49]	IIB-IVa[o+]	575	526	CDDP+5-FU+HU+ pelvic RT+BCT	4y-OS: 66%	0.002*
				CDDP + pelvic RT + BCT	4y-OS: 64%	0.004**
				HU + pelvic RT + BCT	y-OS : 39%	
Keys[o++] [50]	Ib bulky	374	369	CDDP + pelvic RT + BCT + adjuvant hysterectomy	3y-OS: 83%	0.008
				pelvic RT + BCT + adjuvant hysterectomy	3y-OS : 74%	
Peters[o] [51]	IA2-IIA with risk factors after radical hysterectomy	268	263	Adjuvant CDDP + 5-FU + pelvic RT	4-y PFS: 81%	0.01
				Adjuvant pelvic RT	4-y PFS: 63%	

Legend: R, Randomised; E, Evaluable; CDDP, cisplatin; 5-FU, 5-fluorouracil; RT, external irradiation; BCT, brachytherapy ; OS, overall survival; HU, hydroxyurea;PFS, progression-free survival .
o Squamous carcinoma, adenosquamous carcinoma and adenocarcinoma.
+ Histologically negative para-aortic lymph nodes.
++ Histologically or radiologically negative para-aortic lymph nodes.
* Versus HU + RT; ** versus HU + RT.

TAX (at doses up to 50 mg/m^2/week) plus CDDP-based concurrent chemotherapy and pelvic irradiation has been well tolerated in two phase I studies [67,68]. Conversely, in the series of Petera [69] only 4 of out 19 patients were able to complete the planned course of concurrent CDDP and TAX with external irradiation to the pelvis ± para-aortic nodes plus brachytherapy, and in most cases treatment was stopped for haematological toxicity. This poor tolerance was probably due to the frequent use of the extended fields for para-aortic lymph node irradiation.

A phase I study showed that carboplatin [CBDCA] at the dose of 133 mg/m^2/week is a well tolerated and effective radiosensitizer in advanced cervical cancer patients receiving standard pelvic irradiation followed by brachytherapy up to mean doses to points A and B of 85.6 Gy and 62.9 Gy , respectively [70]. The combined use of weekly CBDCA at a dose corresponding to an area under the curve [AUC] of 2 + weekly TAX 60 mg/m^2 concurrent with irradiation appeared to be poorly tolerated due to dose-limiting diarrhoea [71], whereas concurrent weekly CBDCA AUC 1.5 + weekly TAX 50 mg/m^2 and irradiation was found to be feasible and achieved a 2-year progression-free survival of 80% in a series of 15 patients with stage Ib$_2$-IIIb disease [72].

Other agents currently under evaluation for chemoradiation includes irinotecan [73-76], vinorelbine [77] and gemcitabine [78]. For instance, weekly 40 mg/m^2 irinotecan concurrent with pelvic irradiation and brachytherapy obtained 4 complete and 7 partial responses, for an overall response rate of 78.6%, among 14 patients with stage IIIb cervical cancer [76]. Approximately 7% of the women had grade 3 diarrhoea, whereas neither grade 4 toxicity nor treatment-related death occurred.

3. NEOADJUVANT CHEMOTHERAPY FOR ADVANCED CERVICAL CANCER

In the last decade several studies have investigated the role of CDDP-based neoadjuvant chemotherapy in patients with advanced cervical cancer, with clinical complete response rates ranging from 4% to 40.5% mainly dependent on tumour stage and stage [79-102] (Table 4).

Most phase III trials failed to demonstrate a clinical benefit with chemotherapy followed by irradiation versus irradiation alone [79,82-84,93,98-100], probably because of the chemotherapy-induced accelerated tumour clonogen resistant cell repopulation and cross-resistance between irradiation and chemotherapy [103-105]. A meta-analyses of individual data from 18 trials including 2074 patients was performed to compare neoadjuvant chemotherapy followed by irradiation versus irradiation alone [106]. Because of the high level of statistical heterogeneity, the results could not be combined indiscriminately but some interesting observations were drawn by separate analyses of groups of trials. It is noteworthy that trials using CDDP dose-intensities <25 mg/m^2/week demonstrated a significant detrimental effect of neoadjuvant chemotherapy on survival (HR, 1.35; 95% CI, 1.11-1.14; p= 0.002).

Conversely, neoadjuvant chemotherapy followed by radical surgery has achieved satisfactory results in terms of overall survival, [80,81,82,85-90,92,94,95,97,100-102]

Sardi et al. [90] randomly allocated 205 patients with stage Ib squamous cell cervical cancer to receive either primary radical hysterectomy plus adjuvant pelvic irradiation or combination chemotherapy consisting of CDDP (50 mg/m^2 day 1) + vincristine (1 mg/m^2 day 1) + bleomycin (25 mg day 1-3) repeated every 10 days for 3 cycles and followed by radical hysterectomy plus adjuvant pelvic irradiation. After a median follow-up of 67 months, there was a better survival for neoadjuvant chemotherapy arm among patients with tumour diameter >4 cm (80% versus 61%, p< 0.01), whereas there was no survival difference among patients with smaller tumours (82 % versus 77%, p= ns) .

Colombo et al. [94] assessed 100 advanced cervical cancer patients who received six cycles of weekly chemotherapy consisting of CDDP (50 mg/m^2)+ vincristine (1 mg/m^2)+ bleomycin (30 mg 24-hour infusion) prior to radical hysterectomy. A pathological complete response was found in 6 patients, a pathological optimal partial response (residual disease <3 mm) in 22 patients, and a suboptimal partial response in 43 patients, and the patients achieving a pathological complete or an optimal partial response had a significantly longer survival than the others (p= 0.002).

Table 4. Neoadjuvant chemotherapy for advanced cervical cancer: cisplatin-based combination regimen.

Authors	Drug	dose and schedule
Sardi [80, 82, 88-90]	CDDP	50 mg/m^2 day 1
	VCR	1 mg/m^2 day 1 every 10 days x 3 courses
	BLEO	25 mg/m^2 days 1-3
Benedetti [81]	CDDP	100 mg/m^2 day 1
	BLEO	15 mg day 1, 8 every 21 days x 3 courses
	MTX	300 mg/m^2 day 8
Benedetti [102]	CDDP	80 mg/m^2 day 1 every 21 days x 2 courses
	BLEO	15 mg/m^2 days 1,8
Colombo [94]	CDDP	50 mg/m^2 day 1
	VCR	1 mg/m^2 day 1 every 7 days x 6 courses
	BLEO	30 mg day 1
Marth [95]	CDDP	100 mg/m^2 day 1 every 21 days x 2-3 courses
	5-FU	1000 mg/m^2 days 1-5
Sugiyama [96]	CDDP	60 mg/m^2 day 1
	CTP-11	60 mg/m^2 days 1,8, 15 every 28 days x 2-3 courses
Pignata [97]	CDDP	80 mg/m^2 day 1 every 21 days X 3 courses
	VNR	25 mg/m^2 days 1, 8
Zanetta [107] Buda [108]	IFO	5 g/m^2 day 1
	TAX	175 mg/m^2 day 2 every 21 days X 3 courses
	CDDP	75 mg/m^2 day 2
Buda [108]	IFO	5 g/m^2 day 1 every 21 days X 3 courses
	CDDP	75 mg/m^2 day 2
Fossati [109]	TAX	175 mg/m^2 day 1 every 21 days X 3 courses
	CDDP	75 mg/m^2 day 1

Legend CDDP, cisplatin; VCR; vincristine; BLEO, bleomycin; MTX, methotrexate5-FU, 5-fluorouracil; CTT-11, irinotecan; VNR; vinorelbine; IFO, ifosfamide; TAX, paclitaxel.

An Italian multicenter study randomised 441 patients with stage Ib_2-III squamous cell cervical cancer to receive CDDP-based neoadjuvant chemotherapy followed by type III-V radical hysterectomy and pelvic lymphadenectomy or exclusive external irradiation (45 to 50 Gy) followed by brachytherapy (20 to 30 Gy) [101]. As for operated women, adjuvant treatment consisting of external irradiation or chemotherapy was given to patients with positive surgical margins or positive lymph nodes. Both treatments were relatively well tolerated, no treatment-related death occurred, and severe complications affected 32% and 28% of the patients enrolled in the chemosurgical arm and irradiation arm, respectively. The 5-year progression-free survival and 5-year overall survival rates were significantly better for chemosurgical arm among patients with stage Ib_2-IIb disease (59.7 versus 46.7, p= 0.02; and 64.7 versus 46.4, p= 0.005, respectively), whereas no significant differences in 5-year progression-free survival and 5-year overall survival between the two arms were found among stage III patients (41.9% versus 36.4%, p= ns, and, 41.6% versus 36.7%, p= ns, respectively). The more advanced the stage, the larger is the hypoxic and resting phase cell population with reduced chemosensitivity and the chance of developing resistant clones. About one third of failures showed a distant component, and there was no statistically significant difference between the two arms with regard to the pattern of recurrence. These data are in agreement with those reported by Sardi et al. [88-90], thus suggesting that the relatively short duration of neoadjuvant chemotherapy may be not sufficient to control distant micrometastases. The median total dose at point A of 70 Gy was lower than that considered optimal for advanced cervical cancer (80-90 Gy), and moreover brachytherapy was not given to 28% of the patients, mainly because of anatomic reasons.

The usefulness of the addition of TAX to CDDP-based neoadjuvant chemotherapy has been first suggested by Zanetta et al. [107], who showed that the combination of ifosfamide (5 g/m^2 24-hour infusion) + TAX 175 mg/m^2 (3-hour infusion) + CDDP 50-75 mg/m^2 (TIP regimen) achieved a pathological complete response in 16% and a pathological optimal partial response in 18% out of 38 patients with stage Ib_2-IV squamous cell cervical cancer. The SNAP01 (Studio Neo-Adjuvante Portio) Italian Collaborative Study compared TIP regimen versus the combination of ifosfamide 5 g/m^2 + CDDP 75 mg/m^2 (IP regimen) as neoadjuvant chemotherapy followed by radical hysterectomy in 219 patients with locally advanced squamous cell cervical cancer [108]. The pathological optimal response rate (complete + optimal partial) was higher for TIP regimen (48% versus 23%, p= 0 .0003). At a median follow-up of 43.4 months, 79 women experienced disease progression or died, and patients receiving TIP had a lower failure rate (HR, 0.75; 95% CI= 0.48-1.17; p=ns) and a lower death rate (HR, 0.66; 95% CI, 0.39-1.10; p= ns) but the differences were not significant. Grade 3-4 haematological toxicity and neurosensory symptoms were more frequent in TIP arm. There were 4 toxic deaths, 3 in IP arm and one in TIP arm , and of these patients three were older than 70 years and one presented with urological stage IIIb disease. Cox analysis showed that pathological optimal response was an independent predictor of survival (HR, 5.88; 95% CI, 2.50-13.84; p< 0.0001). The SNAP02 Italian trial is currently comparing TIP regimen with the less toxic combination of TAX 175 mg/m^2 + CDDP 75 mg/m^2 (TP regimen) in order to better define the role of ifosfamide in neoadjuvant chemotherapy [109]. Preliminary analysis of the data on 156 patients revealed that TIP regimen achieved a higher pathological optimal response rate when compared with TP regimen (45% [95% CI, 32-58%] versus 30% [95% CI, 19-42%]), whereas grade 3-4 haematological toxicity occurred more frequently in patients who received the triple drug regimen .

The meta-analysis of data from 872 cervical cancer patients enrolled in 5 trials demonstrated a significant reduction in the risk of death with neoadjuvant chemotherapy followed by surgery versus irradiation (HR, 0.65; 95% CI, 0.53-0.80; p= 0.0004), although there were some differences between the trials in their design and results [106].

4. NEOADJUVANT CHEMOTHERAPY FOLLOWED BY CONIZATION FOR EARLY-STAGE CERVICAL CANCER

Vaginal radical trachelectomy with laparoscopic pelvic lymphadenectomy is considered to be an oncologically safe, fertility-preserving surgery in accurately selected stage Ia_2-Ib_1 cervical cancer patient, associated with a 4% failure rate and a 2.5% death rate [110-114]. Tumour diameter >2 cm and lymph-vascular space involvement are the most important risk factors for recurrence. Fertility rates after this operation are good. Over 400 cases of women submitted to radical trachelectomy have been reported in the literature with 100 live births [112]. Overall, there is a 16% rate of first trimester losses, a 4–10% rate of second trimester losses, a 16–19% rate of premature deliveries, and approximately two thirds of pregnant women take home a baby [113]. Another conservative option for these patients is represented by neoadjuvant chemotherapy followed by conization and laparoscopic pelvic lymphadenectomy [115,116]. Andrade et al. [115] administered chemotherapy consisting of bleomycin (30 mg day 1) + CDDP (50 mg/m^2 days 2-3) to a woman with stage IIa cervical cancer, who afterwards refused radical surgery and disappeared. Five months later she returned to the clinic with a 2 month –pregnancy, and she ultimately delivered an healthy baby at 38 weeks by cesarean section, during which neither palpable para-aortic nor pelvic lymph nodes were found. The patient was disease-free after 37 months from delivery. Kobayashi [116] reported the case of a young woman with stage Ib_1 squamous cell cervical cancer who received 4 cycles of combination chemotherapy consisting of CDDP (10 mg/m^2 days 1–7)+ bleomycin (5 mg/m^2 days 1–7)+ vincristine (0.7 mg/m^2 day 7)+ mitomycin-C (7 mg/m^2, day 7) at 4-week intervals. Then she underwent a cold-knife conization with endocervical and endometrial curettage, that revealed a pathological complete response. The patient became pregnant two years later, delivered an healthy infant, and she was disease-free after an interval of 48 months.

5. CHEMOTHERAPY FOR PERSISTENT, RECURRENT OR METASTATIC CERVICAL CANCER

CDDP is the most extensively studied single- agent in patients with persistent, recurrent or metastatic cervical cancer, with response rates of 18 to 31% approximately, a median duration of response of 4 to 6 months, and a median overall survival of 7 months [35-

37,43,117-120] (Table 5). A GOG randomised trial compared CDDP 50 mg/m^2 every 21 days versus CDDP 100 mg/m^2 every 21 days versus CDDP 20 mg/m^2 days 1-5 every 21 days in 497 patients [118]. The corresponding response rates were 20.7%, 31.4%, and 25.0%, respectively, the median progression-free interval ranged from 3.7 to 4.6 months, and the median overall survival ranged from 6.1 to 7.1 months. CDDP at 100 mg/m^2 single- dose achieved a higher response rate than CDDP at 50 mg/m^2 dose (p= 0.015), while producing no improvement in the clinical outcome and causing a greater myelosuppression and nephrotoxicity. CBDCA obtained a 15-28% response rate, but this drug has never been compared with CDDP in a randomised trial [121,122]. Other single-agents with response rates higher than 15% against cervical cancer are reported in the Table 5 [33-42,120,123,124].

Table 5. Single -agents in persistent, recurrent or metastatic cervical cancer.

	Response rates
Cisplatin	18-31%
Carboplatin	15-28%
5-fluorouracil	16%
Ifosfamide	11-30%
Vinorelbine	17-18%
Paclitaxel	17%
Topotecan	19%
Irinotecan	21%

CDDP-based combination chemotherapy achieves a approximately 50% response rate, with increased toxicity profile and without any clear survival advantage when compared with single-agent CDDP [125-131]. Responses are more frequent in non-irradiated than in irradiated sites. For instance, a randomised phase III trial of the European Organisation for Research and Treatment of Cancer [EORTC] showed that the combination of vindesine (3 mg/m^2 day 1) + CDDP (50 mg/m^2 day 1) + bleomycin (15 mg 24-hour infusion days 2-4) + mitomycin C (8 mg/m^2 at alternate cycles) induced an higher response rate (42% versus 25%, p= 0.006), without any impact on survival, when compared with single -agent CDDP 50 mg/m^2 in patients with disseminated squamous cell cervical cancer [131].

In a randomised GOG trial, the combination of CDDP 50 mg/m^2 + IFO 5 g/m^2 obtained a higher response rate (31.1% versus 17.8%, p= 0.004), a longer progression-free survival (p= 0.003) and a greater toxicity, but no improvement in overall survival with respect to with CDDP 50 mg/m^2 [128]. In a phase II GOG trial TAX 135-170 mg/m^2 + CDDP 75 mg/m^2 achieved a 46.3% response rate among 41 patients, with a median progression-free interval of 5.4 months and median overall survival of 10.0 months [129]. A phase III randomised study is currently comparing this regimen versus single-agent CDDP.

A GOG trial randomly allocated 294 patients with stage IVb or recurrent or persistent cervical cancer to receive either CDDP 50 mg/m^2 every 3 weeks or topotecan 0.75 mg/m^2 days 1-3 + CDDP 50 mg/m^2 day 1 every 3 weeks [132]. Combination chemotherapy had a higher response rate (27% versus 13%, p= 0.004), a longer median progression-free survival

(4.6 versus 2.9 months; p= 0.014) and a longer median overall survival (9.4 versus 6.5 months; p= 0.017), associated with a more frequent grade 3-4 haematological toxicity. This is the first randomised phase III trial demonstrating a survival advantage for CDDP-based combination chemotherapy versus single agent-CDDP. A phase I trial of weekly topotecan on pretreated epithelial ovarian cancer patients showed a lower haematological toxicity with respect to the stardard 5-day regimen [133]. A weekly schedule of CDDP + topotecan would be of interest for future studies in advanced cervical cancer.

Prior GOG studies in patients with nonsquamous cervical cancers (adenocarcinoma, adenosquamous carcinoma, undifferentiated carcinoma) detected some drugs with antineoplastic activity against these histological types, such as TAX (31%) [134], CDDP (20%) [135], oral etoposide (11.9%) [136], 5-FU and high–dose leucovorin (14%) [137] and ifosfamide (15.0%) [138]. Recently, GOG published the results of two phase II trials in which vinorelbine (30 mg/ m^2 days 1 and 8 every 3 weeks) and gemcitabine (800 mg/m^2 days 1, 8 and 15 every 4 weeks) achieved an objective response only in 7.1 % out of 28, and, respectively, in 4.5% out of 19 patients with persistent, recurrent or metastatic nonsquamous cervical cancer [139,140]. In 2003 the GOG has decided to include adenocarcinoma and adenosquamous carcinoma in phase III trials of persistent or recurrent cervical cancer, thus discontinuing having separate studies for squamous and nonsquamous histologies.

In a pilot study on women with advanced or recurrent disease, the combination of taxotere 60 mg/m^2 + CBDCA AUC6 obtained an objective response in 70% out of the 10 patients with squamous cell carcinoma and in 86% out of the 7 patients with nonsquamous cell carcinoma, with grade 3-4 neutropenia being the most common severe side effect [141].

6. MOLECULARLY TARGETED AGENTS FOR PERSISTENT, RECURRENT OR METASTATIC CERVICAL CANCER

Most of the responses to chemotherapy in patients with persistent, recurrent or metastatic cervical cancer are partial and short-lived, thus encouraging the research of novel drugs and new combinations also including molecularly targeted agents (Table 6) [142-145].

Table 6. Molecularly targeted therapies in cervical cancer.

Antiangiogenic agents	TPN-470 (analogue of fumagillin)
	IFN-α
	Bevacizumab
Apoptosis inducers	Proteasome inhibitors
	rh TRAIL
Telomerase inhibitors	siRNA specific for hTERT

Legend: IFN-α, interferon –α; rhTRAIL, human recombinant tumour- necrosis factor- related apoptosis inducing ligand; siRNA, small interfering RNA; hTERT, catalytic subunit of human telomerase reverse transcriptase.

6.1. Antiangiogenic Agents

Tumour angiogenesis involves the synthesis by tumour cells of proangiogenic factors, which trigger the proliferation of endothelial cells, the release of proteolytic enzymes, the extensive endothelial membrane remodelling with tubule and loop vessel formation, and the recruitment of pericytes which stabilize the new vessels [142]. One of the most important proangiogenic factors is vascular endothelial growth factor [VEGF], a dimeric glycoprotein of which at least four isoforms have been identified. The biological effects of VEGF are mediated by receptor tyrosine kinases, which differ considerably in signaling properties [146]. Cervical cancer expresses different proangiogenic activators [142]. For instance, increased mRNA for VEGF, basic- fibroblast growth factor [b-FGF] and matrix metalloproteinase [MMP]-9 [147], increased microenvironmental interleukin [IL]-6 [148], and increased platelet-derived endothelial cell growth factor (PD-ECGF) expression have been detected in this malignancy [149]. PD-ECGF is thymidine phosphorylase, a key enzyme in the activation of fluoropyrimidines such as 5-FU, and the evaluation of PD-ECGF expression may be important in designing future chemotherapy trials.

TNP-470, an analogue of the naturally secreted antibiotic fumagillin of Aspergillus fumigatus fresenius, is a vasculotoxin able to inhibit endothelial cell proliferation therby reducing the synthesis of proangiogenuc factors such as VEGF and b-FGF [150-152]. This agent, that has been found to inhibit angiogenesis in vitro and in vivo, entered clinical development as an anti-angiogenic agent for cancer in 1992 and it is currently under evaluation in phase I/II trials in different malignancies [153]. A phase I trial of intravenous TNP-470 (at increasing doses starting from 9.3 mg/m^2) every other day for 28 days, followed by a 14-day rest period, was conducted in 18 patients with metastatic squamous cell cervical cancer [154]. The dose-limiting toxicity level was seen at 71.2 mg/m^2 and the recommended dose for phase II studies was 60 mg/m^2 three times a week. The main toxicity was neurological, with grade 3 ataxia. One patient with lung relapse achieved a complete response within 3 months of treatment initiation, and the drug was given for 18 months until the patient developed chemical hepatitis, which resolved upon therapy discontinuation. She remained disease-free for over 7 years.

Interferon [IFN]-α and IFN-β inhibit angiogenesis through downregulation of IL-8, MMP-9, b-FGF and VEGF gene transcription [155,156]. Retinoids are potent inhibitors of epithelial carcinogenesis through modulation of cell proliferation, differentiation and apoptosis, and synergistic antitumour effects of a combination of interferons and retinoic acid have been demonstrated on different human tumour cells in vitro and in vivo [157-161]. Lippman et al. [162] achieved 1 complete response and 12 partial responses, for an overall response rate of 50% and with a minimal toxicity, among 26 patients with untreated, locally advanced squamous cell cervical cancer who were given oral 13-cis-retinoic acid 1 mg/kg and subcutaneous IFN-α 6 million units daily for at least 2 months. However, retinoids + IFN-α and retinoids + IFN-α + CDDP obtained response rates ranging from 0 to 8% [163-166] and from 18 to 21% [167,168], respectively, in women with recurrent or metastatic squamous cell cervical cancer. Given these unsatisfactory results, IFN-α has probably very little activity in recurrent disease, although long-term stable disease has been sometimes observed [142].

Bevacizumab is an anti- VEGF monoclonal antibody approved for the first-line treatment of metastatic colon-rectal cancer [169,170]. Several ongoing trials are investigating the therapeutic potential of this antibody in other malignancies [171,172]. Bevacizumab is being studied in cervical cancer patients in the GOG protocol 227C [142].

6.2. Apoptosis Inducers

The induction of apoptosis, through the activation of death-receptor-mediated pathway or the inhibition of proteasome, may represent an interesting experimental treatment option for recurrent or metastatic cervical cancer [143,144]. In cervical carcinogenesis, the human papilloma virus [HPV] E6 gene product enhances proteasome-mediated p53 degradation. Hougardy et al. [144] found that, besides restoring normal wild-type p53 levels, the proteasome inhibitor MG132 (carbobenzoxyl-L-leucyl-L-leucyl-L-leucinal) could sensitize HPV-positive cervical cancer cell lines to apoptosis induction by human recombinant tumour- necrosis factor- related apoptosis inducing ligand [rh TRAIL], through   death receptor upregulation and X-linked inhibitor of apoptosis [XIAP] inactivation. Combining proteasome inhibitors with rhTRAIL may be useful for cervical cancer treatment.

6.3. Telomerase Inhibitors

The telomerase is a ribonucleoprotein enzyme complex that uses its own integral RNA as a template for synthesis of telomeric repeats to compensate for the normal loss of terminal DNA sequences during mitosis [173]. The expression of catalytic subunit of human telomerase reverse transcriptase [hTERT] has a great prognostic relevance for different human malignancies [174-176], and in addition this enzyme could represent a novel target for cancer treatment [177,178]. Using retroviral delivery of small interfering RNA (siRNA) specific for hTERT, Nakamura et al. [145] inhibited telomerase activity in cervical cancer cell lines. Cells lacking hTERT expression entered replicative senescence after a considerable number of cell divisions, and moreover these cells were more sensitive to ionizing radiation and chemotherapeutic agents, such as topoisomerase inhibitors or bleomycin, when compared with control cells. Therefore siRNA-based strategy could be applied to the development of novel telomerase inhibitors, that might be used in combination with radiotherapy and/ or chemotherapy.

7. CONCLUSIONS

CDDP-based concurrent chemoradiation is the standard treatment for patients with locally advanced cervical cancer. However, CDDP-based neoadjuvant chemotherapy followed by radical hysterectomy is able to achieve satisfactory results in terms of survival in patients with stage Ib2-IIb disease, and a randomised trial of EORTC (55994) is currently comparing these two treatment modalities [102].

Neoadjuvant chemotherapy followed by conization and laparoscopic pelvic lymphadenectomy could represent a rational therapeutic option, alternative to vaginal radical trachelectomy with laparoscopic pelvic lymphadenectomy, for accurately selected patients with early- stage disease who desire to maintain their fertility.

CDDP is the most active single-agent in patients with persistent, recurrent or metastatic cervical cancer, with response rates of 18 to 31% and with a median survival of 7 months. A recent phase III trial demonstrated a survival advantage for a CDDP-based combination chemotherapy, i.e. CDDP + topotecan, versus single-agent CDDP in these patients [132]. The doses of topotecan used (0.75 mg/m^2 for 3 days every 3 weeks) were considerably lower than those given with the stardard schedule for this drug (1.5 mg/m^2 for 5 days every 3 weeks), and additional trials with higher dose topotecan should be taken into consideration.

Nowadays molecularly targeted therapies are extensively tested in patients with epithelial ovarian cancer [179-184] and endometrial cancer [185-187]. As for cervical cancer, apoptosis inducers, telomerase inhibitors, and antiangiogenic agents represent attractive investigational options for the management of patients with persistent, recurrent or metastatic disease.

8. REFERENCES

[1]   Parkin DM, Bray F, Ferlay J, Pisani P. Estimating the world cancer burden: Globocan 2000. *Int J Cancer* 2001; 4: 153–6

[2]   Bax A, Voigt RR, Coronel CC, Putter H, de Bie Leuving Tjeenk RM, van Marwijk HW.Incidence of cervical carcinoma in a high-risk, non-screened area results of a retrospective analysis on the Dutch Caribbean Antilles from 1983 to 1998. *West Indian Med J* 2004; 53: 150-4.

[3]   Adewole IF, Benedet JL, Crain BT, Follen M. Evolving a strategic approach to cervical cancer control in Africa. *Gynecol Oncol.* 2005; 99 (Suppl.): S209-12.

[4]   Emembolu JO, Ekwempu CC. Carcinoma of the cervix uteri in Zaria: etiological factors. *Int J Gynaecol Obstet* 1988; 26: 265–9.

[5]   Jemal A, Tiwari RC, Murray T, Ghafoor A, Samuels A, Ward E, Feuer EJ, Thun MJ; American Cancer Society. Cancer statistics, 2004. *CA Cancer J Clin* 2004; 54: 8-29.

[6]   Benedet JL, Odicino F, Massoneive P, Beller U, Creasman WT, Heintz APM, Ngan HYS, Pecorelli S. Carcinoma of the uterine cervix. *Int J Obstet Gynecol* 2003; 83 (Suppl.): 41-78.

[7]   Landoni F, Maneo A, Colombo A, Placa F, Milani R, Perego P, Favini G, Ferri L, Mangioni C. Randomized study of radical surgery versus radiotherapy for stage Ib-IIa cervical cancer. *Lancet.* 1997; 350: 535-40.

[8]   Perez CA, Grigsby PW, Lockett MA, Chao KS, Williamson J. Radiation therapy morbidity in carcinoma of the uterine cervix: dosimetric and clinical correlation. *Int J Radiat Oncol Biol Phys.* 1999; 44: 855-66.

[9]   Landoni F, Maneo A, Cormio G, Perego P, Milani R, Caruso O, Mangioni C. Class II versus class III radical hysterectomy in stage IB-IIA cervical cancer: a prospective randomized study. *Gynecol Oncol* 2001; 80: 3-12.

[10] Gonzalez Gonzalez D, Ketting BW, van Bunnigen B, van Dijk JD. Carcinoma of the uterine cervix stage IB and IIA: results of postoperative irradiation in patients with microscopic infiltration in the parametrium and/or lymph node metastasis. *Int J Radiat Oncol Biol Phys* 1989; 16: 389–95.

[11] Alvarez RD, Soong SJ, Kinney WK, Reid GC, Schray MF, Podratz KC, Morley GW, Shingleton HM. Identification of prognostic factors and risk groups in patients found to have nodal metastasis at the time of radical hysterectomy for early-stage squamous carcinoma of the cervix. *Gynecol Oncol* 1989; 35: 130-5. .

[12] Fuller AF Jr, Elliott N, Kosloff C, Hoskins WJ, Lewis JL Jr. Determinants of increased risk for recurrence in patients undergoing radical hysterectomy for stage IB and IIA carcinoma of the cervix. *Gynecol Oncol* 1989; 33: 34–9.

[13] Delgado G, Bundy B, Zaino R, Swvin B, Creasman WT. Major E. Prospective surgical–pathological study of disease-free interval in patients with stage IB squamous cell carcinoma of the cervix: a Gynecologic Oncology Group Study. *Gynecol Oncol* 1990; 38; 352–7.

[14] Monk BJ, Cha DS, Walker JL, Burger RA, Ramsinghani NS, Manetta A, DiSaia PJ, Berman ML. Extent of disease as an indication for pelvic radiation following radical hysterectomy and bilateral pelvic lymph node dissection in the treatment of stage IB and IIA cervical carcinoma. *Gynecol Oncol* 1994; 54 : 4–9

[15] Kridelka FJ, Berg DO, Neuman M, Edwards LS, Robertson G, Grant PT, Hacker NF. Adjuvant small field pelvic radiation for patients with high risk, stage IB lymph node negative cervix carcinoma after radical hysterectomy and pelvic lymph node dissection. A pilot study. *Cancer* 1999; 86: 2059-65.

[16] Yeh SA, Wan Leung S, Wang CJ, Chen HC. Postoperative radiotherapy in early stage carcinoma of the uterine cervix: treatment results and prognostic factors. *Gynecol Oncol* 1999; 72: 10–5.

[17] Lai CH, Hong JH, Hsueh S, Ng KK, Chang TC, Tseng CJ, Chou HH, Huang KG. Preoperative prognostic variables and the impact of postoperative adjuvant therapy on the outcomes of Stage IB or II cervical carcinoma patients with or without pelvic lymph node metastases: an analysis of 891 cases. *Cancer* 1999; 85: 1537-46.

[18] Hellebrekers BW, Zwinderman AH, Kenter GG, Peters AA, Snijders-Keilholz A, Graziosi GC, Fleuren GJ, Trimbos JB. Surgically-treated early cervical cancer: prognostic factors and the significance of depth of tumor invasion. *Int J Gynecol Cancer*. 1999; 9: 212-9.

[19] van der Velden J, Samlal R, Schilthuis MS, Gonzalez DG, ten Kate FJ, Lammes FB. A limited role for adjuvant radiotherapy after the Wertheim/Okabayashi radical hysterectomy for cervical cancer confined to the cervix. *Gynecol Oncol*.1999; 75: 233-7.

[20] Ohara K, Tsunoda H, Nishida M, Sugahara S, Hashimoto T, Shioyama Y, Hasezawa K, Yoshikawa H, Akine Y, Itai Y. Use of small pelvic field instead of whole pelvic field in postoperative radiotherapy for node-negative, high-risk stages I and II cervical squamous cell carcinoma. *Int J Gynecol Cancer* 2003; 13: 170-6.

[21]   Einhorn N, Trope C, Ridderheim M, Boman K, Sorbe B, Cavallin-Stahl E. A systematic overview of radiation therapy effects in cervical cancer (cervix uteri). *Acta Oncol* 2003; 42: 546-56.

[22]   Rotman M, Sedlis A, Piedmonte MR, Bundy B, Lentz SS, Muderspach LI, Zaino RJ. A phase III randomized trial of postoperative pelvic irradiation in stage Ib cervical carcinoma with poor prognostic features: follow-up of a Gynecologic Oncology Group study. *Int J Radiat Oncol Biol Phys* 2006 [Epub ahead of print].

[23]   Barter JF, Soong SJ, Shingleton HM, Hatch KD, Orr JW. Complications of combined radical hysterectomy and postoperative radiation therapy in women with early stage cervical cancer. *Gynecol Oncol* 1989; 32: 292–6.

[24]   Fiorica JV, Roberts WS, Greenberg H, Hoffman MS, LaPolla JP, Cavanagh D. Morbidity and survival patterns in patients after radical hysterectomy and postoperative adjuvant pelvic radiotherapy. *Gynecol Oncol* 1990; 36: 343–7.

[25]   Chen SW, Liang JA, Yang SN, Hung YC, Yeh LS, Shiau AC, Lin FJ. Radiation injury to intestine following hysterectomy and adjuvant radiotherapy for cervical cancer. *Gynecol Oncol*. 2004; 95: 208-14.

[26]   Perez CA, Camel HM, Kuske RR, Kao MS, Galakatos A, Hederman MA, Powers WE. Radiation therapy alone in the treatment of carcinoma of the uterine cervix: a 20-year experience. *Gynecol Oncol* 1986; 23: 127-40.

[27]   Montana GS, Fowler WC, Varia MA, Walton LA, Mack Y, Shemanski L. Carcinoma of the cervix, stage III. Results of radiation therapy. *Cancer* 1986; 57:148-54.

[28]   Fyles A, Keane TJ, Barton M, Simm J. The effect of treatment duration in the local control of cervix cancer. *Radiother Oncol* 1992; 25: 273-9.

[29]   Lanciano RM, Pajak TF, Martz K, Hanks JE. The influence of treatment time on outcome for squamous cell cancer of the uterine cervix treated with radiation: a patterns-of-care study. *Int J Radiat Oncol Biol Phys* 1993; 25: 391-7.

[30]   Girinsky T, Rey A, Roche B, Haie C, Gerbaulet A, Randrianarivello H, Chassagne D. Overall treatment time in advanced cervical carcinomas: a critical parameter in treatment outcome. *Int J Radiat Oncol Biol Phys*. 1993; 27: 1051-6.

[31]   Perez CA, Grigsby PW, Castro-Vita H, Lockett MA. Carcinoma of the uterine cervix. Impact of prolongation of overall treatment time and timing of brachytherapy on outcome of radiation therapy. *Int J Radiat Oncol Biol Phys* 1995; 32: 1275-88.

[32]   Perez CA, Fox S, Lockett MA, Grigsby PW, Camel HM, Galakatos A, Kao MS, Williamson J. Impact of dose in outcome of irradiation alone in carcinoma of the uterine cervix: analysis of two different methods. *Int J Radiat Oncol Biol Phys*. 1991; 21: 885-98.

[33]   Blackledge G, Buxton EJ, Mould JJ, Monaghan J, Paterson M, Tobias J, Alcock C, Spooner D, Meanwell CA. Phase II studies of ifosfamide alone and in combination in cancer of the cervix. *Cancer Chemother Pharmacol*. 1990; 26 (Suppl): S12-6.

[34]   Sutton GP, Blessing JA, Adcock L, Webster KD, DeEulis T. Phase II study of ifosfamide and mesna in patients with previously-treated carcinoma of the cervix. A Gynecologic Oncology Group study. *Invest New Drugs*. 1989; 7: 341-3.

[35]   Park RC, Thigpen JT. Chemotherapy in advanced and recurrent cervical cancer: a review. *Cancer* 1993; 71 (Suppl.): 1446-50.

[36]   Omura GA. Chemotherapy for cervix cancer. *Semin Oncol.* 1994; 21: 54-62.

[37]   Thigpen JT, Vance R, Puneky L, Khansur T. Chemotherapy as a palliative treatment in carcinoma of the uterine cervix. *Semin Oncol.* 1995; 22 (Suppl.): 16-24.

[38]   McGuire WP, Blessing JA, Moore D, Lentz SS, Photopulos G. Paclitaxel has moderate activity in squamous cervix cancer. A Gynecologic Oncology Group study. *J Clin Oncol* 1996; 14: 792-5.

[39]   Morris M, Brader KR, Levenback C, Burke TW, Atkinson EN, Scott WR, Gershenson DM. Phase II study of vinorelbine in advanced and recurrent squamous cell carcinoma of the cervix. *J Clin Oncol*.1998; 16: 1094-8.

[40]   Lhomme C, Vermorken JB, Mickiewicz E, Chevalier B, Alvarez A, Mendiola C, Pawinski A, Lentz MA, Pecorelli S. Phase II trial of vinorelbine in patients with advanced and/or recurrent cervical carcinoma: an EORTC Gynaecological Cancer Cooperative Group Study. *Eur J Cancer* 2000; 36:194-9.

[41]   Bookman MA, Blessing JA, Hanjani P, Herzog TJ, Andersen WA. Topotecan in squamous cell carcinoma of the cervix: a phase II study of the Gynecologic Oncology Group. *Gynecol Oncol* 2000;77: 446-9.

[42]   Friedlander M, Grogan M; US Preventative Services Task Force. Guidelines for the treatment of recurrent and metastatic cervical cancer. *Oncologist* 2002; 7: 342-7.

[43]   Eifel PJ, Rose PG. Chemotherapy and radiation therapy for cervical cancer. In "*American Society of Clinical Oncology. 2000 Educational Book*" (Perry MC Ed), Thirty-Sixth Annual Meeting, May 19-23, 2000, New Orleans, LA, 199-206.

[44]   Milas L. Chemoradiation interactions: Potential of newer chemotherapeutic agents. In "*American Society of Clinical Oncology. 2000 Educational Book* " (Perry MC Ed), Thirty-Sixth Annual Meeting, May 19-23, 2000, New Orleans, LA, 207-13.

[45]   Hreshchyshyn MM, Aron BS, Boronow RC, Franklin EW 3rd, Shingleton HM, Blessing JA. Hydroxyurea or placebo combined with radiation to treat stages IIIB and IV cervical cancer confined to the pelvis. *Int J Radiat Oncol Biol Phys* 1979; 5: 317-22.

[46]   Piver MS, Barlow JJ, Vongtama V, Blumenson L. Hydroxyurea: a radiation potentiator in carcinoma of the uterine cervix. A randomized double-blind study. *Am J Obstet Gynecol* 1983; 147: 803-8.

[47]   Whitney CW, Sause W, Bundy BN, Malfetano JH, Hannigan EV, Fowler WC Jr, Clarke-Pearson DL, Liao SY. Randomized comparison of fluorouracil plus cisplatin versus hydroxyurea as an adjunct to radiation therapy in stage IIB-IVA carcinoma of the cervix with negative para-aortic lymph nodes: a Gynecologic Oncology Group and Southwest Oncology Group study. *J Clin Oncol*. 1999; 17:1339-48.

[48]   Morris M, Eifel PJ, Lu J, Grigsby PW, Levenback C, Stevens RE, Rotman M, Gershenson DM, Mutch DG. Pelvic radiation with concurrent chemotherapy compared with pelvic and para-aortic radiation for high-risk cervical cancer. *N Engl J Med* 1999; 340: 1137-43.

[49]   Rose PG, Bundy BN, Watkins EB, Thigpen JT, Deppe G, Maiman MA, Clarke-Pearson DL, Insalaco S. Concurrent cisplatin-based radiotherapy and chemotherapy for locally advanced cervical cancer. *N Engl J Med* 1999; 340: 1144-53.

[50] Keys HM, Bundy BN, Stehman FB, Muderspach LI, Chafe WE, Suggs CL 3rd, Walker JL, Gersell D. Cisplatin, radiation, and adjuvant hysterectomy compared with radiation and adjuvant hysterectomy for bulky stage IB cervical carcinoma. *N Engl J Med* 1999; 340: 1154-61.

[51] Peters WA 3rd, Liu PY, Barrett RJ 2nd, Stock RJ, Monk BJ, Berek JS, Souhami L, Grigsby P, Gordon W Jr, Alberts DS. Concurrent chemotherapy and pelvic radiation therapy compared with pelvic radiation therapy alone as adjuvant therapy after radical surgery in high-risk early-stage cancer of the cervix. *J Clin Oncol* 2000; 18: 1606-13.

[52] Rotman M, Pajak TF, Choi K, Clery M, Marcial V, Grigsby PW, Cooper J, John M. Prophylactic extended-field irradiation of para-aortic lymph nodes in stages IIB and bulky IB and IIA cervical carcinomas. Ten-year treatment results of RTOG 79-20. *JAMA* 1995; 274: 387-93.

[53] National Cancer Institute: Clinical Announcement. Bethesda, MD, United States Department of Health and Human Services, Public Health Service, February 1999

[54] Rose PG. Chemoradiotherapy: the new standard care for invasive cervical cancer. *Drugs* 2000; 60: 1239-44.

[55] Pearcey R, Brundage M, Drouin P, Jeffrey J, Johnston D, Lukka H, MacLean G, Souhami L, Stuart G, Tu D. Phase III trial comparing radical radiotherapy with and without cisplatin chemotherapy in patients with advanced squamous cell cancer of the cervix. *J Clin Oncol* 2002; 20: 966-72.

[56] Green J, Kirwan J, Tierney J, Vale C, Symonds P, Fresco L, Williams C, Collingwood M. Concomitant chemotherapy and radiation therapy for cancer of the uterine cervix. *Cochrane Database Syst Rev.* 2005; 20: CD002225.

[57] Lanciano R, Calkins A, Bundy BN, Parham G, Lucci JA 3rd, Moore DH, Monk BJ, O'Connor DM. Randomized comparison of weekly cisplatin or protracted venous infusion of fluorouracil in combination with pelvic radiation in advanced cervix cancer: a gynecologic oncology group study. *J Clin Oncol* 2005; 23: 8289-95.

[58] Westermann AM, Jones EL, Schem BC, van der Steen-Banasik EM, Koper P, Mella O, Uitterhoeve AL, de Wit R, van der Velden J, Burger C, van der Wilt CL, Dahl O, Prosnitz LR, van der Zee J. First results of triple-modality treatment combining radiotherapy, chemotherapy, and hyperthermia for the treatment of patients with stage IIB, III, and IVA cervical carcinoma. *Cancer* 2005;104: 763-70.

[59] Rowinsky EK, Cazenave LA, Donehower RC. Taxol: a novel investigational antimicrotubule agent. *J Natl Cancer Inst* 1990; 82: 1247-59.

[60] Tishler RB, Schiff PB, Geard CR, Hall EJ. Taxol: a novel radiation sensitizer. *Int J Radiat Oncol Biol Phys.* 1992;22: :613-7.

[61] Geard CR, Jones JM, Schiff PB. Taxol and radiation. *J Natl Cancer Inst Monogr* 1993; (15): 89-94.

[62] Jaakkola M, Rantanen V, Grenman S, Kulmala J, Grenman R. In vitro concurrent paclitaxel and radiation of four vulvar squamous cell carcinoma cell lines. *Cancer.* 1996; 77:1940-6.

[63] Rodriguez M, Sevin BU, Perras J, Nguyen HN, Pham C, Steren AJ, Koechli OR, Averette HE. Paclitaxel: a radiation sensitizer of human cervical cancer cells. *Gynecol Oncol* 1995; 57:165-9.

[64]   Geard CR, Jones JM. Radiation and taxol effects on synchronized human cervical carcinoma cells. *Int J Radiat Oncol Biol Phys* 1994; 29: 565-9.

[65]   Erlich E, McCall AR, Potkul RK, Walter S, Vaughan A. Paclitaxel is only a weak radiosensitizer of human cervical carcinoma cell lines. *Gynecol Oncol* 1996; 60: 251-4.

[66]   Cerrotta A, Gardan G, Cavina R, Raspagliesi F, Stefanon B, Garassino I, Musumeci R, Tana S, De Palo G. Concurrent radiotherapy and weekly paclitaxel for locally advanced or recurrent squamous cell carcinoma of the uterine cervix. A pilot study with intensification of dose. *Eur J Gynaecol Oncol* 2002; 23: 115-9.

[67]   Chen MD, Paley PJ, Potish RA, Twiggs LB. Phase I trial of taxol as a radiation sensitizer with cisplatin in advanced cervical cancer *Gynecol Oncol* 1997; 67: 131-6.

[68]   Pignata S, Frezza P, Tramontana S, Perrone F, Tambaro R, Casella G, Ferrari E, Iodice F, De Vivo R, Ricchi P, Tramontana F, Silvestro G. Phase I study with weekly cisplatin-paclitaxel and concurrent radiotherapy in patients with carcinoma of the cervix uteri. *Ann Oncol* 2000; 11: 455-9.

[69]   Petera J, Odrazka K, Frgala T, Spacek J. External beam radiotherapy and high-dose brachytherapy combined with cisplatin and paclitaxel in patients with advanced cervical carcinoma. *Gynecol Oncol* 2005; 99: 334-8.

[70]   Duenas-Gonzalez A, Cetina L, Sanchez B, Gomez E, Rivera L, Hinojosa J, Lopez-Graniel C, Gonzalez-Enciso A, de la Garza J. A phase I study of carboplatin concurrent with radiation in FIGO stage IIIB cervix uteri carcinoma. *Int J Radiat Oncol Biol Phys* 2003; 56: 1361-5.

[71]   de Vos FY, Bos AM, Gietema JA, Pras E, Van der Zee AG, de Vries EG, Willemse PH. Paclitaxel and carboplatin concurrent with radiotherapy for primary cervical cancer. *Anticancer Res* 2004; 24: 345–8.

[72]   Rao GG, Rogers P, Drake RD, Nguyen P, Coleman RL. Phase I clinical trial of weekly paclitaxel, weekly carboplatin, and concurrent radiotherapy for primary cervical cancer. *Gynecol Oncol* 2005; 96: 168-72.

[73]   Chen AY, Choy H, Rothenberg ML. DNA topoisomerase I-targeting drugs as radiation sensitizers. *Oncology (Williston Park)*. 1999;13 (Suppl.): 39-46.

[74]   Choy H, MacRae R. Irinotecan and radiation in combined-modality therapy for solid tumors. *Oncology (Williston Park)*. 2001;15 (Suppl.): 22-8.

[75]   Tanaka T, Yukawa K, Umesaki N. Combination effects of irradiation and irinotecan on cervical squamous cell carcinoma cells in vitro. *Oncol Rep*. 2005; 14: 1365-9.

[76]   Suntornpong N, Pattaranutaporn P, Chanslip Y, Thephamongkhol K. Concurrent radiation therapy and irinotecan in stage IIIB cervical cancer. *J Med Assoc Thai* 2003; 86: 430-5.

[77]   Mundt AJ, Rotmensch J, Waggoner SE, Yamada D, Langhauser C, Fleming GF. Phase I trial of concomitant vinorelbine, paclitaxel, and pelvic irradiation in cervical carcinoma and other advanced pelvic malignancies. *Gynecol Oncol* 2001; 82: 333-7.

[78]   Hernandez P, Olivera P, Duenas-Gonzalez A, Perez-Pastenes MA, Zarate A, Maldonado V, Melendez-Zajgla J. Gemcitabine activity in cervical cancer cell lines. *Cancer Chemother Pharmacol* 2001; 48: 488-92.

[79]   Chauvergne J, Rohart J, Heron JF, Ayme Y, Berlie J, Fargeot P, George M, Lebrun-Jezekova D, Pigneux J, Chenal C, et al. Randomized trial of initial chemotherapy in 151 locally advanced carcinoma of the cervix (T2b-N1, T3b, MO) *Bull Cancer* 1990; 77: 1007-24.

[80]   Sardi J, Sananes C, Giaroli A, Maya G, di Paola G. Neoadjuvant chemotherapy in locally advanced carcinoma of the cervix uteri. *Gynecol Oncol* 1990; 38: 486-93.

[81]   Benedetti Panici PL, Scambia G, Baiocchi G, Greggi S, Ragusa G, Gallo A, Conte M, Battaglia F, Laurelli G, Rabitti C, et al. Neoadjuvant chemotherapy and radical surgery in locally advanced cervical cancer. Prognostic factors for response and survival. *Cancer* 1991; 67: 372-9.

[82]   Sardi J, Sananes C, Giaroli A, Bayo J, Rueda NG, Vighi S, Guardado N, Paniceres G, Snaidas L, Vico C, et al. Results of a prospective randomized trial with neoadjuvant chemotherapy in stage IB, bulky, squamous carcinoma of the cervix. *Gynecol Oncol.* 1993; 49:156-65.

[83]   Tattersall MH, Lorvidhaya V, Vootiprux V, Cheirsilpa A, Wong F, Azhar T, Lee HP, Kang SB, Manalo A, Yen MS, et al. Randomized trial of epirubicin and cisplatin chemotherapy followed by pelvic radiation in locally advanced cervical cancer. Cervical Cancer Study Group of the Asian Oceanian Clinical Oncology Association. *J Clin Oncol.* 1995; 13: 444-51.

[84]   Sundfor K, Trope CG, Hogberg T, Onsrud M, Koern J, Simonsen E, Bertelsen K, Westberg R. Radiotherapy and neoadjuvant chemotherapy for cervical carcinoma. A randomized multicenter study of sequential cisplatin and 5-fluorouracil and radiotherapy in advanced cervical carcinoma stage 3B and 4A. *Cancer* 1996; 77: 2371-8.

[85]   Leone B, Vallejo C, Perez J, Cuevas MA, Machiavelli M, Lacava J, Focaccia G, Ferreyra R, Suttora G, Romero A, Castaldi J, Arroyo A, Rabinovich M. Ifosfamide and cisplatin as neoadjuvant chemotherapy for advanced cervical carcinoma. *Am J Clin Oncol* 1996;19: 32-5.

[86]   Bolis G, van Zainten-Przybysz I, Scarfone G, Zanaboni F, Scarabelli C, Tateo S, Calabrese M, Parazzini F. Determinants of response to a cisplatin-based regimen as neoadjuvant chemotherapy in stage IB-IIB invasive cervical cancer. *Gynecol Oncol* 1996; 63: 62-5.

[87]   Lai CH, Hsueh S, Chang TC, Tseng CJ, Huang KG, Chou HH, Chen SM, Chang MF, Shum HC. Prognostic factors in patients with bulky stage IB or IIA cervical carcinoma undergoing neoadjuvant chemotherapy and radical hysterectomy. *Gynecol Oncol* 1997; 64: 456-62.

[88]   Sardi J, Giaroli A, Sananes C,. Rueda N.G,. Vighi S, Ferreira M,. Bastardas M,. Paniceres G, Di Paola G. Randomized trial with neoadjuvant chemotherapy in stage IIIB squamous carcinoma cervix uteri: an unexpected therapeutic management. *Int J Gynecol Cancer* 1996; 6: 85-93.

[89]   Sardi J, Sananes C, Giaroli A, Bermúdez A, Ferreira MH, Soderini AH, Snaidas L, Guardado N, Anchezar P, Ortiz OC, di Paola GR. Neoadjuvant chemotherapy in cervical carcinoma stage IIB: a randomized controlled trial. *Int J Gynecol Cancer* 1998; 8: 441-50.

[90]   Sardi JE, Giaroli A, Sananes C, Ferreira M, Soderini A, Bermudez A, Snaidas L,
        Vighi S, Gomez Rueda N, di Paola G. Long-term follow-up of the first randomized
        trial using neoadjuvant chemotherapy in stage Ib squamous carcinoma of the cervix:
        the final results. *Gynecol Oncol* 1997; 67: 61-9.

[91]   Serur E, Mathews RP, Gates J, Levine P, Maiman M, Remy JCNeoadjuvant
        chemotherapy in stage IB2 squamous cell carcinoma of the cervix. *Gynecol Oncol*
        1997; 65: 348-56.

[92]   Benedetti-Panici P, Greggi S, Scambia G, Amoroso M, Salerno MG, Maneschi F,
        Cutillo G, Paratore MP, Scorpiglione N, Mancuso S. Long-term survival following
        neoadjuvant chemotherapy and radical surgery in locally advanced cervical cancer.
        Eur J Cancer. 1998; 34: 341-6.

[93]   Kumar L, Grover R, Pokharel YH, Chander S, Kumar S, Singh R, Rath GK,
        Kochupillai V. Neoadjuvant chemotherapy in locally advanced cervical cancer: two
        randomised studies. *Aust N Z J Med* 1998; 28: 387-90.

[94]   Colombo N, Gabriele A, Lissoni A, Secchione F, Zanetta G, Pellegrino A, Maneo A,
        Floriani I, Landoni F Neoadjuvant chemotherapy (NACT) in locally advanced uterine
        cervical cancer (LAUCC): correlation between pathological response and survival.
        Proc. Am. Soc. Clin. Oncol. 1998; 17: abstr. 1359.

[95]   Marth C, Sundfor K, Kaern J, Trope C. Long-term follow-up of neoadjuvant cisplatin
        and 5-fluorouracil chemotherapy in bulky squamous cell carcinoma of the cervix.
        Acta Oncol 1999; 38: 517-20.

[96]   Sugiyama T, Nishida T, Kumagai S, Nishio S, Fujiyoshi K, Okura N, Yakushiji M,
        Hiura M, Umesaki N. Combination therapy with irinotecan and cisplatin as
        neoadjuvant chemotherapy in locally advanced cervical cancer. *Br J Cancer.* 1999;
        81: 95-8.

[97]   Pignata S, Silvestro G, Ferrari E, Selvaggi L, Perrone F, Maffeo A, Frezza P, Di
        Vagno G, Casella G, Ricchi P, Cormio G, Gallo C, Iodice F, Romeo F, Fiorentino R,
        Fortuna G, Tramontana S. Phase II study of cisplatin and vinorelbine as first-line
        chemotherapy in patients with carcinoma of the uterine cervix. *J Clin Oncol* 1999; 17:
        756-60.

[98]   Herod J, Burton A, Buxton J, Tobias J, Luesley D, Jordan S, Dunn J, Poole CJ.A
        randomised, prospective, phase III clinical trial of primary bleomycin, ifosfamide and
        cisplatin (BIP) chemotherapy followed by radiotherapy versus radiotherapy alone in
        inoperable cancer of the cervix. *Ann Oncol* 2000; 11: 1175-81.

[99]   Symonds RP, Habeshaw T, Reed NS, Paul J, Pyper E, Yosef H, Davis J, Hunter R,
        Davidson SE, Stewart A, Cowie V, Sarkar T. The Scottish and Manchester
        randomised trial of neo-adjuvant chemotherapy for advanced cervical cancer. *Eur J
        Cancer* 2000; 36: 994-1001.

[100]   Gadducci A, Cosio S, Cionini L, Genazzani AR. Neoadjuvant chemotherapy and
        concurrent chemoradiation in the treatment of advanced cervical cancer. *Anticancer
        Res.* 2001; 21: 3525-33.

[101]   Benedetti-Panici P, Greggi S, Colombo A, Amoroso M, Smaniotto D, Giannarelli D,
        Amunni G, Raspagliesi F, Zola P, Mangioni C, Landoni F. Neoadjuvant
        chemotherapy and radical surgery versus exclusive radiotherapy in locally advanced

squamous cell cervical cancer: results from the Italian multicenter randomized study. *J Clin Oncol.* 2002; 20: 179-88.

[102]   Benedetti Panici PL, Angioli R. Neoadjuvant chemotherapy in cervical cancer. In *"Chemotherapy for gynaecological neoplasms. Current therapy and novel approaches"* (Angioli R, Benedetti Panici P, Kavanagh JJ, Pecorelli S, Penalver M Eds), Marcel Dekker M, Inc., New York, Basel, 2004: 555-71.

[103]   Withers HR, Taylor JM, Maciejewski B. The hazard of accelera¬ted tumor clonogen repopulation during radiotherapy. *Acta Oncol.* 1988; 27: 131-46.

[104]   Ozols RF, Masuda H, Hamilton TC. Mechanisms of cross-resistance between radiation and antineoplastic drugs. *NCI Monogr.* 1988; (6):159-65.

[105]   Eifel PJ, Rose PG. Chemotherapy and radiation therapy for cervical cancer. In: *"American Society of Clinical Oncology. 2000 Educational Book"* (Perry MC Ed), Thirty-Sixth Annual Meeting, May 19-23, 2000, New Orleans, LA, 199-206.

[106]   Neoadjuvant Chemotherapy for Locally Advanced Cervical Cancer Meta-analysis Collaboration Neoadjuvant chemotherapy for locally advanced cervical cancer: a systematic review and meta-analysis of individual patient data from 21 randomised trials. *Eur J Cancer* 2003; 39: 2470-86.

[107]   Zanetta G, Lissoni A, Pellegrino A, Sessa C, Colombo N, Gueli-Alletti D, Mangioni C. Neoadjuvant chemotherapy with cisplatin, ifosfamide and paclitaxel for locally advanced squamous-cell cervical cancer. *Ann Oncol* 1998; 9: 977-80.

[108]   Buda A, Fossati R, Colombo N, Fei F, Floriani I, Gueli Alletti D, Katsaros D, Landoni F, Lissoni A, Malzoni C, Sartori E, Scollo P, Torri V, Zola P, Mangioni C. Randomized trial of neoadjuvant chemotherapy comparing paclitaxel, ifosfamide, and cisplatin with ifosfamide and cisplatin followed by radical surgery in patients with locally advanced squamous cell cervical carcinoma: the SNAP01 (Studio Neo-Adjuvante Portio) Italian Collaborative Study. *J Clin Oncol* 2005; 23: 4137-45.

[109]   Fossati R, Buda A, Rulli E,. Landoni F, Lissoni A, Colombo N, Zola P, Katsaros D, Grassi R, Mangioni C Randomized trial of neoadjuvant chemotherapy followed by radical surgery in locally advanced squamous cell cervical carcinoma (LASCCC). Comparison of paclitaxel, cisplatin (TP), versus paclitaxel, ifosfamide, cisplatin (TIP): the SNAP-02 Italian collaborative study. *Proc Am Soc Clin Oncol* 2005; 24: abstr 5026.

[110]   Mathevet P, Laszlo de Kaszon E, Dargent D. Fertility preservation in early cervical cancer *Gynecol Obstet Fertil* 2003 ;31: 706-12

[111]   Plante M, Renaud MC, Francois H, Roy M. Vaginal radical trachelectomy: an oncologically safe fertility-preserving surgery. An updated series of 72 cases and review of the literature. *Gynecol Oncol* 2004; 94: 614-23.

[112]   Sheperd JH. Uterus-conserving surgery for invasive cervical cancer. Best Pract Res Clin. *Obstet Gynaecol* 2005;19: 577-90.

[113]   Plante M, Renaud MC, Hoskins IA, Roy M. Vaginal radical trachelectomy: a valuable fertility-preserving option in the management of early-stage cervical cancer. A series of 50 pregnancies and review of the literature. *Gynecol Oncol* 2005; 98: 3-10.

[114]   Burnett AF. Radical trachelectomy with laparoscopic lymphadenectomy: review of oncologic and obstetrical outcomes. *Curr Opin Obstet Gynecol* 2006; 18: 8-13.

[115]   Andrade JM, Marana HR, Mangieri LF, Matthes AC, Cunha SP, Bighetti S. Successful preservation of fertility subsequent to a complete pathologic response of a squamous cell carcinoma of the uterine cervix treated with primary systemic chemotherapy. *Gynecol Oncol* 2000; 77: 213-5.

[116]   Kobayashi Y, Akiyama F, Hasumi K. A case of successful pregnancy after treatment of invasive cervical cancer with systemic chemotherapy and conization. *Gynecol Oncol* 2006; 100: 213-5.

[117]   Thigpen T, Shingleton H, Homesley H, Lagasse L, Blessing J. Cis-platinum in treatment of advanced or recurrent squamous cell carcinoma of the cervix: a phase II study of the Gynecologic Oncology Group. *Cancer* 1981; 48: 899-903.

[118]   Bonomi P, Blessing JA, Stehman FB, DiSaia PJ, Walton L, Major FJ. Randomized trial of three cisplatin dose schedules in squamous-cell carcinoma of the cervix: a Gynecologic Oncology Group study. *J Clin Oncol* 1985; 3: 1079-85.

[119]   Thigpen JT, Blessing JA, DiSaia PJ, Fowler WC Jr, Hatch KD. A randomized comparison of a rapid versus prolonged (24 hr) infusion of cisplatin in therapy of squamous cell carcinoma of the uterine cervix: a Gynecologic Oncology Group study. *Gynecol Oncol* 1989; 32: 198-202.

[120]   Cadron I, Vergote I. Chemotherapy for recurrent and advanced cervical cancer. In *"Chemotherapy for gynaecological neoplasms. Current therapy and novel approaches"* (Angioli R, Benedetti Panici P, Kavanagh JJ, Pecorelli S, Penalver M Eds) Marcel Dekker M, Inc., New York, Basel, 2004: 589-607.

[121]   Arseneau J, Blessing JA, Stehman FB, McGehee R. A phase II study of carboplatin in advanced squamous cell carcinoma of the cervix (a Gynecologic Oncology Group Study). *Invest New Drugs* 1986; 4: 187-91.

[122]   McGuire WP 3rd, Arseneau J, Blessing JA, DiSaia PJ, Hatch KD, Given FT Jr, Teng NN, Creasman WT. A randomized comparative trial of carboplatin and iproplatin in advanced squamous carcinoma of the uterine cervix: a Gynecologic Oncology Group study. *J Clin Oncol* 1989; 7: 1462-8.

[123]   Verschraegen CF, Levy T, Kudelka AP, Llerena E, Ende K, Freedman RS, Edwards CL, Hord M, Steger M, Kaplan AL, Kieback D, Fishman A, Kavanagh JJ. Phase II study of irinotecan in prior chemotherapy-treated squamous cell carcinoma of the cervix. *J Clin Oncol.* 1997; 15: 625-31.

[124]   Muderspach LI, Blessing JA, Levenback C, Moore JL Jr. A phase II study of topotecan in patients with squamous cell carcinoma of the cervix: a gynecologic oncology group study. *Gynecol Oncol.* 2001; 81: 213-5.

[125]   Friedlander M, Kaye SB, Sullivan A, Atkinson K, Elliott P, Coppleson M, Houghton R, Solomon J, Green D, Russell P, et al. Cervical carcinoma: a drug-responsive tumor--experience with combined cisplatin, vinblastine, and bleomycin therapy. *Gynecol Oncol* 1983; 16: 275-281.

[126]   Buxton EJ, Meanwell CA, Hilton C, Mould JJ, Spooner D, Chetiyawardana A, Latief T, Paterson M, Redman CW, Luesley DM, et a.l Combination bleomycin, ifosfamide, and cisplatin chemotherapy in cervical cancer. *J Natl Cancer Inst.* 1989; 81: 359-61.

[127] Brader KR, Morris M, Levenback C, Levy L, Lucas KR, Gershenson DM. Chemotherapy for cervical carcinoma: factors determining response and implications for clinical trial design. *J Clin Oncol.* 1998; 16: 1879-84.

[128] Omura GA, Blessing JA, Vaccarello L, Berman ML, Clarke-Pearson DL, Mutch DG, Anderson B.Randomized trial of cisplatin versus cisplatin plus mitolactol versus cisplatin plus ifosfamide in advanced squamous carcinoma of the cervix: a Gynecologic Oncology Group study. *J Clin Oncol.* 1997; 15: 165-71.

[129] Rose PG, Blessing JA, Gershenson DM, McGehee R. Paclitaxel and cisplatin as first-line therapy in recurrent or advanced squamous cell carcinoma of the cervix: a gynecologic oncology group study. *J Clin Oncol.*1999;17: 2676-80.

[130] Sugiyama T, Yakushiji M, Noda K, Ikeda M, Kudoh R, Yajima A, Tomoda Y, Terashima Y, Takeuchi S, Hiura M, Saji F, Takahashi T, Umesaki N, Sato S, Hatae M, Ohashi Y. Phase II study of irinotecan and cisplatin as first-line chemotherapy in advanced or recurrent cervical cancer. *Oncology* 2000; 58: 31-7.

[131] Vermorken JB, Zanetta G, De Oliveira CF, van der Burg ME, Lacave AJ, Teodorovic I, Boes GH, Colombo N. Randomized phase III trial of bleomycin, vindesine, mitomycin-C, and cisplatin (BEMP) versus cisplatin (P) in disseminated squamous-cell carcinoma of the uterine cervix: an EORTC Gynecological Cancer Cooperative Group study. *Ann Oncol* 2001;12: 967-74.

[132] Long HJ 3rd, Bundy BN, Grendys EC Jr, Benda JA, McMeekin DS, Sorosky J, Miller DS, Eaton LA, Fiorica JV; Gynecologic Oncology Group Study.Randomized phase III trial of cisplatin with or without topotecan in carcinoma of the uterine cervix: a Gynecologic Oncology Group Study. *J Clin Oncol* 2005; 23: 4626-33.

[133] Homesley HD, Hall DJ, Martin DA, Lewandowski GS, Vaccarello L, Nahhas WA, Suggs CL, Penley RG. A dose-escalating study of weekly bolus topotecan in previously treated ovarian cancer patients. *Gynecol Oncol.* 2001; 83: 394-9.

[134] Curtin JP, Blessing JA, Webster KD, Rose PG, Mayer AR, Fowler WC Jr, Malfetano JH, Alvarez RD. Paclitaxel, an active agent in nonsquamous carcinomas of the uterine cervix: a Gynecologic Oncology Group Study. *J Clin Oncol* 2001; 19: 1275-8

[135] Thigpen JT, Blessing JA, Fowler WC Jr, Hatch K. Phase II trials of cisplatin and piperazinedione as single agents in the treatment of advanced or recurrent non-squamous cell carcinoma of the cervix: a Gynecologic Oncology Group Study. *Cancer Treat Rep* 1986; 70: 1097-100.

[136] Rose PG, Blessing JA, Buller RE, Mannel RS, Webster KD. Prolonged oral etoposide in recurrent or advanced non-squamous cell carcinoma of the cervix: a Gynecologic Oncology Group study. *Gynecol Oncol* 2003; 89: 267-70.

[137] Look KY, Blessing JA, Valea FA, McGehee R, Manetta A, Webster KD, Andersen WA. Phase II trial of 5-fluorouracil and high-dose leucovorin in recurrent adenocarcinoma of the cervix: a Gynecologic Oncology Group study. *Gynecol Oncol.* 1997; 67: 255-8.

[138] Sutton GP, Blessing JA, DiSaia PJ, McGuire WP. Phase II study of ifosfamide and mesna in nonsquamous carcinoma of the cervix: a Gynecologic Oncology Group study. *Gynecol Oncol.* 1993; 49: 48-50.

[139] Muggia FM, Blessing JA, Waggoner S, Berek JS, Monk BJ, Sorosky J, Pearl ML. Evaluation of vinorelbine in persistent or recurrent nonsquamous carcinoma of the cervix: a Gynecologic Oncology Group Study. *Gynecol Oncol* 2005; 96: 108-11.

[140] Schilder RJ, Blessing J, Cohn DE. Evaluation of gemcitabine in previously treated patients with non-squamous cell carcinoma of the cervix: a phase II study of the Gynecologic Oncology Group. *Gynecol Oncol* 2005; 96: 103-7.

[141] Nagao S, Fujiwara K, Oda T, Ishikawa H, Koike H, Tanaka H, Kohno I. Combination chemotherapy of docetaxel and carboplatin in advanced or recurrent cervix cancer. A pilot study. *Gynecol Oncol* 2005; 96: 805-9.

[142] Rasila KK, Burger RA, Smith H, Lee FC, Verschraegen C.Angiogenesis in gynecological oncology-mechanism of tumor progression and therapeutic targets. *Int J Gynecol Cancer* 2005; 15: 710-26.

[143] Hougardy BM, Maduro JH, van der Zee AG, Willemse PH, de Jong S, de Vries EG. Clinical potential of inhibitors of survival pathways and activators of apoptotic pathways in treatment of cervical cancer: changing the apoptotic balance. *Lancet Oncol* 2005; 6: 589-98.

[144] Hougardy BM, Maduro JH, van der Zee AG, de Groot DJ, van den Heuvel FA, de Vries EG, de Jong S. .Proteasome inhibitor MG132 sensitizes HPV-positive human cervical cancer cells to rhTRAIL-induced apoptosis. *Int J Cancer* 2006; 118: 1892-900.

[145] Nakamura M, Masutomi K, Kyo S, Hashimoto M, Maida Y, Kanaya T, Tanaka M, Hahn WC, Inoue M. Efficient inhibition of human telomerase reverse transcriptase expression by RNA interference sensitizes cancer cells to ionizing radiation and chemotherapy. *Hum Gene Ther*. 2005; 16: 859-68.

[146] Ferrara N, Gerber HP, LeCouter J. The biology of VEGF and its receptors. Nat Med 2003; 9: 669-76.

[147] Van Trappen PO, Ryan A, Carroll M, Lecoeur C, Goff L, Gyselman VG, Young BD, Lowe DG, Pepper MS, Shepherd JH, Jacobs IJA model for co-expression pattern analysis of genes implicated in angiogenesis and tumour cell invasion in cervical cancer. *Br J Cancer* 2002; 87: 537-44.

[148] Wei LH, Kuo ML, Chen CA, Cheng WF, Cheng SP, Hsieh FJ, Hsieh CY. Interleukin-6 in cervical cancer: the relationship with vascular endothelial growth factor. *Gynecol Oncol* 2001; 82: 49-56.

[149] Dobbs SP, Brown LJ, Ireland D, Abrams KR, Murray JC, Gatter K, Harris A, Steward WP, O'Byrne KJ. Platelet-derived endothelial cell growth factor expression and angiogenesis in cervical intraepithelial neoplasia and squamous cell carcinoma of the cervix. *Ann Diagn Pathol* 2000; 4: 286-92.

[150] Ingber D, Fujita T, Kishimoto S, Sudo K, Kanamaru T, Brem H, Folkman J Synthetic analogues of fumagillin that inhibit angiogenesis and suppress tumour growth. *Nature* 1990; 348: 555-7.

[151] Miura S, Emoto M, Matsuo Y, Kawarabayashi T, Saku K. Carcinosarcoma-induced endothelial cells tube formation through KDR/Flk-1 is blocked by TNP-470. *Cancer Lett*. 2004; 203: 45-50.

[152] Wang YQ, Luk JM, Chu AC, Ikeda K, Man K, Kaneda K, Fan ST.TNP-470 blockage of VEGF synthesis is dependent on MAPK/COX-2 signaling pathway in PDGF-BB-activated hepatic stellate cells. *Biochem Biophys Res Commun*. 2006; 341: 239-44.

[153] Kruger EA, Figg WD. TNP-470: an angiogenesis inhibitor in clinical development for cancer. *Expert Opin Investig Drugs* 2000; 9: 1383-96.

[154] Kudelka AP, Levy T, Verschraegen CF, Edwards CL, Piamsomboon S, Termrungruanglert W, Freedman RS, Kaplan AL, Kieback DG, Meyers CA, Jaeckle KA, Loyer E, Steger M, Mante R, Mavligit G, Killian A, Tang RA, Gutterman JU, Kavanagh JJ. A phase I study of TNP-470 administered to patients with advanced squamous cell cancer of the cervix.*Clin Cancer Res* 1997; 3: 1501-5.

[155] McCarty M, Bielenberg D, Donawho C, Bucana C, Fidler I. Evidence for the causal role of endogenous interferon-alpha/beta in the regulation of angiogenesis, tumorigenicity, and metastasis of cutaneous neoplasms. *Clin Exp Metastasis* 2002; 19: 609–15.

[156] von Marschall Z, Scholz A, Cramer T, Schafer G, Schirner M, Oberg K, Wiedenmann B, Hocker M, Rosewicz S. Effects of interferon alpha on vascular endothelial growth factor gene transcription and tumor angiogenesis. *J Natl Cancer Inst* 2003; 95: 437-48.

[157] Kurie JM, Lee JS, Griffin T, Lippman SM, Drum P, Thomas MP, Weber C, Bader M, Massimini G, Hong WK. Phase I trial of 9-cis retinoic acid in adults with solid tumors. *Clin Cancer Res*. 1996; 2: 287-93.

[158] Kolla V, Lindner DJ, Xiao W, Borden EC, Kalvakolanu DV. Modulation of interferon (IFN)-inducible gene expression by retinoic acid. Up-regulation of STAT1 protein in IFN-unresponsive cells. *J Biol Chem*. 1996; 271: 10508-14.

[159] Lindner DJ, Borden EC, Kalvakolanu DV. Synergistic antitumor effects of a combination of interferons and retinoic acid on human tumor cells in vitro and in vivo. *Clin Cancer Res*. 1997; 3: 931-7.

[160] Lancillotti F, Giandomenico V, Affabris E, Fiorucci G, Romeo G, Rossi GB. Interferon alpha-2b and retinoic acid combined treatment affects proliferation and gene expression of human cervical carcinoma cells. *Cancer Res*. 1995; 55: 3158-64.

[161] Ryu S, Kim OB, Kim SH, He SQ, Kim JH.In vitro radiosensitization of human cervical carcinoma cells by combined use of 13-cis-retinoic acid and interferon-alpha2a. *Int J Radiat Oncol Biol Phys* 1998; 41: 869-73.

[162] Lippman SM, Kavanagh JJ, Paredes-Espinoza M, Delgadillo-Madrueno F, Paredes-Casillas P, Hong WK, Holdener E, Krakoff IH. 13-cis-retinoic acid plus interferon alpha-2a: highly active systemic therapy for squamous cell carcinoma of the cervix. *J Natl Cancer Inst* 1992; 84: 241-5.

[163] Lippman SM, Kavanagh JJ, Paredes-Espinoza M, Delgadillo-Madrueno F, Paredes-Casillas P, Hong WK, Massimini G, Holdener EE, Krakoff IH. 13-cis-retinoic acid plus interferon-alpha 2a in locally advanced squamous cell carcinoma of the cervix. *J Natl Cancer Inst*. 1993; 85: 499-500.

[164] Hallum AV 3rd, Alberts DS, Lippman SM, Inclan L, Shamdas GJ, Childers JM, Surwit EA, Modiano M, Hatch KD.Phase II study of 13-cis-retinoic acid plus

interferon-alpha 2a in heavily pretreated squamous carcinoma of the cervix. *Gynecol Oncol* 1995; 56: 382-6.

[165]   Wadler S, Schwartz EL, Haynes H, Rameau R, Quish A, Mandeli J, Gallagher R, Hallam S, Fields A, Goldberg G, McGill F, Jennings S, Wallach RC, Runowicz CD. All-trans retinoic acid and interferon-alpha-2a in patients with metastatic or recurrent carcinoma of the uterine cervix: clinical and pharmacokinetic studies. New York Gynecologic Oncology Group. *Cancer*. 1997; 79: 1574-80.

[166]   Weiss GR, Liu PY, Alberts DS, Peng YM, Fisher E, Xu MJ, Scudder SA, Baker LH Jr, Moore DF, Lippman SM.13-cis-retinoic acid or all-trans-retinoic acid plus interferon-alpha in recurrent cervical cancer: a Southwest Oncology Group phase II randomized trial. *Gynecol Oncol* 1998; 71: 386-90.

[167]   Braud AC, Gonzague L, Bertucci F, Genre D, Camerlo J, Gravis G, Goncalves A, Moutardier V, Viret F, Maraninchi D, Viens P. Retinoids, cisplatin and interferon-alpha in recurrent or metastatic cervical squamous cell carcinoma: clinical results of 2 phase II trials. *Eur Cytokine Netw*. 2002; 13: 115-20.

[168]   Goncalves A, Camerlo J, Bun H, Gravis G, Genre D, Bertucci F, Resbeut M, Pech-Gourg F, Durand A, Maraninchi D, Viens P. Phase II study of a combination of cisplatin, all-trans-retinoic acid and interferon-alpha in squamous cell carcinoma: clinical results and pharmacokinetics. *Anticancer Res*. 2001; 21: 1431-7.

[169]   Marshall J. The role of bevacizumab as first-line therapy for colon cancer. *Semin. Oncol*. 2005; 32 (Suppl): S43-7.

[170]   Hurwitz H, Kabbinavar F. Bevacizumab combined with standard fluoropyrimidine-based chemotherapy regimens to treat colorectal cancer. *Oncology* 2005; 69 (Suppl): 17-24.

[171]   de Gramont A, Van Cutsem E. Investigating the potential of bevacizumab in other indications: metastatic renal cell, non-small cell lung, pancreatic and breast cancer. *Oncology* 2005; 69 (Suppl): 46-56.

[172]   Monk BJ, Choi DC, Pugmire G, Burger RA. Activity of bevacizumab (rhuMAB VEGF) in advanced refractory epithelial ovarian cancer. *Gynecol. Oncol*. 2005; 96: 902-5.

[173]   Morin GB: The human telomere terminal transferase enzyme is a ribonucleoprotein that synthesizes TTAGGG repeats. *Cell 1989*; 59: 521–9.

[174]   Carey LA, Kim NW, Goodman S, Marks J, Henderson G, Umbricht CB, Dome JS, Dooley W, Amshey SR, Sukumar S. Telomerase activity and prognosis in primary breast cancers. *J Clin Oncol* 1999; 17: 3075-81.

[175]   Dome JS, Chung S, Bergemann T, Umbricht CB, Saji M, Carey LA, Grundy PE, Perlman EJ, Breslow NE, Sukumar SHigh telomerase reverse transcriptase (hTERT) messenger RNA level correlates with tumor recurrence in patients with favorable histology Wilms' tumor. *Cancer Res*. 1999; 59: 4301-7.

[176]   Buttitta F, Pellegrini C, Marchetti A, Gadducci A, Cosio S, Felicioni L, Barassi F, Salvatore S, Martella C, Coggi G, Bosari S. Human telomerase reverse transcriptase mRNA expression assessed by real-time reverse transcription polymerase chain reaction predicts chemosensitivity in patients with ovarian carcinoma. *J Clin Oncol* 2003; 21: 1320-5.

[177] Autexier C. Telomerase as a possible target for anticancer therapy. *Chem Biol.* 1999; 6: R299-303.

[178] Bearss DJ, Hurley LH, Von Hoff DD. Telomere maintenance mechanisms as a target for drug development. *Oncogene.* 2000;19: 6632-41.

[179] Bhoola SM, Alvarez RD. Novel therapies for recurrent ovarian cancer management. *Expert. Rev. Anticancer Ther.* 2004; 4: 437-48.

[180] Gordon AN, Schultes BC, Gallion H, Edwards R, Whiteside TL, Cermak JM, Nicodemus CF. CA125- and tumor-specific T-cell responses correlate with prolonged survival in oregovomab-treated recurrent ovarian cancer patients. *Gynecol Oncol* 2004; 94: 340-51.

[181] Kelland LR. Emerging drugs for ovarian cancer. *Expert Opin Emerg Drugs* 2005; 10: 413-24.

[182] Sharma S, Odunsi K. Targeted therapy for epithelial ovarian cancer. *Expert. Opin. Ther. Targets* 2005; 9: 501-13.

[183] Aghajanian C, Dizon DS, Sabbatini P, Raizer JJ, Dupont J, Spriggs DR. Phase I trial of bortezomib and carboplatin in recurrent ovarian or primary peritoneal cancer. *J Clin Oncol* 2005; 23: 5943-9.

[184] Pohl G, Ho CL, Kurman RJ, Bristow R, Wang TL, Shih IeM.. Inactivation of the mitogen-activated protein kinase pathway as a potential target-based therapy in ovarian serous tumors with KRAS or BRAF mutations. *Cancer Res.* 2005; 65: 1994-2000.

[185] Elit L, Hirte H. Current status and future innovations of hormonal agents, chemotherapy and investigational agents in endometrial cancer. *Curr Opin Obstet Gynecol* 2002; 14: 67-73.

[186] Santin AD, Zhan F, Canè S, Bellone S, Palmieri M, Thomas M, Burnett A, Roman JJ, Cannon MJ, Shaughnessy J Jr, Pecorelli S. Gene expression fingerprint of uterine serous papillary carcinoma: identification of novel molecular markers for uterine serous cancer diagnosis and therapy. *Br J Cancer* 2005; 92:1561- 73.

[187] Gadducci A, Cosio S, Genazzani AR. Old and new perspectives in the pharmacological treatment of advanced or recurrent endometrial cancer: Hormonal therapy, chemotherapy and molecularly targeted therapies. *Crit Rev Oncol Hematol.* 2006 Jan 21; [Epub ahead of print]

In: Trends in Cervical Cancer
Editor: Hector T. Varaj, pp. 61-88

ISBN: 1-60021-299-9
© 2007 Nova Science Publishers, Inc.

Chapter III

ANTIHORMONAL AGENTS ON THE CITOTOXICITY INCREASE OF ANTICANCER DRUGS IN CERVICAL CANCER

P. García-López and R. Jurado*

Subdirección de Investigación Básica, Instituto Nacional de Cancerología, Av. San Fernando #22, Tlalpán 14000, Apartado Postal 22026 Mexico, D.F., Mexico.

1. ABSTRACT

Cervical cancer continues to be the major cause of cancer mortality in women in developing countries. Although detection routine screening programs have been implemented since 1975, an increased rate of new cases has also been detected. Some studies have demonstrated a relationship between HPV, cervical intraepithelial neoplasia, and invasive carcinoma of cervix. Additionally, it has been predicted that within 10 years, 66% of all dysplasia -without medical intervention- would progress to carcinoma *in situ*. It is important to bear these data in mind in order to be able to search new alternatives for cervical cancer treatment.

Cisplatin and its derivatives are important drugs in cervical cancer therapy. However, the administration of cisplatin is associated with serious side effects, including nephrotoxic and neurotoxic events. This issue has motivated the search for new agents or new regimens for cisplatin combinations with the purpose of increasing antitumoral activity and decreasing secondary events.

Among the chemosensitizer drugs, antihormonal agents have been used to modulate the cytotoxic activity of antineoplastic agents, principally in hormone-dependent cancers such as breast and prostate cancers. Although the normal cervix is known to respond to steroid sex hormones, hormonal treatments are not frequently employed in cervical carcinoma therapy. In fact, this carcinoma is traditionally considered not to respond to

---

* Correspondence concerning this article should be addressed to Patricia García-López, Ph.D. División de Investigación Básica, Instituto Nacional de Cancerología (INCan), Av. San Fernando # 22, Tlalpán 14000, Apartado Postal 22026, México D.F., México. Phone: (52) (55) 5628-0425,26; Fax: (52) (55) 5628-0432; e-mail: garcia_lopez@salud.gob.mx; pgarcia_lopez@yahoo.com.mx.

antihormonal therapy. We hypothesize that exposure to antihormonal agents for sensitizer cervical cancer cells to the antineoplastic treatment can be independent of steroid-receptors. The importance of antihormonal agents used to modulate the cytotoxic activity of anticancer drugs in cervical cancer will be explored in this article.

2. INTRODUCTION

Pathogenesis and Epidemiology of Cervical Cancer

Cervical cancer is the third most common cancer in women worldwide and continues to be the major cause of cancer deaths for women in underdeveloped countries, representing approximately 25% of cancer-related deaths in Mexican women. Although routine screening programs for its detection have been implemented since 1975, increase of new cases has been detected (Bosch, 2003; Lorincz, 2003). The epidemiology and molecular biology of cervical cancer are well understood, epidemiologic studies have involved a great variety of risk factors associated with cervical cancer; however, it has been postulated that it is a sexually transmitted disease associated with human papillomavirus (HPV). Cervical condyloma induced by HPV is associated with the development both epidermoide and adenocarcinoma cervical cancer.

Since the DNA isolation of the HPV from cervical cancer cells, many researchers have confirmed the role that has these viruses in the pathogenesis of cervical cancer. HPVs are associated with 99% of cervical cancer (Walboomers et al., 1999). Some studies have demonstrated a relationship between HPV, cervical intraepithelial neoplasia, and invasive carcinoma of the cervix. Additionally, it has been predicted that 66% of all dysplasia -without medical intervention- would progress to carcinoma *in situ* within 10 years. There are >100 types of HPVs, but only a sub-set of high-risk viral types induce cervical carcinogenesis (Wilczynski et al., 1988).

HPVs are small double stranded DNA viruses that infect either cutaneous or mucosal epithelia where they can cause epithelial tumours. Papillomaviruses contain a single molecule of circular double-stranded DNA that is about 8 kilobases in length and encodes eight early genes (E1 to E8) and two late genes (L1 and L2). In addition, there is a non-conding regulatory region called the long control region (LCR). In HPV-infected cells, the HPV genome exists as an extrachromosomal DNA circle. In contrasting in HPV-transformed cells from cervical tumors, the viral genome is often integrated into the host genome (Dürst et al., 1985). Integration commonly takes place within the viral E2 gene and results in the loss of the E2 gene product (Baker et al., 1987; Corden et al., 1999), this suggests that the absence of the E2 protein is an important factor in the development of cervical cancer (Schneider-Maunory et al., 1987). In the HPV-associated cervical cancer, two HPV oncogenes, E6 and E7, are commonly up-regulated in their expression, both multifunctional proteins, display transforming properties in tissue culture, including the ability to contribute to the immortalization process.

The genital HPVs can be divided into low risk types such as HPV-6 and HPV-11, and high-risk types such as HPV-16, 18, 31, 33, and 45. The firsts induce benign genital warts and are very rarely associated with malignancies; and the seconds cause lesions that more frequently progress to cervical carcinoma (Lorincz et al., 1992). However, these HPV types have also been detected in non-malignant cervical tissue, and only a small proportion of women with clinically apparent high–risk HPV infection eventually develop cervical carcinoma, possibly because many of these infections may be transient. Of more than 30 HPV types known to infect human genitalia, HPV-16 is most commonly associated with cervical cancer and is found in 50% of tumors. Women who are not diagnosed through screening usually present with advanced disease and cervical cancer. This the major cause of cancer deaths among young women in some developing countries (Walboomers et al., 1999).

Human papillomavirus infection is not sufficient for tumor development, there are other cofactors associated with cervical cancer –such as cigarette smoking, immunodeficiency, possibly the use of oral contraceptives, recurrent infection, early pregnancy, and hormonal status- may play a role in progression to malignancy (Meanwell, 1991). All HPVs latently infect keratinocyte stem cells in the basal layer of the stratified epithelium; however, while low risk HPVs start to replicate in cells that are still proliferating, the replicate phase of high risk HPVs infection is confined to more differential cells that have already left the cell cycle.

Chemotherapy of Cervical Cancer

Currently, approaches for treating of cancer carcinoma have limited success; consequently, 5 year survival rates for women with this cancer remain low. It is estimated that 500,000 women annually will develop cervical cancer, and 200,000 women die every year from cervical cancer. The prognosis for patients with cervical cancer is dependent of the stage of disease at diagnosis. Cervical cancer is staged using the International Federation of Gynecology & Obstetrics Staging System (FIGO). Routine Pap screening is able to detect precancerous lesions in the cervix (cervical intraepithelial neoplasia) and carcinoma in situ. Preinvasive disease is generally managed through the ablative or excisional procedures such as loop electrosurgical excision procedure, conization, or cryosurgery (Herzog, 2003).

For stages IA to IB disease, radical abdominal hysterectomy and pelvic lymphadenectomy are the standard of care for the surgical treatment of cervical cancer. Early invasive disease (stages IA, IB, and small stage IIA with no parametrial involvement) can be successfully treated with radical hysterectomy or radiotherapy with reported 5-year survival rates in the range of 80–90%. Standard therapy for large locally invasive cervical cancer, including stage Ib2 has been radiotherapy. Radiotherapy has been the standard treatment for patients with advanced cervical cancer and selected patients with early stage disease. However, advanced disease (stages IIB2–IV) is rarely managed surgically because of regional involvement and a high relapse rate. Also, about 50% of advanced disease cases are unresectable. Radiotherapy alone or in combination with chemotherapy, is used to treat these patients. However, current treatment approaches are often ineffective and the 5-year survival rates for patients with stage IIB, III, or IVA tumors are 65, 40, and <20%, respectively (Herzog, 2003; Fiorica 2003; Schilder and Stehman, 2003).

The role of chemotherapy in the treatment of cervical cancer, including the use of new active agents is the actual tendency of therapy because the radiotherapy fails to control the progression of cervical cancer in 35–90% of women with locally advanced disease.

The rationale for combining chemotherapy with radiation is to eradicate systemic micrometastases, which are not eradicated by local radiation. In addition, cisplatin based chemotherapy may synergize with radiation by inhibiting the repair of radiation induced sublethal damage and by sensitizing hypoxic cells to radiation damage (Herzog, 2003).

The concomitant administration of cisplatin based chemotherapy with radiotherapy improves survival rates significantly compared with radiotherapy alone in patients with early stage or locally advanced cervical cancer. For example, the estimated 5-year survival in patients with cervical cancer stages IIB through IVA, with a tumor diameter of at least 5 cm or involvement of pelvic lymph nodes, who were treated with radiotherapy plus cisplatin and 5-fluorouracil was 73%, compared with 58% in patients who received radiotherapy alone. These studies strongly suggest that cisplatin based chemotherapy in cervical cancer patients requiring radiotherapy.

Despite this improvement in the efficacy of treatment, most patients with advanced cervical cancer experience recurrent or persistent disease. Persistent and recurrent cervical cancers are not usually responsive to irradiation therapy. In the other hand, metastases are common in patients with advanced cervical cancer; chemotherapy is an important component of treatment. However, response rates with current chemotherapy regimens are commonly in the range of 20–30% and median survival is approximately 12–14 months (Fiorica, 2003). Several phase II studies have demonstrated that chemotherapy before either radiotherapy or surgery produce a high response rates in patients who had not previously received chemotherapy.

The addition of concurrent chemotherapy to radiotherapy improves the outcome, and is now the standard of care for patients with locally advanced cervical cancer and for those patients with early stage disease and high risk factors (Schilder & Stehman, 2003). The use of concurrent chemoradiation has reduced the overall mortality rate by nearly 50 %. Even in the patients with recurrent cervical cancer or in those women with disseminated disease, recent results with combination chemotherapy suggest major improvement.

The majority of patients considered for combined chemotherapy are those who had failed prior therapy including radiation (Thigpen, 2003).

Although many agents are available, the standard single agent treatment is cisplatin, usually given at a dose of 50 mg/m^2. Response rates of 17–38% have been reported in patients with advanced or recurrent cervical cancer treated with cisplatin; however, these responses are partial and the median overall survival is about 6-7 months (Fiorica, 2003).

The majority of studies of cytotoxic therapy have been realized in squamous cell carcinoma which account for more than 80 % of all cases. Twenty one anticancer agents have been proved in cervical squamous cancer obtaining a response rate of 15 % or grater. The most commonly used are the following:

Three platinum compounds (cisplatin, carboplatin, and iproplatin) have been used in squamous carcinoma of the cervix and produced response rates of 23 %, 15 %, and 11 % respectively. Cisplatin is clearly active against squamous cell carcinoma of the cervix at a dose of 50 mg per m2, given every three weeks. The toxicity of the other two compounds is less than cisplatin but also its citotoxicity.

Ifosfamide acts as a classic alkylating agent. In patients with carcinoma of the cervix and no prior chemotherapy, the response rate is of 31 % to 50 % even if they were prior radiotherapy treated and they have a prolongation of the median progression-free interval (4.6 versus 3.2 months) compared with cisplatin alone. In patients who have received prior chemotherapy, the response rate was only of 8 %. Ifosfamide thus has clear activity in patients with no prior chemotherapy (Fiorica, 2003; Thigpen, 2003).

Dibromodulcitol is a halogenated sugar that acts primarily as an alkylating agent. It has been reported a response rate of 15 % to 29 % in patients with no prior chemotherapy thus showing significant activity in carcinoma of the cervix.

Doxorubicin is an antibiotic who has activity in squamous cell carcinoma of the cervix, showing a 20 % response rate. Doxorubicin is an anthracycline antibiotic which has a wide range of clinical activities. The mechanism of cytotoxicity and the exact intracellular target remains controversial. The target of intracellular drug is intranuclear much of which is intercalated in the DNA. Although DNA intercalation has been felt to be the principle cytotoxic mechanism, more recent evidence suggests that inhibition of topoisomerase-II may play a more important role. Additionally, other cytotoxic actions including helicase inhibition have recently been noted (Rose, et al 2006; Thigpen, 2003).

Taxanes, paclitaxel and docetaxel are important antitumor drugs with a unique mechanism of action: they inhibit microtubule from disassembled. The taxanes bind to a subunit of the tubulin heterodimers that form cellular microtubules; the binding of the taxanes accelerates the polymerization of tubulin, effectively stabilizing and inhibiting the depolymerization of the microtubules. Nocodazole and the vinca alkaloids in contrast inhibit the polymerization of the tubulin heterodimers, in turn preventing the formation of microtubules. The taxanes currently in clinical use are effective against a broad spectrum of human tumors, in particular, ovarian, lung and breast cancers. They have demonstrated a significant activity against many solid tumors as single agent or as an agent combined with other chemotherapeutic agents.

In advanced or recurrent cancer of cervix, Gynecologic Oncology Group conducted phase II trial which demonstrated a moderate activity of paclitaxel with the result of 17% response. In another NCI-supported study, the activity of paclitaxel with the result of 21% partial response was shown in advanced or recurrent cancer of the cervix. Other study report that paclitaxel with previously radiated squamous cell carcinoma produced a 17 % response to 170 mg per m2 once every 3 weeks. After these trials, paclitaxel is widely applied against cervical cancer (Lee et al 2005; Thigpen, 2003).

Gemcitabine (2', 2' -difluorodeoxycytidine) is an antineoplastic agent that inhibits DNA synthesis, resulting in apoptosis. In addition to its established uses in pancreatic and non-small-cell lung cancer, the drug has been shown in clinical trials to be active against a wide variety of solid tumors and, in vitro, is cytotoxic to cervical cancer cell lines at plasma levels similar to those achieved clinically.

As a single agent, gemcitabine has demonstrated little activity as first- or second-line therapy for recurrent or advanced-stage cervical cancer (Mutch & Bloss, 2003).

In view of the limited success of current treatment approaches in patients with advanced disease, the use of a number of new chemotherapy agents has been investigated in clinical trials.

Topotecan has shown promise in a number of clinical trials in cervical cancer patients. This agent, currently licensed for the treatment of recurrent ovarian cancer, inhibits the topoisomerase I enzyme, causing double-stranded DNA breaks during replication which lead to cell death. Topotecan has a significant cytotoxic effect in several squamous cell cancer cell lines of the cervix uteri and vulva, including the C-33, Caski, and CAL-39 cell lines. The cytotoxic activity of topotecan was superior to that of cisplatin in the C-33 and Caski cell lines.

Results of clinical trials with this new agent, in a study who included patients with a measurable cervical cancer lesion received 1.2 mg/m^2 topotecan administered by intravenous (iv) infusion over 30 min for 5 consecutive days, the overall response rate was 18%. The principal toxicity was hematologic; however, all reported incidences of these events were controllable and there were no toxicity related withdrawals. The toxicity levels observed in clinical trials of topotecan in patients with cervical cancer are similar to those observed in patients with relapsed ovarian cancer and are not significantly different from levels observed with other chemotherapy agents (Fiorica, 2003). Also topotecan produces a 19 % response rate with previously radiated squamous cell carcinoma.

Combination treatments with two or more agents can produce higher overall response rates than single agents but are associated with increased toxicity.

Combination chemotherapy improves response rate as it was reported by several studies, also it has been stated that combination chemotherapy is essential if systemic treatment is to have a major impact on survival in patients with squamous cell carcinoma of the cervix.

Platinum based combinations are consistently actives and yield high response rates, particularly in patients with no prior radiation. Response rate in cisplatin combined therapy improves when it is combined from 18 % to 21 % with dibromodulcitol, 31 % with ifosfamide, and 36 % with paclitaxel, and there is a superior progression free survival with no differences in overall survival (Thigpen, 2003).

The combination of cisplatin and ifosfamide has shown a higher response rate, but this was achieved at the cost of considerably greater toxicity and there was no clear impact on overall survival. Concomitant administration of topotecan enhanced the cytotoxic activity of cisplatin, etoposide, and paclitaxel in some cell lines. In addition to its cytotoxic effects, topotecan also has radiation sensitizing activity in vitro in a number of human cancer cell lines. The augmentation of cisplatin activity is thought to occur through inhibition of DNA repair, suggesting that the concomitant administration of these two agents might be advantageous compared with either agent alone. These observations have prompted the instigation of a number of clinical trials of topotecan in cervical cancer patients (Fiorica, 2003).

The combination of cisplatin – doxorubicin results highly toxic when studied in 75 - 100 mg/m^2 in a phase I study, where myelosuppression was dose limiting. There is actually a liposomal doxorubicin (Doxil) preparation which is a polyethylene glycol liposomal encapsulation of doxorubicin. This results in an alteration of the pharmacokinetics in comparison to the parent compound. Specifically, there is minimal hematologic toxicity.

Additionally, there is a prolonged circulation time, reduced clearance, a smaller volume of distribution, and limited uptake by the reticulo endothelial system. The liposomal encapsulation of doxorubicin significantly alters the toxicity profile of doxorubicin and in particular the myelotoxicity is considerably reduced. In animals using ovarian xenografts in nude mice, liposomal doxorubicin has resulted in a greater tumor to normal tissue drug uptake and an improved therapeutic index. A report of the pegylated liposomal doxorubicin in combination with carboplatin has demonstrated a 38% response rate among patients with squamous cervix carcinoma cell. Liposomal doxorubicin was well tolerated with minimal myelosuppression and no treatment related deaths (Rose, et al 2006).

In phase II trials, the combination of paclitaxel - cisplatin for metastatic cervical carcinoma has demonstrated response rates as high as 45–50%. A phase III trial by the Gynecologic Oncology Group demonstrated that cisplatin-paclitaxel not only improves response rate over single agent cisplatin, but also progression free survival in patients with FIGO stage IVB, recurrent or persistent squamous cell carcinoma of the cervix. Even in patients previously treated with chemo-radiation, carboplatin-paclitaxel has reasonable activity, is well tolerated, and can be delivered at full dose (Tinker, 2005).

Both in vitro and in vivo studies have shown that gemcitabine and cisplatin act synergistically against cancer cells, suggesting that combining them might lead to greater antitumor activity than would be expected simply by adding the cytotoxic effects of each drug alone. A neoadjuvant regimen based on low doses of gemcitabine combined with cisplatin and followed with definitive surgery or radiotherapy can yield very high overall response rates and prolonged survival. The response rate is higher among patients who had not received radiation therapy previously (57%) than among those who had (30%). Progression-free survival is 1.9 months and overall survival, 4.9 months. The relatively low toxicity of the regimen is very encouraging (Mutch and Bloss, 2003).

Chemotherapy agents are less effective in patients who have already received previous courses of chemotherapy because of relative or absolute drug resistance to the previous treatments. Response rates of >15% can be achieved in chemotherapy naive patients but are lower in previously treated patients. In addition, radical surgery and irradiation both lead to deterioration in the local vasculature, further reducing effects of systemically administered chemotherapy agents.

There is evidence from a number of studies that combination chemotherapy with cisplatin and pelvic irradiation improves progression free survival. This may be due to inhibition of the repair of radiation induced damage, initiation of proliferation, and reduction in the fraction of hypotoxic cells resistant to radiation (Fiorica, 2003).

As with other drugs that have been evaluated in patients with advanced or recurrent cervical cancer, gemcitabine is most active in those who have not had prior chemotherapy or radiation. Concomitant gemcitabine/radiation regimen obtained results with 89% of complete response, and 5% of partial response with a remarkable disease free survival of 84 %, and overall survival of 100% (Mutch and Bloss, 2003).

Other drugs used include at least other 13 agents with a response rate of 15 % or greater, opening the possibility for the development of effective combination chemotherapy.

3. Participating of Steroid Hormones in Cervical Cancer

Hormones can be classified generally into two broad groups: nonsteroidal as amino acids, peptides, and polypeptides, which usually requires cell-membrane localized receptors that regulated second messengers such as cAMP (Adenoside Mono Phosphate cycle) to mediate their action; and steroidal, which bind directly to intracellular receptors to mediate their action. Some examples of steroid hormones include estrogen, androgen, glucocorticoids, mineralocorticoids, and progestin.

Estrogens are endogenous hormones with numerous physiological actions. The most potent naturally estrogen in humans is 17β-estradiol, followed by estrone (E1) and estriol (E3). Estradiol, estrone and estriol are derived from androgenic precursors (androstenedione or testosterone) trough aromatization of the A-ring. Estradiol is oxidized reversibly to estrone, and both estradiol and estrone can be converted to estriol (Birkhauser, 1996). Estradiol is the predominant estrogen during the premenopausal period, and is mainly secreted by the ovaries. After menopause, the main estrogen is estrone. Estrone is synthesized in adipose tissue from adrenal dehydroepiandrosterone.

The biological activity of estrogen is mediated through a specific high-affinity estrogen receptor (ER) located within cell nuclei. The mechanism of action of ER is similar to that of other nuclear receptors. In the absence of hormone, the receptor is sequestered within the nuclei of target cells in a multiprotein inhibitory complex. The binding of ligand induces an activating conformational change within ER, an event that promotes homodimerization and high affinity binding to specific nucleotide sequences termed estrogen response elements (EREs) present in target genes, and these interactions increases, or in some cases decreases, transcription of hormone-regulated genes (Tasai and O`Malley, 1994). In addition to the classic ligand-mediated activation pathway, it has been shown that ER can be activated in the absence of ligand by grow factors or other agents that elevate intracellular cAMP levels (Aronica and Katzenellenbogen, 1993; Ignar-Trowbridge et al., 1993)

In the case of the progesterone, the biological actions are mediated primarily by its progesterone receptor (PR), a member of superfamily of intracellular receptor that mediates the nuclear effects of steroid hormones, thyroid hormone, and the non-nutritional vitamins A and D. The mechanism of action of PR is similar to that of other steroid receptors. In the absence of progesterone, the receptor is transcriptionally inactive and remains sequestered in a large complex of heat shock proteins (HSPs) as HSP-90, HSP-70 (Tsai and O`Malley, 1994). On hormone binding, the receptor undergoes a conformational change, resulting in the dissociation from heat shock proteins, translocations to the nucleus, and dimerization and binding to progesterone responsive elements (PREs) within the promoter regions of target genes (Beato et al., 1995; Mangelsdorf et al., 1995).

Studies reported by Beatson in 1896 were the first that showed that estrogens possess a growth-stimulating effect on breast tumors and that tumor growth could be reduced by removal of the ovaries. There are evidences that involved the association of increased serum estrogens, or estrogen excretion, with postmenopausal breast cancer. Mammary tissues accumulate serum estrogens to concentrations significantly higher than those present in serum (Miller, 1997). Besides, breast tissues also synthesize estrogens trough a pathway similar to that peripheral adipose tissues (Birkhauser, 1996). There are data that show that normal, benign, and malignant breast tissue in postmenopausal women contain concentrations of 17 β-estradiol up to 10-fold higher than those seen in serum (Drafta et al., 1983; Edery et al., 1981). This property of the estrogens, demonstrated by innumerable research studies, has acquired clinical significance in the pharmacological suppression of estrogen production in breast cancer. Estrogen receptor and progesterone receptor status is a well recognized prognostic indicator in women with breast carcinoma, patients with ER-positive tumors have a significantly higher response to antiestrogens than patients with ER-poor or ER-negative tumors. Expression of the progesterone receptor also has been implicated as predictor of response, this likely related to ability of estrogens to induce its expression. Concurrent expression of both ER and PR is often associated with a higher response than in ER-positive, but PR-negative, tumors. So in women with breast carcinoma, hormone receptor status is routinely used as a guide for design therapy.

In the case of the uterine cervix normally responds to stimuli by female sex hormones, which seem to be regulated by mechanisms similar to those proposed for varies target organs. The normal cervix is a hormone-dependent tissue and it has been shown to contain estrogen and progesterone receptors (Terenius et al., 1974; Sanborn et al., 1976; Fujiwara et al., 1997). However, for cervical carcinoma tissues, estrogen and progesterone receptors have also been noted to be present but in a lower percentage than reported for breast and endometrial carcinoma. In fact, there are controversial data suggesting that ER and PR status may be of importance in women with invasive adenocarcinoma of the cervix.

An example showing the importance of steroids on the development of cervical cancer relapse is the fact that not all women infected with HPV develop cervical cancer, HPV infection alone is insufficient for tumor development, and like other cancers, the etiology of cervical neoplasia is a multistep process involving other cofactors. One of these factors can be the sex steroid hormones. The role of estrogens in the development of cervical carcinoma has been widely debated (Piper, 1985). The widespread oral contraceptives use by women in the 1960s and 1970s was associated with an increase in the incidence of cervical dysplasia, however, this idea was abandoned when it was observed that the use of oral contraceptives and the increased risk of HPV exposure was due to a lack of concomitant use of barrier methods. However, some studies have documented that synergism may exist between steroid hormones and HPV in the pathogenesis of cervical cancer; specifically, in vitro studies have demonstrated that the estrogen can enhance the transcription of HPV-16 E6 and E7 oncogenes (Khare et al., 1997; Tewari et al., 2000). In fact, it is know that 17B-estradiol stimulates the proliferation on CaSKi and HeLa cells at the concentration of 1×10^{-6} M. Antiestrogens, such as tamoxifen, also showed a similar stimulatory growth effect at low concentrations ($0,1 \times 10^{-6}$M) in Hela cells. However, in HPV-negative cervical cancer such as C33A, the stimulation of cell proliferation by estradiol was not exhibited. These experimental data provide evidence to demonstrate that HPV might play an important role in the hormonal stimulation of cell growth (Kim et al., 2000).

In addition, glucocorticoids have also been shown to enhance the efficiency and frequency of transformation of rodent cell by HPV16 (Brisson et al., 1994; Laga et al., 1992) and together with progestorone can enhance HPV gene expressions through of hormone response elements (Chan et al., 1989; Mittal et al., 1993). Several reports have linked the use of oral contraceptives with a higher risk of being HPV positive and there is an elevated risk of developing cervical cancer with increased duration of oral contraceptives use (Brinton et al., 1986; Hildeshein et al, 1990; Munoz et al., 1994). In addition, pregnant patients had a significantly higher positive rate for HPV infection (Bosch et al., 1995; Fife et al., 1996). These experimental and clinical studies suggest an important link between steroid homones, high-risk HPV infection, and the development of cervical carcinoma.

Nonetheless, contrasting findings have been reported on the clinical behaviour respect to steroid receptor expression in cervical tumors. Most studies have shown that the content of steroid hormone receptors has not prognostic value for survival (Hunter et al., 1987; Fujiwara et al., 1997; Martin et al., 1986). However, there are data that demonstrate that ER and PR can have prognostic value and might be related to better survival (Gao et al., 1983). Potish et al., (1986) and Twiggs et al., (1987) found that in squamous carcinomas, a higher incidence of ER-positive and PR-positive tumors in comparison with the adenosquamous carcinoma type; while other authors observed no difference between these two types (Gao et al., 1983; Hunter et al., 1987).

Some studies suggest that the number of cervical adenocarcinomas affecting young women in their 20s and 30s may have increased (Parazzini et al., 1990; Peters et al., 1986). In Mexico, it has also been observed that the adenosquamous type is more frequently observed in younger women, while squamous carcinoma predominates in postmenopausal women (Mohar et al., 1993; Ramirez et al., 1987). These data suggest that hormonal profile may participate in histological differentiation and perhaps in the biological behaviour of cervical cancer.

There are experimental data supporting that steroid hormones have the ability to increase the transcription of the oncoproteins E6 and E7 of HPV-16 and HPV-18 (Brake and Lambert, 2005; Kim et al., 2000) the two subtypes most associated with cervical cancer, and part of the therapeutic strategies in the cervical cancer are focused in reducing the transcription of these viral oncoproteins to get the reversion or amelioration of the malignant phenotype even though cervical carcinoma is traditionally considered not to be responsive to antiestrogens (Scambia et al., 1990; Von knebel Doeberitz et al., 1992). However, tamoxifen is only antiestrogen that has been used in this type of cancer, and it is known that this drug has agonist effect in the lower genital tract and it has established an association between the use of tamoxifen in breast cancer and the subsequent development of endometrial carcinoma (Friedrich et al; 1998; Mourits et al., 2002; Tan-Chiu et al., 2003). Indeed, it has been shown that tamoxifen at a low concentration ($10^{-9} M$) causes stimulation of cell proliferation in a cervical cancer cell line (SFR cell line) that does not contain the estrogen receptor (ER) (Hwang et al., 1992). As well, short-term administration of estrogens to cervical carcinoma patients produces an increase in tumor proliferation (Bhattacharya et al., 1997), the potential therapeutic value of pure antiestrogen and antiprogestin on cervical carcinoma justify to be studied on cervical carcinoma.

4. ANTIHORMONAL TREATMENT AS CHEMOSENSITIZER DRUGS

Among the chemosensitizer drugs, antiestrogens such as tamoxifen and ICI 182,780; and antiprogestins as mifepristone have been used to modulate the cytotoxic activity of antineoplastic agents such as doxorubicin, paclitaxel and cisplatin among others.

Role of the Antiestrogen Tamoxifen as a Possible Chemosensitizar

Tamoxifen is a non steroidal estrogen antagonist. In 1985, tamoxifen was approved by the Food and Drug Administration (FDA) as adjuvant therapy with chemotherapy in postmenopausal women with node-positive breast cancer, in 1989 was approved for the use in the treatment of premenopausal women with ER-positive advance breast cancer; and in 1990, approval was obtained for pre- and postmenopausal patients who had node-positive and ER-positive breast cancer. Thus, up to date, it is the most prescribed drug for the treatment of breast cancer and it has been the "gold standard" selective estrogen receptor modulator. However, the use of tamoxifen is limited by the development resistance; the tumors become resistant in metastatic breast cancer after average treatment duration of only 10-12 months.

Some studies have shown that tamoxifen sensitizes the effect of cisplatin in several cell lines. For example, it has been demonstrated that in head and neck squamous cell carcinoma, tamoxifen alone induces a transient G_1 arrest that greatly sensitizes the cells to apoptosis induced by cisplatin (Tavassoli et al., 2002). Recently, it has also been demonstrated that tamoxifen increases the apoptotic effect of cisplatin in primary endometrial cell cultures (Drucker et al., 2003). Following these results, a phase I trial of tamoxifen in combination with cisplatin in patients with lung cancer was done, and it was concluded that a regimen of high-dose tamoxifen in combination with cisplatin can be safety administered, since it did not show any hematological toxicity (Perez et al., 2003).

Tamoxifen has been commonly used for all stages of breast carcinoma. However, several authors have established an association between the use of tamoxifen in breast cancer and the subsequent development of endometrial carcinoma (Friedrich et al, 1998; Mourits et al., 2002; Tan-Chiu et al., 2003), and thromboembolic events (Fisher et al, 1994). Moreover, it has been shown that tamoxifen at a low concentration ($10^{-9} M$) causes stimulation of cell proliferation in a cervical cancer cell line (SFR cell line) that does not contain estrogen receptor (ER) (Hwang et al., 1992). Therefore, these data suggest the possibility that others antiestrogens may be effective as chemosensitizers in the chemotherapy of cervical carcinoma.

Role of the Antiestrogen ICI 182,780 as a Possible Chemosensitizer

The novel pure antiestrogen, ICI 182,780, is an analogue of estradiol that differs substantially from tamoxifen in terms of the chemical, pharmacologic, and biologic properties. This agent has not intrinsic estrogen–agonist activity and, therefore, is considered a pure antiestrogen. It has advantages over tamoxifen because it is devoid of estrogen agonist activity and its affinity with the ER is approximately 100 times greater than that of tamoxifen (Howell et al., 1994). Studies examining the mode of action have shown that the activity of the ER is completely attenuated by ICI 182,780; there are multiple changes in the ER function as impaired dimerization, increase turnover, and disrupted nuclear localization. Thus, not only is ER blocked functionally, but cellular levels of ER are reduced markedly by ICI 182,780.

It has been used in postmenopausal patients with breast cancer, and clinical results have confirmed that it has useful activity against breast cancer (De Friend et al., 1994), as well as a safety profile that includes reduced adverse effects such as headache and nausea (Thomas et al., 1994). Additionally, there is no evidence of agonist activity in the endometrium of postmenopausal women (Addo et al., 2002). Consequently it has been increasingly used against breast cancer (Cummings, 2002). In accordance with findings of De Vincenzo et al. (1996), in MCF-7 cells and their doxorubicin-resistant variant (MCF-7 ADR), ICI 182,780 increases the effect of doxorubicin, suggesting the participating of the Pgp drug-efflux pump. Also has been reported that this pure steroidal antiestrogen can increase the activity of cisplatin in an estrogen receptor negative ovarian cancer cell line (A2780 WT) and its cisplatin-resistant variant (A2780 CP3). The mechanism involved is not dependent of the cell cycle or apoptosis (Ercoli et al., 2000).

In a work realized by our group (Garcia-Lopez et al., 2004), using in vitro assays, we demonstrated that ICI 182,780 combined with cisplatin was able to enhance cytotoxicity in three cervical cancer cell lines (HeLa, SiHa and CaSki). These cervical carcinoma cells were chosen for the study because they contain the human papillomavirus type 18 (HeLa) and Type 16 (SiHa and CaSki) genotypes, which have been shown in multi-institutional studies to account for >65% of all HPVDNA-positive invasive cervical carcinomas. Moreover, these cells were selected because they represent different histological subtypes; HeLa cells derived from an adenocarcinoma, SiHa cells from a squamous carcinoma, and CaSki cells from an epidermoid cervical carcinoma. The cisplatin was chosen because it is not a substrate for Pgp drug-efflux pump (Nooter and Stoter et al., 1996), and in relation to the studies of De Vincenzo et al. (1996), in MCF-7 cells and their doxorubicin-resistant variant (MCF-7 ADR), ICI 182,780 increases the effect of doxorubicin, suggesting the participation of the P-glycoprotein (Pgp) drug-efflux pump. Therefore, we wanted to study the activity of the drug combination independent of Pgp and in a type of cancer that does not respond to hormonal treatment as cervical carcinoma.

In our studies we found that in the cervical cancer cell lines used, ER and PR gene levels were relatively low compared to those observed in MCF-7 cells. These findings are in accordance with clinical data that show that this type of tumor exhibits low or undetectable level of ER and PR as determined by immunohistochemical and ligand-binding-assays (Hahnel et al., 1979). Although the level of ER and PR gene expression in cervical cancer was low, the levels were enough to demonstrated that ICI 182, 780 effectively down-regulate ER and PR genes in HeLa and SiHa cells, suggesting that these effects were partially responsible for cisplatin sensitization in both cells. It is also important to mention that HeLa cells are considered one of the most sensitive cervical cancer cell lines to cisplatin effect, and SiHa as one of the most resistant cells to this drug. We found a synergistic citotoxic effect more evident in HeLa cells, with approximately 18 times higher potency in comparison to alone cisplastin. However, SiHa and CaSki, resulted in a pontetiation of up to 4.5 fold. These results may be associated to the fact that HeLa cells are adenocarcinoma cells and adenocarcinomas tumors are more likely to hormonally sensitive. It has been reported that estrogens may induce physiological effects at the membrane level, such as synthesis and cyclin expression, indicating that a large amount of cells may respond to estrogenic actions in the absence of its intracellular cognate receptors (Marino et al., 2002). Therefore, chemosensitivity to cisplatin following exposure to ICI 182, 780 in SiHa and CaSki may be related with these mechanisms.

It is known that derivatives of platin such as cisplatin and carboplatin are fixed covalently to DNA forming cisplatin–DNA adducts. This damage is eliminated by the nucleotide excision repair system of the DNA. It has also been demostrated that the high-mobility group (HMG) domain proteins such as HMG1 bind specifically to major cisplatin adducts and that the platinum-DNA-protein complex is involved in mediating cisplatin cytotoxicity by blocking nucleotide excision repair of the damage (Huang et al., 1994). There is an inverse correlation between HMG1 and the ability of cells to repair damage both in vivo and in vitro. Moreover, it has been reported that HMG1 is also able to facilitate the interaction of steroid hormone receptors such as ER and PR with their cognate DNA binding sites (He et al., 2000) In relation to our results, we hypothesize, that exposure to ICI 182,780 could lead to increase in HMG1 expression and therefore to sensitization of ER+ and PR + cells, such as CaSki cells, to the treatment with cisplatin.

In our study we also demonstrated that the combination of ICI 182,780 and cisplatin induced significant increase in G2/M phase of cell cycle in the cervical cancer cells, previous studies have also shown that doxorubicin combined with ICI 82,780 induces G_2/M blockage in MCF-7 breast cancer cells, so this pure antiestrogen is more effective than tamoxifen in inducing G_2/M arrest (De Vincenzo et al., 1996). In the other hand, cervical cancer cell lines in the G2/M phase of the cell cycle are believed to be more radiosensitive that those in G_0/G_1 phase (Hornback et al., 1994) due to the failure of this checkpoint, genomic instability can be produced resulting in hypersensitivity to radiation. Thus the combination of ICI 182,780 and cisplatin simultaneously with radiotherapy could effectively increase the antiproliferative effect and improve the treatment of cervical cancer.

Other mechanisms that could be involved in the synergistic antiproliferative effect of cisplatin and ICI 182, 780 are those independent of ER, such as decreasing the insulin-like growth factor receptor (IGF-1) (Chan et al, 2001; Huynh et al 1996) and decreasing transforming-growth factor-beta (TGF-beta) (Lackey et al., 2000) or loss of c-fos expression (Hyder et al., 1997). These findings suggest that this pure antiestrogenic compound could be a promising agent to be tested in combination with cisplatin not only in patients with cervical carcinoma, but also in those who are undergoing cisplatin therapy.

ICI 182,780, in addition to be a pure antiestrogen, has also been shown to have antiprogestin activity in human breast cancer cell lines (Rosenberg et al., 2000), as well produces a significant loss in PR expression in tumors and in cell proliferation-related antigen, Ki67 (De Friend et al., 1994). In clinical studies, the effects of three different doses of ICI 182,780 and one dose of tamoxifen on cellular ER and PR levels were examined in postmenoupausal women with primary breast cancer. The doses used were either a single intramuscular injection of ICI 182,780 (50, 125 or 250 mg), or 20 mg of oral tamoxifen, daily for 14-21 days. In this study was demonstrated a dose-dependent reduction in ER ands PR levels; in contrast, tamoxifen treatment produced significant increases in PR levels, possibly due to its estrogen agonist effect (Roberstson et al, 2001).

Role of the Antiprogestin Mifepristone (RU-486) as a Possible Chemosensitizer

As it has mentioned in this chapter, an important event in the malignant progression of cervical intraepithelial neoplasia appears to be the up-regulation of high-risk HPV expression. The steroid hormones have been linked to the progression from malignant in HPV positive lesions. In presence of glucocorticoids and progesterone, the GREs (glucocorticoids response elements) can enhance the transcription of E6-E7 increasing both cell proliferation and tumor growth of cervical tumor cells. According with these studies the glucocorticoid or progesterone antagonists can be used in the treatment of a variety of hormone-dependent tumors (Kettel et al., 1998; Rocereto et al., 2000). These antagonists include compound such as mifepristone, which is a progesterone receptor and glucocorticoid receptor antagonist. In presence of progesterone, mifepristone acts as competitive receptor antagonist, but it is a partial agonist with weak activity when is present alone. It has been widely used as the first-line drug for the termination of early pregnancy (Mahajan et al., 1997).

Biological actions of progesterone are mediated primarily by the progesterone receptor, a member of the nuclear receptor superfamily of transcription factors (Tsai et al 1994; Beato et al., 1995; Mangelsdorf et al.,1995). In the absence of progesterone, the receptor exists in a transcriptional inactive form associated with heat shock proteins (Smith and Toft, 1993). On hormone binding, the receptor undergoes a conformational change, resulting in dissociation from heat shock proteins, translocation to the nucleus, and dimerization and binding to progesterone responsive elements (PREs) within the promoter regions of target genes (Tsai et al., 1994, Beato et al., 1995, Mangelsdorf et al., 1995). When bound to the PRE, the receptor can modulate target gene transcription by directly contacting components of the transcriptional machinery (Ing et al., 1992) or indirectly by means of coactivators, such as steroid receptor coactivator-1 (SRC-1) (Onate et al., 1995) and p300/CBP (CREB-binding protein) (Smith et al., 1996). Progesterone antagonists are synthetic pharmaceutical agents that suppress the transcriptional activity of the natural steroid agonist, progesterone.

Mifepristone acts at the receptor level, binding strongly to progesterone and antiglucocorticoid receptors; its binding affinity for progesterone and glucocorticoid receptors is approximately five times greater than progesterone, and three times greater than dexametasone. Mifepristone, like progesterone, enters to target cell and reaches its receptors; however, it operate differently to progesterone producing conformational changes in the receptor. When the progesterone occupying its receptor in the nucleus may modify the receptor's shape and binding to chromatin, this binding leads to gene transcription and protein synthesis. Mefepristone antagonizes these effects by occupying the receptor without stimulating gene transcription (Spitz et al., 1993; Christian–Maitre et al., 2000). The early metabolism of mifepristone is characterized by rapid demethylation and hydroxylation. The three metabolites as the parental mifepristone retain considerable affinity toward human progesterone and glucocorticoid receptors. Thus, the combined pool of mifepristone plus its metabolites seems to be responsible for the biological actions of mifepristone (Attardi et al., 2004).

Interestingly, recent studies have proved that mifepristone could effectively inhibit the proliferation of PR-positive breast cancer (Liang et al., 2003; El Etreby et al., 1998), ovarian cancer (Rose and Barnea, 1996; Rocereto et al., 2000), endometrial cancer (Schneider et al., 1998), prostate cancer (El Etreby et al., 2000), and gastric cancer (Li et al., 2004).

Despite several reports showing that mifepristone can inhibit human cell growth only limited information is available on the basic mechanism of this effect. Some in vitro and in vivo mechanisms involved in the antiproliferative effects of mifepristone, in the case of the breast cancer, show that mifepristone induces growth arrest and cell death stimulating the activation of caspase-3, -8, and -9 in ER+ PR+, antiestrogen-resistant breast cancer cell (Gaddy et al., 2004). It is known that traditionally, caspase-8 activation is used as an indicator of activation of the extrinsic pathway of apoptosis, whereas caspase-9 activation indicates involved of the intrinsic mitochondrial pathway of apotosis (Kaufmann and Earnshow 2000). The cross-talk between these two death pathways, in part is mediated by caspase-3 activation. Once activated, caspase-3 can amplify apotosis by activating caspase-8 or -9 (Slee et al., 1999; Fujita et al., 2001).

In the case of the endometrial cell proliferation regulation by mifepristone is suggested an antioxidant mechanism by the mifepristone (Murphy et al., 2000). It has been reported an induction of apoptosis through up-regulation of NF-kB (Han and Sidell et al., 2003), one of the early response transcription factors that play a important role in the regulation of genes that are involved in the cascade of events leading to cellular apoptosis (Barkett and Gilmore 1999). The up-regulation of NF-kB in endothelial cells stimulates apotosis by 75% (Matsushita et al., 2000). Simultaneously to a marked increase in NF-kB activity is present an overexpression of Bax oncogen, protein involved in to promote apotosis and down-regulation of Bcl-2, this gene has been shown to rescue cell from apotosis.

It is also known that mifepristone can down-modulate the overexpression of two proteins involved in drug resistance as P-gp and MRP (Multidrug Resistance Protein) in MRP-overexpressing lung tumor GLC4/Sb30 cells (Payen et al., 1999); and induced apoptosis in human LNCaP prostate cancer cells by regulating the expression of apoptosis control gene Bcl-2 and TGFbeta$_1$ proteins (El Etreby et al., 2000); mifepristone has also shown a potent reversal effect on MDR in human gastric adenocarcinoma SGC-7901 cells via inhibiting the function of MRP and P-gp, and modulating the expression of Bcl-2 and Bax proteins (Li et al., 2004).

Other interesting mechanism described for mifepristone is its ability to modulate the activity of antitumor compound such as doxorubicin and vinka alkaloids. There is evidence that some endogenous compounds as steroid hormones also interact with P-gp (Yang et al., 1989). Corticosteroids and mineralocorticoids are substrates for P-gp transport (Ueda el al., 1992). Moreover, some steroid antagonist, such as tamoxifen and toremifen, also interfere with P-gp function, the features that usually describing to these modulators agents are the hydrophobicity and presence of phenyl rings (Hait and Aftab 1992). These properties are also characteristics of antiprogestin mifepristone. Therefore, it has been reported that mifepristone enhance doxorubicin cellular accumulation in resistant human leukaemia cells K562 and RHCL rat hepatoma cells (Lecureur et al., 1994) suggesting a inhibitory effect on P-gp function related to direct interactions with drug binding sites on P-gp, mechanism of action that has already been demonstrated for others chemosensitizers agents, including verapamil and cyclosporine (Ford and Hait 1990).

Recently it has been shown that mifepristone enhances the chemosensitivity of cisplatin in resistant ovarian cancer cell line COC1 (Qin and Wang 2002); finding consistent with the data by Liu et al (2003), showing in a mouse model bearing xenografted cisplatin-resistant ovarian carcinoma, a significantly greater inhibition rates of the tumors in the combined treatment in comparison with alone cisplatin treatment. These effects possibly are due to regulating of Bcl-2 and Bax protein expressions.

5. NEW PRECLINICAL ADVANCES OF THE ANTIPROGESTIN MIFEPRISTONE IN THE CHEMOSENSITAZING OF CISPLATIN IN CERVICAL CANCER

Cisplatin is one of the most commonly used drugs in cervical carcinoma; however, the side effects as nephrotoxicity, ototoxicity, neuropathy, and mylosuppression; and intrinsic and acquired resistance to cisplatin are major limitations in the use of this drug. The lack of efficacy is generally multifactorial and has been shown to be due to reduced drug accumulation, inactivation by thiol containing species, increased repair/tolerance of platinum-DNA adducts, and alterations in proteins involved in apotosis. It is important to mention that pharmacological agents who are able to modulate any of the above parameters could partially restore the sensitivity to cisplatin; therefore, is important to identify new compound that modulate the cisplatin cytotoxicity in cervical carcinoma, in which cisplatin-based chemotherapy has been the mainstay of treatment since the activity of regimens based on cisplatin was demonstrated.

To date there are not clear data that establishing the participation of mifepristone in the modulation of antineoplastic drug in human cervical carcinoma. In our group we are studying the combination of mifepristone and cisplatin on cervical carcinoma. The aim of the study presented here is to investigate whether mifepristone in combination with cisplatin could act synergistically on the citotoxicity increase in cervical carcinoma; therefore, we propose the analysis of the cisplatin-mifepristone combination as a pharmacological tool to get a synergistic association that permit to potentiate the antiproliferative effect of cisplatin without increasing the serious side effects. Our research, in this chapter, shows the results obtained both *in-vitro* and *in-vivo* using a human cervical cancer cell line HeLa. In an effort to correlate the mechanism of action of this antiprogestin in the modulation of ciplatin activity, we evaluated the intracellular cisplatin accumulation both in the presence and in the absence of mifepristone.

Mifepristone and Cisplatint Treatment *In-Vitro*

We used the HeLa human cervical cell line obtained from ATCC (Rockville, Md.). The effect of mifepristone on proliferation of cell exposed to cisplatin was evaluated using the XTT assay (sodium 3' - [1-(phenylamino-carbonyl) - 3,4 - tetrazolium]–bis (Roche Molecular Biochemicals) [4]. The assay was based on the cleavage of the yellow tetrazolium salt XTT to form an orange formazan dye by metabolic active cells. The treatment was cisplatin alone or the combination of cisplatin plus mifepristone. Measurement of spectrophotometric absorbance samples was carried out using a microtiter plate ELISA reader at 492 nm.

The cells were conditioned for 4 days with 10 μM mifepristone. Control cells were only exposed to vehicle (final ethanol concentration never exceeded 1% in treated and control samples). At the end of the incubation period, the culture medium was removed and fresh medium with various amounts of cisplatin (0.1-330 μM) was added for 4 h. After simultaneous and individual exposure to the drugs, the cells were cultivated for 24 hours. Cell proliferation was evaluated using the XTT-assay before mentioned. Mean concentration in each set of 3-4 wells was measured by triplicate. The percentage of growth inhibition was calculated and IC_{50} values (concentration of drug to achieve 50% growth inhibition) were obtained graphically from the survival curves distribution.

Synergism or drug additivity can be determined by calculating the combination index (CI) using de equation: $CIx=(D_1/Dx_1)+(D_2/Dx_2)+alfa(D_1)(D_2)/(Dx_1)(Dx_2)$. CIx represents the CI value for X% effect. Dx_1 and Dx_2 are the doses of agents 1 and 2 required to exert X% effect alone, whereas D_1 and D_2 represent the doses of agents 1 and 2 that elicit the same x% effect in combination with the other agent respectively. Alfa describes the type of interaction: alfa=0 for mutually exclusive drugs (similar mechanisms of action), alfa=1 for mutually non-exclusive drugs (independent modes of action), the equation was resolved for alfa=1. CI=1 indicates additivity, CI<1 synergism and CI>1 antagonism.

Growth inhibition experiments Citotoxicity is expressed as percentage growth inhibition of HeLa cells treated with cisplatin for 4 h, or cisplatin in combination with mifepristone pre-treatment (Fig. 1). The antiproliferative effect of cisplatin (0.1-330 μM) was potentiated in combination with mifepristone (10 μM). The IC_{50} of cisplatin in combination with mifepristone was lower (14.2 μg/mL) than that of cisplatin alone (34.2 μg/mL). To determine whether the combination effect of mifepristone and cisplatin was synergistic or additive, the CI was determined using the equation before mentioned. The CI obtained showed that the interaction of mifepristone and cisplatin was synergistic throughout of the dose of 10 and 33 μg/mL.

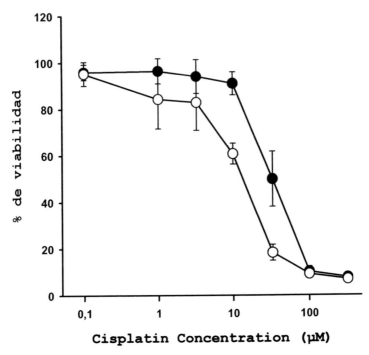

Figure 1. Representative growth inhibition curves of HeLa cells exposed to cisplatin alone (●) and in combination with mifepristone at 10 μM (○). Cells were exposed to mifepristone for 4 days followed by cisplatin for 4 h. After treatment, the effect was evaluated at 24 h. All growth inhibition assays were repeated in triplicate in at least three independent experiments. Values are the means ± SEM.

Intracellular Cisplatin Accumulation

In the preparation of the cell samples, HeLa cervix cancer cell line were plated at 1×10^5 cells /mL in specific medium supplemented as above was described. After 24 h the medium was replaced with fresh medium containing cisplatin alone for 4 h to a final concentration of 33μg/m or in combination with mifepristone (10 μM). As control non-exposed cells were treated with vehicle and cultured for the same period. The cells were harvested after 24 h and washed twice with PBS. After that they were counted with a haemocytometer and lysed with buffer (Tris 100 mM, EDTA 5 mM, NaCl 200 mM, SDS 0.2%, at pH 8) by 3 h at 55°C. The intracellular concentration of cisplatin was estimated by High Performance Liquid Chromatograpic method previously reported (Lopez-Flores et al., 2004). Briefly, the homogenate was ultrafiltrated, derivatized with DDTC in 0.1 N NaOH, samples were incubated in a 37°C water bath for 15 min, and extracted with 80 μl chloroform by vortexing at maximal speed for 1 min. The two layers were separated by centrifugation at 10,000 rpm for 5 min. Finally, 20 μl of chloroform layer was injected into the chromatographic system.

The results of intracellular levels of cisplatin indicated that mifepristone increased cellular cisplatin retention. The concentration used of mifepristone of 10 μM was able to enhance cisplatin accumulation by approximately 2-fold, this dose of mifepristone is in the range of plasma concentration usually observed in humans after oral administration of the drug (Kartner et al., 1985).

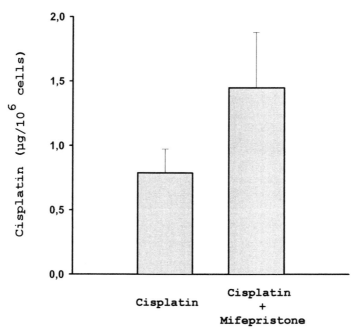

Figure 2. Effect of mifepristone on cisplatin accumulation in HeLa cells. The cells were incubated with 33 μg/mL of cisplatin for 4 h either alone or in presence of 10 μM of mifepristone. The intracellular cisplatin levels were then determined using the HPLC method. The values are the mean ± SEM of three independent experiments.

Mifepristone and Cisplatin Treatment *In-Vivo*

For xenograft model in nude mice we used female *nu/nu* mice (National Institute of Nutrition, Mexico City) between 6-8 weeks of age, they were kept in a pathogen-free environment and fed *ad lib*. The protocol for animal experiments was approved by the ethic committee of National Institute of Cancerology (Mexico, City). The *nu/nu* mice were subcutaneously injected with 6×10^6 HeLa cells in a flank. Once tumors were approximately 5 mm x 5 mm, the animals were treated with a subcutaneous injection of mifepristone 2 mg/kg/day for 3 day previously to the administration of cisplatin (3 mg/kg daily on days 1 through 3). The control animals received only the vehicle. The tumor volumes were measured with a caliper and calculated using the following formule: $\pi[\text{width}^2 \, (mm) \times \text{length} \, (mm)]/4$. The tumor growth was followed by 8 weeks.

The measurement of the tumor volume revealed a reduction of tumor growth in cisplatin-treatment alone and mifepristone-treatment alone with regarding to control animals; however, the tumor growth-inhibiting effect was more evident when the mice were treated with the combination of cisplatin and mifepristone (Fig. 3), revealing an effect modulator of mifepristone on cisplatin activity *in-vivo*. These findings are consisted with previous reports that show an improvement of antitumor effect of cisplatin against human ovarian carcinoma cells by mifepristone *in-vivo* (Liu Y et al., 2003).

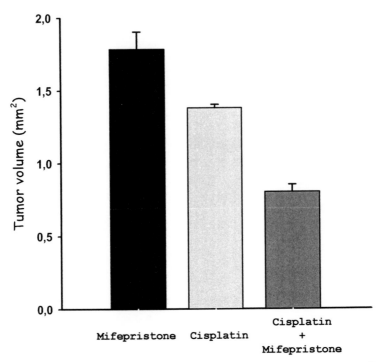

Figure 3. Effects of mifepristone, cisplatin, and mifepristone plus cisplatin on growth of HeLa tumor in nude mice after 8 weeks, the drug-treatments were indicated in the text. Data are expressed as the mean of 8 animals ± S.E.M.

6. CONCLUSION

Even when there are many antihormonal agents used in the treatment of patients with cancer, the primary use of these agents is in hormonally responsive cancer such as breast, prostate or ovarian cancer. However, due to the structural properties, they become attractive drugs as modulator agents of chemotherapeutic drugs in several carcinomas. Aside from the action mechanism of antihormonal agents described in this chapter, there is evidence that not all effects of steroid hormones are mediated via the regulation of genomic or transcriptional events, the importance of these nontranscriptional actions in cervical carcinoma is not known; in fact, it is important to mention that these nontranscriptional mechanisms could be involved in the action of antihormonal agents as chemosensitizers of chemotherapeutics drugs in cervical carcinoma. Taking into account that this carcinoma is traditionally considered to not respond to antihormonal therapy, the understanding of the mode of action of antihormonal compounds will allow the development of new treatment strategies to improve patients outcome with cervical carcinoma.

ACKNOWLEDGMENT

This work was support by CONACYT (México), grants I35551-M and P44176-M .

7. REFERENCES

Addo, S; Yates, RA; Laight A. A phase 1 trials to assess the pharmacology of the new oestrogen receptor antagonist fulvestran on the endometrium in healthy postmenopausal volunteers. *Br J Cancer*, 2002 87:1354-1359.

Attardi, BJ; Burgenson, J; Hild, SA; Reel, JR. In vitro antiprogestational/ antiglucocorticoid activity and progestin and glucocorticoid receptor binding of the putative metabolites and syntetic derivatives of CDB-2914, CDB-4124, and mifepristone. *J Steroid Biochem Mol Biol*, 2004 88:277-288.

Aronica, SM; Katzenellenbogen, BS. Stimulation of estrogen receptor-mediated transcription and alteration in the phosphorylation state of the rat uterine estrogen receptor by estrogen, cyclic adenosine monophosphate, and insulin-like growth factor-I. *Mol Endocrinol*, 1993 7:743-52

Barket, M; Gilmore, TD. Control of apoptosis by Rel/NF-KB transcription factors. *Oncogene*, 1999 18:6910-6924

Baker, CC; Phelps, WC; Lindgren, V; Braun, MJ; Gonda, MA; Howley, PM. Structural and transcriptional analysis of human papillomavirus type 16 sequences in cervical carcinoma cell lines. *J Virol*, 1987 61:962-97.

Beato, M; Herrlich, P; Schutz, G. Steroid hormone receptors: many actors in search of a plot. *Cell*, 1995 83:851-857

Beatson, GT. On the treatment of inoperable cases of carcinoma of the mamma: Suggestion from a new method of treatment, with illustrative cases. *Lancet*, 1896 ii:104-107

Bhattacharya, D; Redkar, A; Mitra, I; Sutuaria, U; MacRae, KD. Oestrogen increase S-phase fraction and estrogen and progesterone receptors in human cervical cancer in vivo. *Br J Cancer*, 19975 7:554-558

Bosch, FX; Manos, MM; Muñoz, N; Sherman, M; Jansen, AM; Peto, J; Schiffman, MH; Moreno, V; Kurman, R; Shah, KV. Prevalence of human papillomavirus in cervical cancer, a worldwide perspective: International biological study on cervical cancer (IBSCC) study group. *J Natl Cancer Inst*, 1995 81:796-802

Bosch, FX. Epidemiology of human papillomavirus infections: new option for cervical cancer prevention. *Salud Publica Mex*, 2003 45:S326-S329

Birkhauser, MH. Chemistry, Physiology, and Pharmacology of sex steroids. *J Cardiovasc Pharmacol*, 1996 28:S1-S13

Brake, T; Lambert, P. Estrogen contributes to the onset, persistence, and malignant progression of cervical cancer in a human papillomavirus-transgenic mouse model. *Proc Natl Acad Sci USA*, 2005 102:2490-2495.

Brinton, LA; Huggins, GR; Lehman, HF;, Mallin, K; Savitz, DA; Trapid, E; Rosenthal, J; Hoover, R. Long-term use of oral contraceptives and risk of invasive cervical cancer. *Int J Cancer*, 1986 38:339-344.

Chan, TW; Pollak, M; Huynh, H Inhibition of insulin-like growth factor signaling pathways in mammary gland by pure antiestrogen ICI 182,780. *Clin Cancer Res*, 2001 7:2545-2554

Chan, WK; Klock, G; Bernhardt, HU. Progesterone and glucocorticoid response elements occur in the long control regions of several human papillomaviruses involved in anogenital neoplasia. *J Virol*, 1989 63:3261-3269.

Christin-Maitre, S; Bouchard, P; Spitz, IM. Drug Therapy: medical termination of pregnancy. *N Engl J Med*, 2000 342:946-56

Corden, SA; Sant-Cassia, LJ; Easton, AJ; Morris, AG. The integration of HPV-18 DNA on cervical carcinoma. *Mol Pathol*, 1999 52:275-278.

Cummings, FJ. Envolving uses of hormonal agents for breast cancer therapy. *Clin Ther*, 2002 24:C3-C25

DeFriend, DJ; Howell, A; Nicholson, RI; Anderson, E; Dowsett, M; Mansell, RE. Investigation of a new pure cancer. *Cancer Res*, 1994 54:408-414

De Vincenzo, R; Scambia, G; Benedetti, PP; Fattorasi, A; Bonanno, G; Ferlinic, C; Isola, G; Pernisco, S; Mancuso, S. Modulatory effects of tamoxifen and ICI 182, 780 on Adriamycin resistance in MCF-7 human breast cancer cells. *Int J Cancer*, 1996 68:340-348.

Drafta, D; Priscu, A; Neacsu, E; Gangura, M; Schindler, AE; Stroe, E; Anghel, C; Panaitescu, G. Estradiol and progesterone receptor levels in human breast cancer in relation to cytosol and plasma estrogen level. *J Steroid Biochem* 1983, 8:459-63.

Drucker, L; Stackieviez, R; Radnay, J; Shapiro, H; Cohen, I; Yarkoni, S. Tamoxifen enhances apoptotic effect of cisplatin on primary endometrial cell cultives. *Anticancer Res*, 2003 23:1549-1554.

Durst, M; Kleinheinz, A; Hotz, M; Gissmann, L. The physical state of human papillomavirus type 16 DNA in benign and malignant genital tumours. *J Gen Virol* 1985 66:1515-22.

Edery, M; Goussard, J; Dehennin, L; Scholler, R; Reiffsteck, J; Drosdowsky, MA. Endogenous oestradiol-17beta concentration in breast tumours determined by mass fragmentography and by radioimmunoassay: relationship to receptor content. *Eur J Cancer*, 1981 17:115-20.

El Etreby, MF; Liang, Y; Wrenn, RW; Schoenlein, PV. Additive effect of mifepristone and tamoxifen on apoptotic pathways in MCF-7 human breast cancer cells. *Breast Cancer Res Treat*, 1998 51: 149-168

El Etreby, MF; Liang, Y; Johnson, MH; Lewis, RW. Antitumor activity of mifepristone in the human LNCaP, LNCaP-C4, and LNCaP-C4-2 prostate cancer models in nude mice. *Prostate*, 2000 42: 99-106

Ercoli, A; Battaglia, A; Raspaglio, G; Fattorossi, A; Alimonti, A; Petrucci, F; Carola, S; Mancoso, S; Scambia, G. Activity of cisplatin and ICI 182,780 on estrogen receptor negative ovarian cancer cells: cell cycle and cell replication rate perturbation, Chromatin texture alteration and apoptosis induction. *Int J Cancer*, 2000 85:98-103

Fife, KH; Katz, BP; Roush, J; Handy, VD; Brown, DR;, Hansell, R. Cancer associated Human papillomavirus types are selectively increased in the cervix of women in the first trimester of pregnancy. *Am J Obstet Gynecol*, 1996 174:1487-1493.

Fiorica, JV. The role of topotecan in the treatment of advanced cervical cancer. *Gynecol Oncol*, 2003 90:S16-21.

Fisher, B; Constantino, JP; Redmond, CK; Fisher, ER; Wickerham, DL; Cronin, WM; Endometrial cancer in tamoxifen-treated breast cancer patients: findings from the

National Surgical Adjuvant Breast and breast Project (NSA BP) B-14. *J Natl Cancer Inst*, 1994 86:527-537.

Ford, JM; Hait, WN. Pharmacology of drugs that alter multidrug resistance in cancer. *Pharmacol Rev*, 1990 42:155-99.

Friedrich, M; Mink, D; Villena-Heinsen, C; Woll-Hermann, A; Schmidt, W. Tamoxifen and proliferation of vaginal and cervical epithelium in postmenopausal women with breast cancer. *Eur J Obstet Gynecol Reprod Biol*, 1998 80:221-225.

Fujita, E; Egashira, J; Urase, K; Kuitda, K; Mommi, T. Caspase-9 processing by caspase-3 via feedback amplification loop in vivo. *Cell Death*, 2001 8:335-344

Fujiwara, H; Tortoledo-Luna, G; Mitchell, MF; Koulos, JP; Wright, TC Jr.. Adenocarcinoma of the cervix. Expression and clinical significance of estrogen and progesterone receptors. *Cancer*, 1997 79:505-512.

Gaddy, VT; Barrett, JT; Delk, JN; Kallab, AM; Porter, AG; Schoenlein, PV. Mifepristone induces growth arrest, caspase activation, and apoptosis of estrogen receptor-expressing, antiestroogen-resistant breast cancer cell. *Clin Cancer Res*, 2004 10:5215-5225.

Gao, YL; Twiggs, LB; Leung, BS; Yu, WC; Potish, R; Okagaki, T; Adcock, L; Prem KA. Cytoplasmic estrogen and progesterone receptors in primary cervical carcinoma: clinical and histopatologic correlates. *Am J Obstet Gynecol*, 1983 146:299-306.

Garcia-Lopez, P; Rodriguez-Dorantes, M; Perez-Cardenas, E; Cerbon, M; Mohar-Betancourt, A. Synergistic effects of ICI 182,780 on the cytoxicity of cisplatin in cervical carcinoma cell lines. *Cancer Chemother Pharmacol*, 2004 53:533-540.

Hait, WN; Aftab, DT. Rational design and pre-clinical pharmacology of drugs for reversing multidrug resistance. *Biochem Pharmacol*, 1992 43:103-107

Hahnel, R; Martin, JD; Masters, AM; Ratajezak, KT; Twaddle, E. Oestrogen receptors and blood hormone levels in cervical carcinoma and other gynecological tumors. *Gynecol Oncol*, 1979 8:226-233

Hand, S; Sidell, N. RU486-induced growth inhibition of human endometrial cells involves the nuclear factor-kappa B signaling pathway. *J Clin Endocrinol Metab*, 2003 88:713-719.

He, Q; Liang, CH; Lippard, SJ. Steroid hormones induce HMG1 overexpression and sensitize breast cancer cells to cisplatin and carboplatin. *Proc Natl Acad Sci*, 2000 97:5768-5772

Herzog, TJ. New approaches for the management of cervical cancer. *Gynecol Oncol*, 2003 90: S22–S27.

Hildeshein, A; Reeves, WC; Brinton, L; Lavery, C; Brenes, M; DeLa Guardia, ME; Godoy, J; Rawls, WE. Association of oral contraceptive use and human papillomaviruses in invasive cancers. *Int. J Cancer*, 1990 45:860-864.

Hornback, NB; Shen, RN; Sutton, GP; Shidnia, H; Kaiser, HE. Synergistic cytotoxic and antitumor effects of irradiation and taxol on human HeLa cervix carcinoma and mouse B16 melanoma cells. *In vivo*, 1994 8:819-823.

Howell, A; Osborne, CK; Morris, CH; Wakeling, AE. ICI 182 780 (Faslodex), Development of a novel, "pure" antiestrogen. *Cancer*, 2000 89:817-825

Huang, JC; Zamble, DB; Reardon, JT; Lippard, ST; Sancar, A. HMG-domain proteins specifically inhibit the repair of the major DNA adduct of the anticancer drug cisplatin by human excision nuclease. *Proc Natl Acad Sci*, 1994 91:10394-10398.

Hunter, R; Longcope, C; Keough, P. Steroid hormone receptors in carcinoma of the cervix. *Cancer*, 1987 60:392-396.

Huynh, H; Nickerson, T; Pollak, M; Yang X. Regulation of insulin-like growth factor I receptor expression by the pure Antiestrogen ICI 182,780. *Clin Cancer Res*, 1996 2:2037-2042.

Hwang, JY; Lin, BY; Tang, FM; Yu, WC. Tamoxifen stimulates human papillomavirus type 16 gene expression and cell proliferation in a cervical cancer cell line. *Cancer Res*, 1992 52:6848-6852.

Hyder, S; Chiappetta, C; Murthy, L; Stancel, G. Selective inhibition of estrogen–regulated gene expression in vivo by the pure antiestrogen ICI 182,780. *Cancer Res*, 1997 57:2547-2549.

Ignar-Trowbridge, DM; Teng, CT; Ross, KA; Parker, MG; Korach, KS; McLachlan, JA. Peptide growth factors elicit estrogen receptor-dependent transcriptional activation of an estrogen-responsive element. *Mol Endocrinol*, 1993 7:922-8.

Ing, NH; Beekman, JM; Tsai, SY; Tsai, MJ; O'Malley, BW. Members of the steroid hormone receptor superfamily interact with TFIIB (S300-II). J Biol Chem, 1992 267: 17617-17623.

Kaufmann, SH; Earnshaw, WC. Induction of apoptosis by cancer chemotherapy. *Exp Cell Res*, 2000 256:42-9.

Kartner, N; Evernden-Porelle, D; Bradley, G; Ling, V. Detection of P-glycoprotein in multidrug-resistant cell lines by monoclonal antibodies. *Nature*, 1985 316:820-823.

Ketter, LM; Murphy, AA ; Morales, AJ; Yen, SS. Preliminary reports on the treatment of endometriosis with low-dose mifeprostone (RU486) *Am J Obstet Gynecol* 1998 178:1151-1156.

Khare, S; Pater, MM; Tang, SC; Pater, A. Effect of glucocorticoid hormones on viral gene expression, growth, and dysplastic differentiation in HPV16-immortalized ectocervical cells. *Exp Cell Res*, 1997 232:353-360.

Kim, CJ; Um, S; Kim, TY; Kim, E; Park, TC; Kim, SJ; Namkoong, SE; Park, JS. Regulation of cell growth and HPV genes by exogenous estrogen in cervical cancer cells. *Int J Gynecol Cancer*, 2000 10:157-164.

Lackey, BR; Gray, SL; Henricks, DM. Synergistic approach to cancer therapy: exploiting interactions between anti-estrogens, retinoids, monoterpenes and tyrosine kinase inhibitors. *Med Hypotheses*, 2000 54:832-836

Laga, M; Icenogle, JP; Marsella, R; Manoka, AT; Nzila, N; Ryder, RW; Vermund, SH; Heyward, WL; Nelson, A; Reeves; WC. Genital papillomavirus infection and cervical dysplasia –opportunistic complications of HIV infection. *Int J Cancer*, 1992 50:45-48.

Lecureur, V; Fardel, O; Guillouzo, A. The antiprogestatin drug RU 486 potentiates doxorubicin cytotoxicity in multidrug resistant cells through inhibition of P-glycoprotein function. *FEBS Lett*, 1994 355:187-91.

Lee, KH; Yim, EK; Kim, CJ; Namkoong, SE; Um, SJ; Park, JS.. Proteomic analysis of anti-cancer effects by paclitaxel treatment in cervical cancer cells. *Gynecol Oncol* 2005. 98:45-53.

Li DQ, Wang ZB, Bai J, Zhao J, Wang Y, Hu K, Du YH. Effects of mifepristone on proliferation of human gastric adenocarcinoma cell line SGC-7901 in vitro. *World J Gastroenterol*, 2004 10:2628-2631.

Liang, Y; Hou, M; Kallab, AM; Barrett, JT; El Etreby, F; Schoenlein, PV. Induction of antiproliferation and apoptosis in estrogen receptor negative MDA-231 human breast cancer cells by mifepristone and 4-hydroxytamoxifen combination therapy: a role for TGFbeta1. *Int J Oncol*, 2003 23: 369-380.

Liu, Y; Wang, LL; Deng, Y. Enhancement of antitumor effect of cisplatin against human ovarian carcinoma cells by mifepristone in vivo. *Di Yi Jun Yi Da Xue Xue Bao*, 2003 23:242-4.

Lopez-Flores, A; Jurado, R; Garcia-Lopez, P. A high-performance liquid chromatographic assay for determination of cisplatin in plasma, cancer cell, and tumor samples. *J pharmacol Toxicol Methods*, 2005 52:366-372.

Lorincz, AT. Screening for cervical cancer: new alternatives and research. *Salud Publica Mex*, 2003,45:S376-387.

Lorincz, AL; Reid, R; Jonson, AB; Greenberg, MD; Lancaster, W; Kurman, RJ. Human papillomavirus infection of the cervix: relative risk associations of 15 common anogenital types. *Obstet Gynecol*, 1992 79:328,

Mahajan, DK; London, SN. Mifepristone (RU486): a review. Fertil Steril, 1997 68: 967-976

Mangelsdorf, DJ; Thummel, C; Beato, M; Herrlich, P; Schutz, G; Umesono K; Blumberg, B; Kastner, P; Mark, M; Chambon, P; Evans, RM. The nuclear receptor superfamily: the second decade Cell, 1995 83:835-839.

Marino M, Acconcia F, Bresciani F, Weisz A, Trentalance A (2002) Distinct nongenomic signal transduction pathways controlled by 17B-estradiol regulate DNA synthesis and cyclin D1 gene transcription in HepG2 cells. *Mol Biol Cell* 13:3720-3729.

Martin, JD; Hahnel, R; Mc Cartney, AJ; DeKlerk, N. The influence of estrogen and progesterone receptors on survival in patients with carcinoma of the uterine cervix. *Gynecol Oncol*, 1986 23:329-335.

Matsushita, H; Morishita, R; Nata, T; Aoki, M; Nakagami, H; Taniyama, Y; Yamamoto, K; Higaki, J; Yasufumi, K; Ogihara, T. Hypoxia-induced endothelial apoptosis through nuclear factor-kappaB (NF-kappaB)-mediated bcl-2 suppression: in vivo evidence of the importance of NF-kappaB in endothelial cell regulation. *Cir Res,* 2000 86:974-81.

Meanwell, CA. The epidemiology and etiology of cervical cancer. In:Blackledge GRP, Jordan JA, Shingleton HM, eds. *Textbook of gynecologic oncology*. Philadelphia: WB Saunders, 1991:250.

Miller, WR. Uptake and synthesis of steroid hormones by the breast. *Endocr Related Cancer*, 1997 4:307-311.

Mittal, R; Tsutsumi, K; Pater, A; Pater, MM. Human papillomavirus type 16 expression in cervical keratinocytes: role of progesterone and glucocorticoid hormones. *Obstet Gynecol*, 1993 81:5-12.

Mohar, A; Frias, M; Beltran, A; Mora, T; Solorza, G; Herrera, A; Ramírez, J. Epidemiología descriptiva del cancer cervico uterino. Instituto Nacional de Cancerología 1985-1991. *Rev Inst Nal Cancerol (Mex)*, 1993 39:1849-1854.

Mourits, MJ; Hollema, H; De Vries, EG; Ten-Hoor, KA; Willemse, PH; VanDer Zee, AG.) Apoptosis and apoptosis-associated parameters in relation to tamoxifen exposure in postmenopausal endometrium. *Hum Pathol*, 2002 33:341-346.

Muñoz, N; Bosch, FX; de Sanjose, S; Shah, KV. The role of HPV is the etiology of cervical cancer. *Mutat. Res*, 1994 305:293-301.

Murphy, AA; Zhou, MH; Malkapuram, S; Santanam, N; Parthasarathy, S; Sidell, N. RU486-induced growth inhibition of human endometrial cells. *Fertil Steril*, 2000,74:1014-9.

Mutch, DG; Bloss, JD. Gemcitabine in cervical cancer. *Gynecol Oncol* 2003 90:S8-15.

Nooter, K; Stoter, G. Molecular mechanisms of multidrug resistance in cancer chemotherapy. *Pathol Res Pract*, 1996 192:768-780.

Onate, SA; Tsai, SY; Tsai, MJ; O'Malley, BW. Sequence and characterization of a coactivator for the steroid hormone receptor superfamily. *Science*, 1995 270: 1354-1357

Parazzini, F; LaVecchia, C. Epidemiology of adenocarcinoma of the cervix. *Gynecol Oncol*, 1990 39:40-46.

Payen, L; Delugin, L; Courtois, A; Trinquart, Y; Guillouzo, A; Fardel, O. Reversal of MRP-mediated multidrug resistance in human lung cancer cells by the antiprogestatin drug RU486. *Biochem Biophys Res Commun*, 1999 258: 513-518.

Perez, EA; Gandara, DR; Edelman, MJ; O'Donnell, R; Lauder, IJ; DeGregorio, M. Phase I trial of high-dose tamoxifen in combination with cisplatin in patients with lung cancer and other advanced malignancies. *Cancer Invest*, 2003 21:1-6.

Peters, RK; Chao, A; Mack, TM; Thomas, D; Bernstein, L; Henderson, BE. Increased frequency of adenocarcinoma of the uterine cervix in young women in Los Angeles Country. *J Natl Cancer Inst*, 1986 1986:423-8.

Piper, JM. Oral contraceptives and cervical cancer. *Gynecol Oncol*, 1985 22:1-14.

Potish, RA; Twiggs, LB; Adcock, LL; Prem, K; Savage, JE; Leung, BS. Prognostic importance of progesterone and estrogen receptors in cancer of the uterine cervix. *Cancer*, 1986 58:1709-1713.

Qin, TN; Wang, LL. Enhanced sensitivity of ovarian cell line to cisplatin induced by mifepristone and its mechanism. *Di Yi Jun Yi Da Xue Xue Bao*, 2002 22:344-6.

Ramirez, J; Luévano, E; Mora, A; Solorza, G; Alcal, J; Verduzco, L; Guadarama, R; Beltran, A. Carcinoma cervico uterino: Análisis epidemiológico de 140 casos. *Rev Inst Nal Cancerol (Mex)*, 1983 3:417-442.

Roberstson, JF; Nicholson, RI; Bundred, NJ; Anderson, E; Rayter, Z; Dowsett, M; Fox, JN; Gee, JM; Webster, A; Wakeling, AE; Morris, C; Dixon, M. Comparison of the short-term biological effects of 7á-[9-(4,4,5,5,5-pentafluoropenthylsulfinyl)-nonyl]estra-1,3,5,(10)-triene-3,17 beta-diol (faslodex) versus tamoxifen in postmenopausal women with primary breast cancer. *Cancer Res*, 2001 61: 6739-6746.

Rocereto, TF; Saul, HM; Aikins, JA Jr; Paulson, J. Phase II study of mifepristone (RU486) in refractory ovarian cancer. *Gynecol Oncol*, 2000 77: 429-432.

Rose, FV; Barnea, ER. Response of human ovarian carcinoma cell lines to antiprogestin mifepristone. *Oncogene*, 1996 12: 999-1003.

Rose, PG; Blessing, JA; Lele, S; Abulafia, O. Evaluation of pegylated liposomal doxorubicin (Doxil) as second-line chemotherapy of squamous cell carcinoma of the cervix: A phase

II study of the Gynecologic Oncology Group. *Gynecol Oncol*, 2006 [Epub ahead of print].

Rosenberg-Zand, RS; Grass, L; Magklara, A; Jenkins, DJ; Diamandis, EP.) Is ICI 182,780 an antiprogestin in addition to being an antiestrogen?. Breast Cancer Res Treat, 2000 60:1-8.

Sanborn, BM; Held, B; Kuo, HS. Hormonal action in human cervix-II. Specific progestogen binding proteins in human cervix. *J Steroid Biochem*, 1976 7:665-672.

Scambia, G; Panici, B; Baiochi, G; Battaglia, F; Ferrandina, G; Greggi, S; Mancuso, S. Steroid hormone receptors in carcinoma of the cervix: look of response to an antiestrogen. *Gynecol Oncol*, 1990, 37:323-326.

Schilder, JM; Stehman, FB. Stage Ia - IIa cancer of the cervix. *Cancer J*, 2003 9:395-403.

Schneider, CC; Gibb, RK; Taylor, D; Wan, T; Gercel-Taylor, C. Inhibition of endometrial cancer cell lines by mifepristone (RU 486*). J Soc Gynecol Investig*, 1998 5: 334-338.

Schneider-Maunory, S; Croissant, O; Orth, G. Integration of human papillomavirus type 16 DNA sequences: a possible early event in the progression of genital tumors. *J Virol*, 1987 61:3295-3298.

Slee, EA; Harte, MT; Kluck, RM; Wolf, BB; Casiano, CA; Newmeyer, DD; Wang, HG; Reed, JC; Nicholson, DW; Alnemnri, ES; Green, DR; Martin, SJ. Ordering the cytocrome c-eliminated caspase cascade: hierarchial activation of caspase -2,-3,-6,-7,-8, and 10 in caspase -9-dependent manner. *J Cell Biol*, 1999 144:281-292.

Smith, CL; Onate, SA; Tsai, MJ, O'Malley, BW. *Proc. Natl. Acad. Sci. USA*, 1996 93: 8884-8888.

Smith, DF; Toft, DO. Steroid receptors and their associated proteins. *Mol Endocrinol*, 1993 7:4-11.

Spitz, IM; Bardin, CW. Mifepristone (RU486), a modulator of progestin and glucocorticoid action. *N Engl J Med*, 1993 329:404-12.

Tan-Chiu, E; Wang, J; Costantino, JP; Paik, S; Butch, C; Wickerham, DL; Fisher, B; Wolmark, N. Effects of tamoxifen on benign breast disease in women at high risk for breast cancer. *J Natl Cancer Inst*, 2003 95:302-307.

Tavassoli, M; Soltaninia, J; Rudnicka, J; Mashanyare, D; Johnson, N; Gaken, J. Tamoxifen inhibits the growth of head and neck cancer cells and sensitizes these cells to cisplatin induced apoptosis: role of TGF-beta1. *Carcinogenesis*, 2002 23:1569-1575.

Terenius, L; Lindell, A; Persson, BH. Binding of estradiol-17-beta to human cancer tissue of the female genital tract. *Cancer Res*, 1971 31:1895-1898.

Tewari, KS; Taylor, JA; Liao, SY; DiSaia, PJ; Burger, R; Monk, B; Hughes, CC; Villarreal, LP. Development and assessment of a general theory of cervical carcinogenesis utilizing a severe combined immunodeficiency murine-human xenograft model. *Gynecol Oncol*, 2000 77:137-148.

Thigpen, T. The role of chemotherapy in the management of carcinoma of the cervix. *Cancer J*, 2003 9:425-432.

Thomas, EJ; Walton, P; Thomas, NM; Dowsett, M. The effects of ICI 182,780, a pure anti-estrogen, on the hypothalamic-pituitary-gonadal axis and on endometrial proliferation in pre-menopausal women. *Hum Reproduction*, 1994 9:1991-1996.

Tinker, AV; Bhagat, K; Swenerton, K; Hoskins, PJ. Carboplatin and paclitaxel for advanced and recurrent cervical carcinoma: the British Columbia Cancer Agency experience. *Gynecol Oncol*, 2005 98:54-58.

Tsai, MJ; O'Malley, BW. Molecular mechanism of action of steroid/thyroid receptor superfamily members. *Ann Rev Biochem*, 1994 63:451-486.

Twiggs, S; Potish, R; Leung, B; Carson, L; Adcock, L; Savage, J; Prem, K. Cytosolic estrogen and progesterone receptors as prognostic parameters in stage IB cervical carcinoma. *Gynecol Oncol,* 1987 28:156-160.

Ueda, K; Okamura, N; Hirai, M; Tanigawara, Y; Saeki, T; Kioka, N; Komano, T; Hori, R. Human P-glycoprotein transports cortisol, aldosterone, and dexamethasone, but not progesterone. *J Biol Chem*, 1992 267:24248-52.

Von Knebel Doeberitz, M; Bauknecht, T; Bartsch, D; ZurHausen, H. Influence of chromosomal integration on glucocorticoid regulated transcription of growth -stimulating papillomavirus genes E6/E7 in cervical carcinoma cells. *Proc Natl Acad Sci USA*, 1991 88:1411-1415.

Von Knebel Doeberitz, M; Rittmuller, ; Zur Hausen, H; Durst, M. Inhibition of tumorigenicity of cervical cancer cells in nude mice by HPV E6/E7 anti-sense RNA. *Int J Cancer*, 1992 51:831-834.

Walboomers, JM; Jacobs, MV; Manos, MM; Bosch, FX; Kummer, JA; Shah, KV, Snijders, PJ; Peto, J; Meijer CJ; Munoz, N. Human papillomavirus is a necessary cause of invasive cervical cancer worldwide. *J Pathol*, 1999 189:12-19.

Wilczynski, SP; Bergen, S; Walker, J; Liao, SY; Pearlman, LF. Human papillomaviruses and cervical cancer: analysis of histopathologic features associated with different viral types. *Hum Pathol*, 1988 19:697-704.

Yang, CP; DePinho, SG; Greenberger, LM; Arceci, RJ; Horwitz, SB. Progesterone interacts with P-glycoprotein in multidrug-resistant cells and in the endometrium of gravid uterus. *J Biol Chem*, 1989 264:782-8.

In: Trends in Cervical Cancer
Editor: Hector T. Varaj, pp. 89-96

ISBN: 1-60021-299-9
© 2007 Nova Science Publishers, Inc.

Chapter IV

NOVEL GENTLE THERAPEUTIC TRENDS FOR PATIENTS OF UTERINE CERVICAL CANCER

Jiro Fujimoto[*], Hideki Sakaguchi, Hiroshi Toyoki, Israt Jahan, Syed Mahfuzul Alam, Eriko Sato and Teruhiko Tamaya

Department of Obstetrics and Gynecology, Gifu University School of Medicine
1-1 Yanagido, Gifu City 501-1194, Japan.

ABSTRACT

In uterine cervical cancers, lymph node metastasis, recognized as a common form of metastasis, and recurrence after curative resection are critical to patient prognosis. The growth of secondarily spreading and initial recurrent lesions must be suppressed to improve patient prognosis. Chemotherapy and radiation are often not very specific to cancer cells, and it produces severe effects on even normal cells, especially bone marrow and renal cells. On the other hand, anti-angiogenic therapy is specific to the rapidly growing vascular endothelial cells in tumors, without any effect on slow growing vascular endothelial cells and other normal cells. Therefore, anti-angiogenic therapy should be an excellent strategy to suppress the growth of secondarily spreading and initial recurrent lesions. However, if an angiogenic factor is suppressed by anti-angiogenic therapy for a long period, another angiogenic factor might be induced by an alternately linked angiogenic pathway, which is recognized as tolerance. Therefore, we have studied the expression manner of angiogenic factors and one angiogenic transcription factor in uterine cervical cancers, and herein introduce novel gentle therapeutic trends for patients of uterine cervical cancers.

---

[*] Correspondence concerning this article should be addressed at Department of Obstetrics and Gynecology, Gifu University School of Medicine, 1-1 Yanagido, Gifu City 501-1194, Japan. Phone +81 58 230 6349; Fax +81 58 230 6348; jf@cc.gifu-u.ac.jp.

Keywords: angiogenesis, uterine cervical cancers, basic FGF, VEGF, COX-2, angiopoietin, IL-8, thymidine phosphorylase, HIF-1α, ETS-1.

INTRODUCTION

Angiogenesis is essential for development, growth and advancement of solid tumors [1]. The manner of advancement specific to each tumor is vital to patient prognosis. In uterine cervical cancers, lymph node metastasis, recognized as a common form of metastasis, and recurrence after curative resection are critical to patient prognosis.

When the cluster of cancer cells is smaller than 2 mm in diameter, angiogenesis does not occur. However, when the cluster size reaches 2 mm, angiogenesis inevitably occurs. Thereafter, a new capillary network is rapidly formed to nourish and grow the tumors. Therefore, attaining a diameter of 2 mm is critical to the manner of tumor growth [1]. Unfortunately, when a secondarily spread lesion has been discovered, its size is usually already larger than 2 mm in diameter. This means angiogenesis in the lesion has already begun. Consequently, although detachment and invasion of cancer cells can be suppressed, the growth of the previously formed secondarily spread lesions will not be suppressed. The growth of secondarily spread lesions must be suppressed to improve patient prognosis, and inhibition of angiogenesis should be an excellent strategy to suppress the growth of those secondarily spread lesions. Furthermore, chemotherapy is often not very specific to cancer cells, and it produces severe effects on even normal cells, especially bone marrow and renal cells. On the other hand, anti-angiogenic therapy is specific to the rapidly growing vascular endothelial cells in tumors, without any effect on slow growing vascular endothelial cells and other normal cells.

However, if an angiogenic factor is suppressed by anti-angiogenic therapy for a long period, another angiogenic factor might be induced by an alternately linked angiogenic pathway, which is recognized as tolerance. Therefore, we have studied the expression manner of angiogenic factors with a mediator, and angiogenic transcription factors, and herein introduce new strategies for anti-angiogenic therapy in uterine cervical cancers.

CONCEPT OF TUMOR ANGIOGENESIS

Neovascularization involves two concepts, vasculogenesis and angiogenesis. Vasculogenesis is formation of vascular plexus by differentiation from hemangioblasts to endothelial cells without any existing vascular system. For example, primary vascular plexus is formed from hemangioblasts in fetuses by the process of vasculogenesis. Angiogenesis is formation of new capillary from existing capillary. Angiogenesis occurs in tumors, and supports growth and advancement of tumors.

Angiogenic factors from tumors induce and activate matrix metalloproteinase, plasminogen activator, collagenase, and other enzymes in endothelial cells. The enzymes dissolve the basement membrane of endothelial cells, after which the endothelial cells proliferate and migrate under the influence of angiogenic factors. Angiogenic factors induce production of integrins in the endothelial cells. The endothelial cells then form immature capillary tubes. In normal tissue, the capillary is matured upon being covered with pericytes. However, the pericyte-covering layer of capillaries in tumors, consisting of fewer cells than normal with inferior function, is not very good. Therefore, the unique point is that cancer cells can easily invade to and from the immature capillary. If there is a positive correlation between microvessel density in tumors and the target factor levels, it is plausible that the target factor is an angiogenic factor. The microvessel density is evaluated by counting microvessels using immunohistochemical staining for CD31, CD34 or factor VIII-related antigen specific to the endothelial cells.

The angiogenic factors basic fibroblast growth factor (bFGF), vascular endothelial growth factor (VEGF), cyclooxygenase (COX)-2, angiopoietin (Ang), interleukin (IL)-8, and thymidine phosphorylase (TP) are the main angiogenic factors in cancers of reproductive organ. A brief introduction to each of them follows: bFGF expressed in cancer and stromal cells works on basic angiogenesis. VEGF expressed in cancer cells translocates to endothelial cells to work on sensitive angiogenesis. COX-2 expressed in cancer cells works on angiogenesis associated with tumor growth and advancement. The metabolites of COX-2, prostaglandin (PG)E1 and PGE2, have weak angiogenic activity [2], and PGE1 and PGE2 induce VEGF production in osteoblasts, synovial fibroblasts and macrophages [3-5]. Angs are expressed on vascular endothelial cells. Although Ang-1 induces phosphorylation of the tyrosine kinase domain of tie-2 as a receptor of Ang-1 and Ang-2, Ang-1 does not directly work on proliferation of vascular endothelial cells. In Ang-1 knockout mice, normal vasculogenesis is developed, but incomplete angiogenesis is induced and links to lethal heart dysplasia [6]. On the other hand, although Ang-2 conserves high affinity to tie-2 as Ang-1 does, Ang-2 does not induce phosphorylation of tie-2 tyrosine kinase domain. Conversely, overexpression of Ang-2 inhibits the signal transduction of Ang-1 liked to tie-2. In detail, Ang-1 is constitutively produced from pericytes, and works on stabilization of the interaction of vascular endothelial cells with pericytes. Once an event, for example hypoxia, stimulates Ang-2 production from vascular endothelial and stromal cells near vascular endothelial cells, and angiogenesis is initiated with the dissociation of pericytes and the dissolution of basement membrane of vascular endothelial cells. Furthermore, VEGF with Ang-1 enhances the formation of capillary network, and VEGF with Ang-2 enhances the expansion of capillary network [7]. IL-8 secreted from macrophages works on angiogenesis associated with cancer cell invasion. TP expressed in stromal cells works on specific angiogenesis with enzymatic activity.

Furthermore, angiogenesis is induced by hypoxia with angiogenic transcription factor hypoxia inducible factors (HIF). HIF-1 belongs to the Per-Ahr/Arnt-Sim (PAS) family of basic helix-loop-helix proteins. HIF-1 consists of HIF-1α and HIF-1β (aryl hydrocarbon receptor nuclear translocator), or HIF-2α and HIF-1β as a heterodimer using helix-loop-helix domain [8]. Although HIF-1α is constitutively reduced by proteasome after ubiquitinization of HIF-1α, hypoxia stabilizes and activates HIF-1α [9,10]. On the other hand, HIF-2α is expressed abundantly in various organs under normoxia, although transcriptional activating properties of HIF-2α are similar to those of HIF-1α [11]. HIF-1α may be responsible for VEGF expression mediated by hypoxia, and may be closely related to tumor angiogenesis [12-14]. During angiogenesis, angiogenic transcription factor E26 transformation specific

(ETS)-1 is strongly expressed in vascular endothelial cells and the adjacent interstitial cells [15]. Once angiogenesis has ended, ETS-1 expression is distinctly down regulated [16,17]. The representative angiogenic factors VEGF and bFGF immediately induce ETS-1 expression in the early stage of angiogenesis, while the inhibition of ETS-1 expression leads to suppression of angiogenesis [18,19]. The proteases urokinase type-plasminogen activator (u-PA), matrix metalloprotease (MMP)-1, MMP-3, and MMP-9 conserve an ETS-binding motif, and transcription factor ETS-1 converts vascular endothelial cells to angiogenic phenotypes by inducing proteases u-PA, MMP-1, MMP-3 and MMP-9 and integrinβ3 gene expression [20,21].

Following are the details of the working manners of the various angiogenic factors and angiogenic transcription factors that are closely related with the advancement manners of uterine cervical cancers.

NOVEL GENTLE THERAPEUTIC TRENDS FOR PATIENTS

In uterine cervical cancers, the main manner of angiogenesis is shown in Fig. 1. bFGF levels increase with advancement regardless of histological type. However, the correlation between bFGF levels and poor patient prognosis is not so clear. Therefore, bFGF might be associated with basic angiogenesis to drive uterine cervical cancers in growth and secondarily spreading [22].

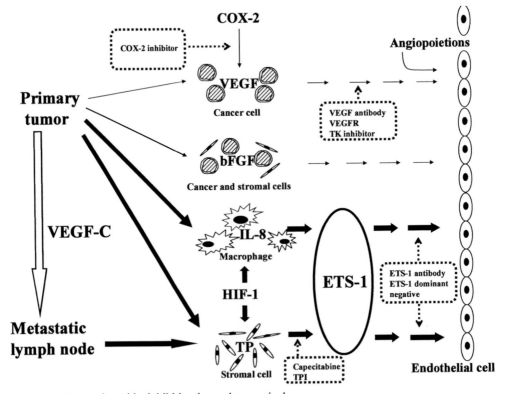

Figure 1. Angiogenesis and its inhibition in uterine cervical cancers.

Among the subtypes of VEGF, the populations of $VEGF_{165}$ and $VEGF_{121}$ are dominant in uterine cervical cancers. The levels of $VEGF_{165}$ and $VEGF_{121}$ are remarkably higher in advanced stage adenocarcinomas of the cervix than in other cases. Thus, the elevation of $VEGF_{165}$ and $VEGF_{121}$ might contribute to the relatively late advancement via angiogenic activity in advanced adenocarcinomas of the cervix [23]. Furthermore, VEGF associated with COX-2 works on advancement of uterine cervical cancers via angiogenesis. Therefore, long-term administration of COX-2 inhibitors might be effective on the suppression of regrowth or recurrence after intensive treatment for advanced uterine cervical cancers. The ratio of Ang-2/Ang-1 increases up to late stage II and correlates with VEGF levels. Therefore, Angs interacted with VEGF might work on angiogenesis in comparatively early stage of uterine cervical cancers. It is very interested in the inhibition of tumor growth by administration of soluble extracellular domain of tie-2 that conserves the binding domain of Ang-1 and Ang-2.

IL-8 levels correlate with microvessel and infiltrated macrophage counts, and the localization of IL-8 is similar to that of CD68 specific to macrophages. The prognosis of patients with high IL-8 was extremely poor. Consequently, IL-8 can be regarded as a prognostic indicator as an angiogenic factor supplied from macrophages in uterine cervical cancers [24]. Although IL-8 mainly works on angiogenesis with advancement in the primary tumor, the suppression of IL-8 might not lead to the efficient inhibition of angiogenesis, because IL-8 is involved in cytokine networks with alternating angiogenic potential.

TP has a wide range of expression and is highly expressed in uterine cervical cancers regardless of clinical stage. The prognosis of patients with high TP in primary tumors is worse than in those with low TP. Hence, it is apparent that TP in uterine cervical cancers plays a role of basic angiogenesis in all processes of advancement of uterine cervical cancers [25]. Furthermore, TP remarkably increased in 8 of 40 metastatic lymph node lesions of uterine cervical cancers, and the prognosis of the patients with high TP in metastatic lymph node lesions was extremely poor. Therefore, TP expressed in stromal cells appears to contribute to the advancement of metastatic lymph nodes after the establishment of metastasis, and is recognized as a prognostic indicator [26]. Incidentally, VEGF-C expressed in cancer cells directly contributes to lymph node metastasis in uterine cervical cancers as a non-angiogenic factor [27]. TP and VEGF-C expressions in metastatic lymph node are keys to evaluating patient prognosis and to building new strategies of anti-angiogenic therapy. In addition, serum TP in patients with uterine cervical cancers reveals positive correlations with clinical stage and tumor size and with the advancement indicators lymph node metastasis, parametrial involvement, and vessel permeation in both squamous cell carcinomas and adenocarcinomas. Therefore, serum TP level is recognized as a novel tumor marker regardless of histopathological type of the uterine cervical cancer [28]. Although VEGF-C expressed in cancer cells directly contributes to lymph node metastasis as a non-angiogenic factor, VEGF-C antibody or inhibitor could suppress the process of lymph node metastasis and lead to better patient prognosis. Since capecitabine is converted to 5-fluorouracil (FU) by TP, resulting in remarkably increased 5-FU levels in metastatic lymph nodes containing high TP levels, with capecitabine as the metabolite, 5-FU might be highly effective on the suppression of metastatic lymph nodes. Additionally, TP inhibitor (TPI) can directly suppress TP activity for angiogenesis in metastatic lymph nodes.

HIF-1α levels correlate with microvessel counts, and the localization of HIF-1α is in the cancer cells. HIF-1α levels correlate with IL-8 and TP levels in uterine cervical cancers, HIF-1α appears to induce IL-8 and TP as an angiogenic mediator, and is recognized as a candidate for a prognostic indicator of uterine cervical cancers. On the other hand, ETS-1 levels correlate with microvessel counts, and the localization of ETS-1 is similar to that of vascular endothelial cells in uterine cervical cancers. ETS-1 levels correlate with IL-8 and TP levels. ETS-1 might work on angiogenesis as an angiogenic transcription factor, and be a prognostic indicator in uterine cervical cancers [29]. Furthermore, ETS-1 antibody and/or dominant-negative ETS-1 can be useful to suppress the linkage of angiogenic factors to ETS-1. Therefore, to avoid inducing alternative angiogenic pathways as a sort of tolerance to an angiogenic inhibitor, the simultaneous suppression of the main target angiogenic factors IL-8 and TP, and the transcription factor ETS-1 might be highly effective.

CONCLUSION

Uterine cervical cancers conserve specific expression manners of various angiogenic factors bFGF, VEGF, COX-2, Ang, IL-8 and TP, and of the angiogenic transcription factors HIF-1α and ETS-1 in specific advancement via angiogenesis with the promotion of lymph node metastasis developed by VEGF-C. The keys to creating new strategies of anti-angiogenic therapy are: (1) The overexpression of TP induced by HIF-1α and linked to ETS-1 in metastatic lymph nodes of uterine cervical cancers. (2) The COX-2 inducible VEGF interacted with Angs in comparatively early stage of uterine cervical cancers. We are looking forward to proceeding with clinical trials of anti-angiogenic agents in advanced-stage patients and after curative resection for uterine cervical cancers.

REFERENCES

[1]   Folkman J: Tumor angiogenesis. *Adv Cancer Res* 1985;43:175-203

[2]   Rochels R: Pathobiochemical aspects of corneal neovascularization. *Fortschr Med* 1984;102:101-102

[3]   Harada S, Nagy JA, Sullivan KA, Thomas KA, Endo N, Rodan GA, Rodan SB: Induction of vascular endothelial growth factor expression by prostaglandin E2 and E1 in osteoblasts. *J Clin Invest* 1994;93:2490-2496

[4]   Sunderkotter C, Steinbrink K, Goebeler M, Bhardwaj R, Sorg C: Macrophages and angiogenesis. *J Leukoc Biol* 1994;55:410-422

[5]   Ben-Av P, Crofford LJ, Wilder RL, Hla T: Induction of vascular endothelial growth factor expression in synovial fibroblasts by prostaglandin E and interleukin-1: a potential mechanism for inflammatory angiogenesis. *FEBS Lett* 1995;372:83-87

[6]   Suri C, Jones PF, Patan S, Bartunkova S, Maisonpierre PC, Davis S, Sato TN, Yancopoulos GD: Requisite role of angiopoietin-1, a ligand for the TIE2 receptor, during embryonic angiogenesis. *Cell* 1996;87:1171-1180

[7]   Asahara T, Chen D, Takahashi T, Fujikawa K, Kearney M, Magner M, Yancopoulos GD, Isner JM: Tie2 receptor ligands, angiopoietin-1 and angiopoietin-2, modulate VEGF-induced postnatal neovascularization. *Circ Res* 1998;83:233-240

[8]   Wang GL, Semenza GL: Purification and characterization of hypoxia-inducible factor 1. *J Biol Chem* 1995;270:1230-1237

[9]   Huang LE, Arany Z, Livingston DM, Bunn HF: Activation of hypoxia-inducible transcription factor depends primarily upon redox-sensitive stabilization of its alpha subunit. *J Biol Chem* 1996;271:32253-32259

[10]   Kallio PJ, Pongratz I, Gradin K, McGuire J, Poellinger L: Activation of hypoxia-inducible factor 1alpha: posttranscriptional regulation and conformational change by recruitment of the Arnt transcription factor. *Proc Natl Acad Asci USA* 1997;94:5667-5672

[11]   Ema M, Taya S, Yokotani N, Sogawa K, Matsuda Y, Fujii-Kuriyama Y: A novel bHLH-PAS factor with close sequence similarity to hypoxia-inducible factor 1alpha regulates the VEGF expression and is potentially involved in lung and vascular development. *Proc Natl Acad Sci USA* 1997;94:4273-4278

[12]   Maxwell PH, Dachs GU, Gleadle JM, Nicholls LG, Harris AL, Stratford IJ, Hankinson O, Pugh CW, Ratcliffe PJ: Hypoxia-inducible factor-1 modulates gene expression in solid tumors and influences both angiogenesis and tumor growth. *Proc Natl Acad Sci USA* 1997;94:8104-8109

[13]   Carmeliet P, Dor Y, Herbert JM, Fukumura D, Brusselmans K, Dewerchin M, Neeman M, Bono F, Abramovitch R, Maxwell P, Koch CJ, Ratcliffe P, Moons L, Jain RK, Collen D, Keshert E: Role of HIF-1alpha in hypoxia-mediated apoptosis, cell proliferation and tumour angiogenesis. *Nature* 1998;394:485-490

[14]   Ryan HE, Lo J, Johnson RS: HIF-1 alpha is required for solid tumor formation and embryonic vascularization. *EMBO J* 1998,17:3005-3015

[15]   Wernert N, Raes MB, Lassalle P, Dehouck MP, Gosselin B, Vandenbunder B, Stehelin D: c-ets proto-oncogene is a transcription factor expressed in endothelial cells during tumor vascularization and other forms of angiogenesis in humans. *Am J Pathol* 1992;140:119-127

[16]   Kola I, Brookes S, Green AR, Garber R, Tymms M, Papas TS, Seth A: The Ets-1 transcription factor is widely expressed during murine embryo development and is associated with mesodermal cells involved in morphogenic process such as organ formation. *Proc Natl Acad Sci USA* 1993;90:7588-7592

[17]   Maroulakou IG, Papas TS, Green JE. Differential expression of ets-1 and ets-2 proto-oncogenes during murine embryogenesis. *Oncogene* 1994;9:1511-1565

[18]   Iwasaka C, Tanaka K, Abe M, Sato Y: Ets-1 regulates angiogenesis by inducing the expression of urokinase-type plasminogen activator and matrix metalloproteinase-1 and the migration of vascular endothelial cells. *J Cell Physiol* 1996;169:522-531.

[19]   Tanaka K, Abe M, Sato Y. Roles of extracelluar signal-regulated kinase 1/2 and p38 mitogen-activated protein kinase in the signal transduction of basic fibroblast growth factor in endothelial cells during angiogenesis. *Jpn J Cancer Res* 1999;90:647-654

[20]   Oda N, Abe M, Sato Y. ETS-1 converts endothelial cells to the angiogenic phenotype by inducing the expression of matrix metalloproteinases and integrin β3. *J Cell Physiol* 1999;178:121-132.

[21]   Sato Y, Abe M, Tanaka K, Iwasaka C, Oda N, Kanno S, Oikawa M, Nakano T, Igarashi T: Signal transduction and transcriptional regulation of angiogenesis. *Adv Exp Med Biol* 2000;476:109-115

[22]   Fujimoto J, Ichigo S, Hori M, Hirose R, Sakaguchi H, Tamaya T: Expression of basic fibroblast growth factor and its mRNA in advanced uterine cervical cancers. *Cancer Lett* 1997;111:21-26

[23]   Fujimoto J, Sakaguchi H, Hirose R, Ichigo S, Tamaya T: Expression of vascular endothelial growth factor (VEGF) and its mRNA in uterine cervical cancers. *Br J Cancer* 1999;80:827-833

[24]   Fujimoto J, Sakaguchi H, Aoki I, Tamaya T: Clinical implications of expression of interleukin 8 related to angiogenesis in uterine cervical cancers. *Cancer Res* 2000;60:2632-2635

[25]   Fujimoto J, Sakaguchi H, Hirose R, Ichigo S, Tamaya T: The expression of platelet-derived endothelial cell growth factor in uterine cervical cancers. *Br J Cancer* 1999;79:1249-1254

[26]   Fujimoto J, Sakaguchi H, Hirose R, Wen H, Tamaya T: Clinical implication of expression of platelet-derived endothelial cell growth factor (PD-ECGF) in metastatic lesions of uterine cervical cancers. *Cancer Res* 1999;59:3041-3044

[27]   Fujimoto J, Toyoki H, Sato E, Sakaguchi H, Tamaya T: Clinical implication of expression of vascular endothelial growth factor-C in metastatic lymph nodes of uterine cervical cancers. *Br J Cancer* 2004;91:466-469

[28]   Fujimoto J, Sakaguchi H, Aoki I, Tamaya T: The value of platelet-derived endothelial cell growth factor as a novel predictor of advancement of uterine cervical cancers. *Cancer Res* 2000;60:3662-3665

[29]   Fujimoto J, Aoki I, Toyoki H, Khatun S, Tamaya T: Clinical implications of ETS-1 related to angiogenesis in uterine cervical cancers. *Ann Oncol* 2002;13:1598-1604

In: Trends in Cervical Cancer
Editor: Hector T. Varaj, pp. 97-123

ISBN: 1-60021-299-9
© 2007 Nova Science Publishers, Inc.

Chapter V

NERVE SPARING RADICAL HYSTERECTOMY FOR THE TREATMENT OF CERVICAL CANCER: NEW RESEARCH ON SURGICAL TECHNIQUES

Francesco Raspagliesi[1], Antonino Ditto[1,*], Francesco Hanozet[1], Fabio Martinelli[1], Eugenio Solima[1], Rosanna Fontanelli[1], Shigeki Kusamura[2] and Flavia Zanaboni[1]

[1]Department of Gynecologic Oncology, Istituto Nazionale Tumori, Milan, Italy;
[2]Department of Surgery, Istituto Nazionale Tumori, Milan, Italy.

ABSTRACT

Five-year survival rates of over 90% have been reported after radical surgery for early cervical cancer. An increasing number of technical modifications have been suggested since this procedure was first described by Wertheim. Changes in the way radical surgery is viewed have led to the idea that benefits from oncological surgery must not be evaluated simply in terms of disease control but also by the functional end-results that may affect the quality of life.

Major causes of radical hysterectomy (RH) morbidity are disturbances in bladder, sexual and rectal functions. These negative sequelaes could derive from damage to the sympathetic and parasympathetic nervous systems.

Yabuki pioneered a nerve-sparing radical hysterectomy (NSRH) technique for cervical cancer to reduce morbidity. In Europe, some investigators have also begun practicing NS surgery, based on studies of the anatomy of the autonomic nervous system of the pelvis. Results have been encouraging.

Raspagliesi et al. reported on 23 cervical cancer patients treated by NSRH. The endpoints were the assessment of the feasibility of the NS technique and the rate of early

---

* Correspondence concerning this article should be addressed to Francesco Raspagliesi, M.D., Istituto Nazionale Tumori, via Venezian 1, 20133 Milan, Italy. Tel: +39/2/23902392; FAX: +39/2/23902349; E-mail: antonino.ditto@istitutotumori.mi.it.

bladder dysfunctions. Two (9%) patients were discharged with self-catheterization and one of them recovered the ability to void her bladder. They concluded that the NSRH technique was feasible, with promising results in terms of preventing early bladder dysfunction.

Recently, the same group of investigators decided to retrospectively compare the safety of the procedure with that of other types of RH. Accordingly class III NSRH was compared with other classes of RH in terms of incidence of early bladder dysfunctions and complications. One hundred and ten patients with cervical cancer were submitted to class II RH (group 1), class III NSRH (group 2) and class III RH (group 3). The groups did not differ significantly in terms of GIII/IV morbidity. Group 1 and 2 presented a prompt recover of bladder function, significantly different from that of the group 3. The class III NSRH is comparable to class II RH and superior to class III RH in terms of early bladder dysfunctions.

There is a deep gap between the information contained in anatomic textbooks and the reality of operating theatre. Despite the growing number of papers addressing the issue of NSRH, with the emergence of several techniques, no consensus has been reached. In this chapter we are going to discuss some landmarks of the neuroanatomy and neurophysiology, highlighting the most significant elements which support the performance of a NS technique in RH.

Keywords: cervical cancer, radical hysterectomy, nerve sparing technique, morbidity

BACKGROUND

Surgical Treatment of Cervical Cancer

Five-year survival rates of over 90% have been reported after radical surgery for early cervical cancer [1]. This relatively good prognosis has directed the attention on quality of life outcomes for survivors. An increasing number of technical modifications have been suggested to radical hysterectomy (RH) to minimize morbidity. Among the various possible complications, serious bladder dysfunction is the most significant and has been reported in up to 10%-32% of patients, depending on the surgical radicality [2,3]. Rectal dysfunction also occurs frequently after RH, but is generally less problematic. Concepts of radical surgery have changed so that benefits from oncological surgery have been evaluated not only in terms of disease control but also in terms of quality of life.

The aim of RH, as with any primary cancer surgery, is to remove the tumor with an adequate margin of normal tissue to ensure complete resection. There are technical variations of RH, although the Piver–Rutledge concept has been widely adopted. The class II RH, later termed a "modified RH", is a procedure in which the uterine vessels are ligated as they cross the ureters. The uterosacral ligaments (USLs) are cut halfway along their length. The medial half of the cardinal ligament (CL) and the upper third of the vagina are removed. Ligating the uterine arteries as they cross the ureters preserves the distal ureteral blood supply and reduces the incidence of vascular necrosis and subsequent fistula formation.

The class III RH is the equivalent to the classical RH described by Wertheim and Meigs. Unlike the class II procedure, the uterine artery is ligated at its origin from the internal iliac artery. Dissection of the ureter is more radical and involves dissection up to the entry point into the bladder. The USLs are resected at their sacral attachments, and likewise the CLs are excised at the pelvic side wall. Up to half of the vagina is also removed (figure 1).

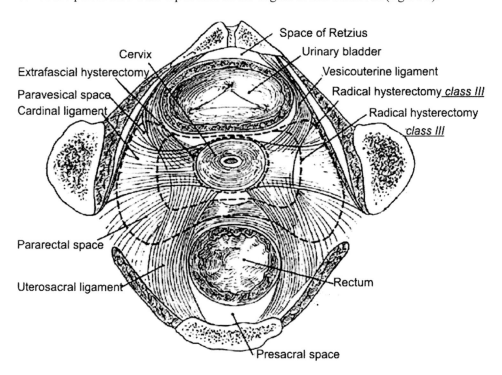

Figure 1: Class 2 radical hysterectomy (RH) versus class 3 RH. Transversal view. Outside line represents class III RH and inside line represents class II RH. The Class III operation includes resection of the entire cardinal ligament. Dissection of the ureter is more radical and involves dissection up to the entry point into the bladder. The USLs are resected near at their sacral attachments.

Parametrectomy is the most technically difficult aspect of RH and is closely related to morbidity. It was hypothesized that the more radical parametrium dissection, the greater the nerve damage and higher the degree of dysfunction [4]. Some authors are of the opinion that the less radical dissections may spare the more lateral portions of the uterine-supporting ligaments and the larger proportion of nerve fibers contained within them, thus resulting in less postoperative morbidity [5]. Other authors indicated that the extent of the vaginal resection may also be related to bladder dysfunction [6,7].

Given that radicality is directly related to morbidity, one raised the hypothesis that the reduction of the extent of the parametrial resection could minimize the postoperative visceral dysfunctions. However, such proposal is debatable. The class II RH for early stage disease was initially conceived to reduce the vascular complications. A number of studies have shown reduced morbidity for modified RH with similar prognosis, when compared with historical controls submitted to class III RH [8,9,10].

Despite these reports, there are concerns regarding the safety and acceptability of preserving the distal parts of the parametrium. Some authors continue to advocate the complete removal of this tissue for all tumor sizes due to the potential existence of randomly distributed parametrial lymph nodes, which may be involved in early tumor spread. Occult parametrial disease has been reported in up to 13-39% after class III RH [11,12,13].

To our knowledge, only one prospective randomized study comparing modified (class II) versus classical (class III) RH was published [14]. In this work 243 patients with stage IB1-IIA cervical cancer were randomized by surgical treatment (class II vs class III RH) and the authors have showed similar recurrence-free and overall survivals between the two arms. The benefit of the class II RH was a statistically significant decrease in the length of the operation and postoperative morbidity, particularly bladder dysfunction. However, adjuvant postoperative radiation therapy was used in 54 and 55% of class II and III RH patients, respectively, so that the effect of the extent of surgical resection may only truly be determined in 46 and 45% of study patients, respectively. Moreover, the study was powered to detect a 20% difference in death and morbidity. In view of the relatively high cure rate for early cervical cancer treated by RH, a larger trial would be needed to detect small differences of this magnitude. Therefore, clearer cut data is required before establishing the results of this study as standard of care of patients affected by cervical cancer.

The ideal surgical management of cervical cancer patients should be also tailored on the basis of prognostic factors. In particular, the surgeon should perform a less radical operation taking into account the tumor size, the nodal spread and the parametrial involvement, which are considered the most important factors linked to prognosis [11,13]. A recent study reports that pre-treatment evaluation of these adverse prognostic factors in patients affected by cervical cancer FIGO stages IA2–IB1 is feasible to determine if a less radical surgery is applicable and safe [15]. Furthermore, in early stage cervical cancer parametrial spread has been reported to be an independent prognostic factor [11] and many studies have evaluated the risk of microscopic parametrial spread relative to primary cervical tumor characteristics. Factors reported to be associated with a low-risk of parametrial disease include: tumor occupying less than one-half of the cervical volume [16], tumor < 2 cm [17], and Tumor < 2cm with no LVSI [18].

Within the discussion concerning the optimal level of radicality of the hysterectomy which is still a matter of controversy a new concept of nerve sparing radical hysterectomy (NSRH) has been developed in order to reduce morbidity without compromising the oncological disease control.

THE CONCEPT AND RATIONALE OF NERVE-SPARING TECHNIQUE

In order to reduce morbidity an increasing number of technical modifications to RH have been suggested since this procedure was first described by Wertheim and Meigs [19].

NSRH may represent another option for reducing bladder and bowel morbidities and indirectly improve quality of life, without compromising radicality [7]. The mechanism for pelvic visceral dysfunction is primarily attributed to the partial impairment of the autonomic nerve supply during the dissection of the vesico-vaginal ligament (VVL), CL and USL as well as the vaginal cuff at RH. However, the available objective data to support this hypothesis are contrasting. The main caveat of NSRH is the weakness of the theoretical background for preventing neurogenic bladder. In fact, the most of the information results from cadaver dissection or by personal intraoperative experiences. Only few studies addressed the issue using a more consistent methodology like direct intraoperative observation of nerve fibers [6] and immunohistochemistry [20].

Bladder, bowel, and sexual dysfunctions caused by iatrogenic lesions of the inferior hypogastric plexus (IHP) are still frequent in pelvic surgery. The preservation of the pelvic autonomic nervous system is technically complex. The nerves are not distinctly seen in the surgical field because of their tiny structure and the depth and narrowness of the pelvis. In addition, confusing anatomical and surgical nomenclature of the structures in this region does not encourage the performance of nerve-sparing (NS) techniques. For instance, current nomenclature for uterine supporting structures uses the term "ligamentum". This term misleadingly suggests the presence of only connective tissue and absence of nervous fibers. In reality, the ligaments of the uterus contain an abundance of autonomic nerves as reported by some authors [20].

Pelvic NS techniques applied in adults are based in large part on microscopic investigations of fetuses, wherein relatively thick nerves are surrounded by little connective tissue [21]. A gross anatomic investigation of the IHP in adults should demonstrate a better macroscopic topography of the autonomic pelvic network. Thus, it should provide a more consistent background for successful dissection and protection of these nerves in adult patients. Unfortunately, detailed descriptions of the pelvic autonomic nerves reported earlier seem to have fallen into disuse [22].

The CL and USL form specific parts of the parametrium when pararectal and paravesical spaces are dissected surgically. Extensive cadaver dissections have shown that the autonomic nerves are closely related to these structures [23] and, in addition, the IHP may extend into the supporting ligaments [20], which therefore contain numerous autonomic nerves and ganglia. Using immunohistochemical techniques, Butler Manuel et al. [24] have shown that significantly more autonomic nerves are cut with RH as compared to a simple hysterectomy. In addition, the same authors investigated the nerve content of lateral 3rd of USL and CL by cross sectional biopsies. They observed that sympathetic, parasympathetic, sensory and sensory motor nerve types are present within CL and USL. Moreover, they concluded that the proportion of each nerve type differs between the CL and USL, and the sympathetic nerves in USL are the single largest nerve type.

Maas [25] investigated the extent and nature of nerve damage in conventional and NSRH. Macroscopic disruption of nerves was assessed through anatomical dissection after conventional and NS surgery on five fixed and one fresh cadaver. Immunohistochemical analysis of surgical margins was performed to confirm nerve damage using a general nerve marker (S100) and a sympathetic nerve marker (anti-tyrosine hydroxylase) within sections of biopsies. Macroscopic evaluation of the anatomical relations between the pelvic autonomic nerves and the surgically important landmarks in RH showed that conventional RH results in the disruption of a substantial part of the pelvic autonomic nerves. The NS modification led to macroscopic reduction in nerve disruption. Microscopic evaluation of the nerve content of the surgical margins confirmed the macroscopic findings. However, the data also showed that the conventional technique did lead to partial nerve damage, but not to total destruction of the pelvic autonomic nervous system. These findings correlate with the clinical observation that symptoms of denervation of pelvic organs might vary in gravity between patients with a history of RH.

Thus, the concept of NS consists of pursuing the preservation of autonomic nerve system of the pelvis without compromising the radicality of the standard surgical procedure. Several surgical strategies have been proposed to achieve such target, in part as the result of fragmentary, and sometimes contradictory data concerning the anatomical distribution of pelvic nerve structures. Following we are going to discuss some landmarks of the neuroanatomy and neurophysiology, highlighting the most significant elements which supports the performance of a NS technique in RH.

NEUROANATOMY

There is a deep gap between the information contained in anatomic textbooks and the reality of operating theatre. The theoretical description of the basic autonomic nerve supply to the pelvis is hardly, if ever, confirmed by the surgeon, during RH. Related information gathered from anatomic studies of cadavers to practical use in the operating room has been slow to occur [23].

The focal point of the pelvic autonomic nervous system is the IHP, which is a bilateral plexus of nerves formed from the hypogastric (sympathetic) nerves and parasympathetic branches from the second, third, and fourth sacral nerves (figure 2). The mechanism for pelvic visceral dysfunction is primarily believed to be partial denervation of the autonomic nerve supply to the viscera during the dissection of the VVL, CL, USL as well as the vaginal cuff at RH. However, there is little objective data to support this hypothesis.

The sympathetic efferent fibers from the twelfth thoracic and first two lumbar segments of the spinal cord run over the lumbo-aortic vessels. They constitute the superior hypogastric plexus at the level of the aorta bifurcation (Figure 2) and the middle hypogastric plexus at the level of the sacral promontory.

Two hypogastric nerves originate at the middle hypogastric plexus and run cranio-caudally and 2 cm medio-dorsally to the ureters, in the posterior and lateral layer of the USL. The sympathetic innervation from the superior hypogastric plexus project to the two IHPs via the bilateral fiber bundles of the hypogastric nerves. In addition, the IHP receives sympathetic input from the sacral splanchnic nerves. Baader et al. [26] observed in cadaver dissection a sacral splanchnic nerve originating from S2 sympathetic ganglion and contributing to the IHP. Sacral splanchnic nerves derived from either S1 or S2 sympathetic ganglia.

The parasympathetic contributions to the IHP derived from sacral ventral rami of more inferior levels. The IHP receives its pelvic splanchnic nerves mainly from either ventral rami S3 or S4. The efferent parasympathetic fibers arise from the second to the fourth sacral roots of the spinal cord (Figure 2). The first 3 cm of the parasympathetic fibers are covered by the pelvic parietal fascia. The parasympathetic fibers cross the pararectal space to reach the IHP. When the pararectal space is developed, two different groups of fibers are identified. The first group runs along the lateral side of the pararectal space to the dorsomedial part of the CL.

The second group is found running from the sacrum along the medial side of the pararectal space, parallel to the USL and over the pelvic floor. All these groups originate at sacral roots reaching the IHP [7].

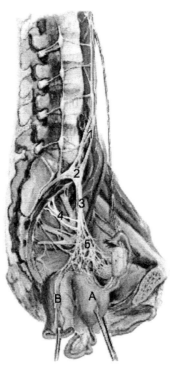

Figure 2: Neuroanatomy of pelvic autonomic nerves. Lateral view. The sympathetic efferent fibers from the twelfth thoracic and first two lumbar segments of the spinal cord run over the lumbo-aortic vessels. They constitute the superior hypogastric plexus (SHP) at the level of the aorta bifurcation. The focal point of the pelvic autonomic nervous system is the inferior hypogastric plexus (IHP), which is a bilateral plexus of nerves formed from the hypogastric (sympathetic) nerves and parasympathetic branches from the second, third, and fourth sacral nerves. (1) Sympathetic trunk; (2) SHP; (3) hypogastric nerves; (4) parasympathetic trunks (5) IHP. (A) Uterus; (B) Rectum.

To sum up, contributions to an IHP arise from three different sources: from the superior hypogastric plexus via the hypogastric nerve, from the sympathetic trunk via sacral splanchnic nerves, and from ventral rami of sacral spinal nerves via pelvic splanchnic nerves. The IHP, otherwise known as the Lee Franchenauser ganglia, is a laminar structure placed in a sagittal plain. It stretches from an area antero-lateral to the rectum, passes the cervix and the vaginal fornix laterally, and extends to the base of the bladder. The IHP is constituted by both sympathetic and parasympathetic fibers. From its origin in the IHP, the pelvic nerve branched out in a web-like fashion, sending multiple branches to the pelvic viscera. Many of these branches pierced the endopelvic fascia to innervate the rectum and bladder.

Besides the origin of the contributing nerves to the IHP, it is important to investigate the exact position of the IHP. The location of the plexus varies largely, the nerve fibers of the IHP are identified in four locations: USL; CL; and a few cases pararectally and in the fold between the urinary bladder and the uterus, respectively. The IHP is positioned immediately lateral to the pelvic organs.

The posterior part of the IHP innervates the superior part of the rectum; the inferior part of the rectum is innervated by inferior branches of the anterior part of the IHP. In addition, fibers accompanying the middle rectal artery after its penetration of the IHP provide innervations to the rectum. Of surgical importance is the finding that the rectum is always innervated on its lateral aspect, but never on its posterior aspect.

NEUROPHYSIOLOGY

The autonomic nerves of the pelvic region are responsible for the neurogenic control of rectal, bladder and sexual function (table 1). The nerves supplying the bladder consist both somatic afferent (sensitive) and efferent (motor) systems, in addition to the autonomic system made up of sympathetic and parasympathetic components. The sympathetic system, seems to inhibit the detrusor muscle, stimulate the sphincter vesicae. Hence, it seems to govern bladder compliance, urinary continence, and the contraction of the small muscles during orgasm. On the other hand, the parasympathetic system, represented by the sacral roots, controls the rectal function, vaginal lubrication, and detrusor contractility [27].

Neurophysiology of micturition. The process of micturition is dependent on the operation of a spinal-bulbospinal reflex which comprises different afferent (sensitive) and efferent (motor) peripheral pathways which are integrated and co-ordinated at spinal and supra-spinal centers [28,29]. Take also part in this process a lot of stimuli arising directly from the urothelium via different mediators such as adenosine 3' phosphate (ATP), nitric oxide (NO) [30,31].

The innervation of urethra and bladder consist of [28,29,30]:

- Sensory afferent nerves especially of the trigone and posterior urethra originating in the thoraco-lumbo-sacral region, traveling via pelvic nerves, seem to carry sensation of filling and pain from bladder;
- Parasympathetic motor fibers arising from S2-S4, traveling via pelvic nerves and ending in ganglion cells of bladder wall, seem to elicit contracting signal to the detrusor and inhibitory signals to the sphincter vesicae;
- Sympathetic afferents and efferents originating in the ganglia at the thoraco-lumbar level, traveling via hypogastric nerve, seem to carry sensation of filling and pain from bladder and seem to inhibit the detrusor and stimulate the sphincter vesicae;
- Somatic afferent and motor nerves of the striated muscle (outer sphincter of bladder) originating in the sacral region, traveling via pudendal nerve, seem to be responsible for the sensation from the outer sphincter and for eliciting signal of contraction and relaxation to it.

The afferent nerves have been identified in the detrusor and also suburothelially, where they form a plexus that lies immediately beneath the epithelial lining [30].

The normal micturition results from a spinal reflex which pathway follows the afferent (sensory, somatic and sympathetic) and efferent (parasympathetic, sympathetic, somatic) nerves. These in turn are controlled by brainstem and cortical facilitating and inhibiting signals. Upon regular myogenic contraction of bladder the stretch reflex arising especially from the distention of the bladder wall and posterior urethra, during the filling phase, powered by signals originating from the urothelium, activates the micturition reflex. It consists in generating contraction of the bladder and relaxation of the inner and outer sphincter of the urethra to achieve the voiding. If the bladder filling is not enough this reflex vanishes in less than a minute, but if the bladder storage is greater the reflex becomes self-maintaining and leads to an higher contraction of the bladder that can be voluntary controlled and inhibited for a while or can lead to voiding. In fact, the outer sphincter is under voluntary control and everyone can "decide" when relax it and let the physiological voiding taking part, but if the micturition reflex is really strong it can itself inhibits the outer sphincter contraction leading to non voluntary voiding [28]. Most of the afferent signals reach the spinal control center by Aδ- and c-fibers during the filling phase, when the sympathoinhibitory drive is active and norepinephrine (NE) increase the compliance of the bladder through β-adrenoreceptor (β-ARs) which activates the adenylyl cyclase cascade whit an increase of cAMP. From the center start the efferent stimuli which major component is the parasympathetic one. Using acetylcholine (Ach) as neurotransmitter this efferent signals led the detrusor to contract and the inner sphincter to relax [29,30].

Table 1. Neurophysiologic autonomic mechanisms.

Via \ Target	Cholinergic (parasympathetic)	Adrenergic (sympathetic)	NANC (non-adrenergic – non-cholinergic)
Detrusor	Contraction	Relaxation	Contraction / Relaxation #
Sphincter vesicae	Relaxation	Contraction	Contraction / Relaxation #
Bladder function	Voiding	Filling	Voiding / Filling #
Sexual arousal (lubrication, swelling, increased vaginal and clitoris blood flow, engorgement, lengthening of vagina)	Facilitatory	Inhibitory	Facilitatory
Bowel smooth muscles	Contraction	Relaxation	Contraction / Relaxation #*
Internal sphincter of rectum	Relaxation	Contraction	Contraction / Relaxation #*
Bowel function	Defecation	Contention	Defecation / Contention #*

\# differs according to the neurotransmitter / neuromodulator acting.
* Both function under control of ENS (enteric nervous system).

The Ach system seems to be the most important one in voiding, but in the contraction play a role also the sympathetic and the nonadrenergic-noncholinergic (NANC) mechanisms.

The Ach acts on the muscarinic receptors on the smooth muscle (detrusor) which is endowed principally with M2 (66%) and M3 (33%) muscarinic receptors. The former one are coupled to Gi family of guanine nucleotide proteins, activation of which would be expected to result in inhibition of adenylyl cyclase, probably resulting in an inhibition of the sympathetic relaxant tone; however other contractile mechanisms are supposed to take part in the process, such as activation of non-specific channel and inactivation of potassium channel. The latter, coupled to Gq proteins, are believed to cause a direct smooth muscle contraction through phosphoinositide hydrolysis and are mainly responsible for the normal micturition contraction. The magnitude of the post-junctional response depends also on the pre-junctional facilitatory (M1) or inhibitory (M2/M4) muscarine receptors modulating Ach release according to the frequency of stimulation [29,30,32].

The adrenergic mechanism may play a role in the contraction via α-adrenoceptores, but the main receptors represented in the bladder are of β-type, especially of β3 type, and are associated with relaxation of the smooth muscle, so playing a role in the filling of the bladder rather than in its voiding [29,32].

The NANC mechanism is still under investigation and up to date there is different evidence of its role on micturition. There are a lot of transmitters that can be evaluated and of those there are evidence on the role of ATP, nitric-oxide (NO), neuropeptydes (VIP, ETs, SP, NKA, NKB, ANG-I, ANG-II), prostanoids, and less knowledge upon γ-Aminobutyric acid, dopamine, enkefalin, serotonin, opioid [30,32].

The ATP, probably released from the stretching of urothelium, seems to play a role in the contraction, acting on P2X receptors (a ion channel family) [30,32].

The NO L-Arginine derived seems to be responsible for the main part of the inhibitory response; it acts via cGMP signaling. It has relaxant effects on bladder and urethra and also serves as a neurotransmitter, according to the findings of nitric oxide synthetase (NOS) in major pelvic ganglion projecting principally to the urethra. It also serves as a neuromodulator, by virtue of its close association with the cholinergic and sympathetic systems [31,32].

The neuropetydes play different role [32]:

-   VIP (vasoactive intestinal peptide): is a neuromodulator that has different activity from contraction to relaxation in relation to different stimulations;
-   ETs (endothelines): are neuromodulators which induce contraction of the detrusor (ET-1 and ET-3 via ETa receptor);
-   SP (substance P), NKA (neurokinin A), NKB (neurokinin B), all together called tachykinins, of which the most potent is NKA, which plays a role in contraction via NK2 receptor, and is L-type Calcium channels dependent (sensitive to nifedipine);
-   ANG I and II (angiotensins): may act as neuromodulator via ANG II receptor, contracting the urinary bladder;
-   Prostanoids: probably act as neuromodulator of afferent and efferent neurotransmission.

So up to date there is still a lot to understand upon the mechanism of regulation of the micturition and further studies are needed to clarify the pathways, neurotransmitters and neuromodulators involved in this process.

Neurophysiology of sexual function in women: peripheral pathways. Up to date little is known about the mechanisms of sexual response in human and the major part of these are derived from animal studies [33].

The physiology of desire, arousal and orgasm is dependent on both central and peripheral stimuli, the former ones especially playing a role in modulating, via facilitatory or inhibitory (serotoninergic projections) signals, the latter ones, which act through spinal reflex mechanism dependent on interneurons. All the mechanisms are also under the control of hormonal status, which is implicated in the modulating of both neurotransmission and status of genital organs [33].

The major pathways implicated in sexual function are [33,34,35,36]:

- Facilitatory and sensory parasympathetic fibers originating from the sacral roots, traveling via pelvic nerve and ending in the vagina (especially the anterior vaginal wall and fornix), clitoris (via cavernous nerve), cervix and body of the uterus;
- Inhibitory and sensory sympathetic fibers originating at the thoraco-lumbar level (T12-L3), traveling via the hypogastric nerve and the paravertebral sympathetic chain, and ending in all the pelvic organs (ovaries included), with a particular role in conveying pain sensation from the uterus;
- Somatic sensory and motor fibers originating in the sacral plexus, traveling via the pudendal nerve and ending in the striated perineal muscles, the bulbospongiosus, ischiocavernous, external anal and urethral sphincter, and clitoris;
- Vagal pathways which conveys sensory information and remains active also after spinal transection.

During sexual response several spinal reflexes are involved, leading to genital swelling and lubrication, increased vaginal and clitoris blood flow, engorgement, lengthening of vagina. Most of them are elicited by pudendal afferents and the majors outflow channels are coordinated somatic, which can voluntary enhance arousal [33], and autonomic activities. Of these reflexes investigations have been pointed on [33,34]:

- The bulbocavernous reflex: a polysynaptic response, elicited by light touch pudendal sensory fibers which activated contraction of perineal striated muscles (circumvaginal muscles, levator ani, external urethral sphincter) via pudendal motor nerves, and bladder activity inhibition via the clitoris sensory which lead to pelvic (relaxation of detrusor) and hypogastric (contraction of bladder neck) response;
- Another reflex involving vaginal and clitoral cavernosal autonomic stimulation which gives rise to an engorgement of clitoris and vagina, a lengthening of vagina and increased blood flow.

All of these effects take part thanks to different neurotransmitter and neuromodulator which exact role is up to date under investigation.

We know that there is a rich cholinergic innervations, but the exact role of acetylcholine is uncertain [33], it is possible that it plays a role in vaginal muscle contraction and a minor role in modifying vaginal blood flow [35]. The noradrenergic effects are supposed to be inhibitory [35].

A great role is also played by NANC system. There are a lot of mediators contained in human genitalia nerves, such as VIP (vasoactive intestinal polypeptide), NO (nitric oxide), NPY (neuropeptyde P), PACAP (pituitary adenylate cyclase-activating polypeptide), SP (substance P), CGRP (calcitonine gene-related peptide), PHM (peptide histidine methionine) [33]. Of these the most investigate are VIP, which plays a role in regulation of vaginal blood flow and lubrication [33,34], and NO interested in regulation of vaginal smooth muscle tone [33] and vasodilatation [36].

Over these mechanisms the hormonal status of the women plays an important role, which acts as a regulator of the response to different stimuli modifying the sensibility of target organs. For example estrogens seem to modulate blood flow by regulating NOS (nitric oxide syntetase) and VIP in the vagina [33].

Neurophysiology of lower bowel tract: continence and defecation. The neurophysiology of gut differs from the neurophysiology of urinary tract and genitalia because it is a compound of two different system strictly interrelated: the CNS (central nervous system) and the ENS (enteric nervous system). [37,38,39] The latter one also called "brain in the gut" or "enteric minibrain" contains sensory-neurons, interneurons and motoneurons which are organized to act independently of CNS. They control motility, secretion and blood flow of gut. The ENS acts through different neurotransmitters and neuromodulators such as : a) acetylcholine and substance P which stimulate muscle contraction;b) acetylcholine and VIP responsible for evoking secretion; c) ATP, VIP, NO (nitric oxide), PACAP (pituitary adenylate cyclase-activating polypeptide) implicated as inhibitory neurotransmitters [37,38,40].

The control of CNS on this independent system takes part with [37,41]:

- Parasympathetic afferent and efferent fibers via sacral pelvic nerve, which seems to increment smooth muscle contraction, increase peristaltic movement and relax internal sphincter;
- Somatic afferent and efferent fibers traveling via pudendal nerves, ending in the striated muscle of the perineum (levator ani, coxigeal muscle, external anal sphincter) which play a role in the voluntary control of defecation and continence;
- Sympathetic fibers that seem to have an inhibitory effects on rectal muscles;
- Vagal afferent, directly from sensory neurons sensible to mechanical or chemical stimuli, and efferent, ending in the interneurons of ENS with both excitatory or inhibitory effects on motility and excitatory effects over secretion.

All this components participate in an integrated network of signals, also involving emotional stimuli [41], that controls the mechanism of continence and defecation. In fact, upon a myogenic basal tone of the musculature of the digestive tract due to a self excitable electrical syncytium of interstitial cells of Cajal (ICCs) [37,38], the intrinsic reflex of defecation can be evoked. When feces reach the rectum a stretch stimulus in the myoentheric plexus starts which leads to an increased peristalsis and when the wave reach the anus the inhibitory recto-anal stretch reflex inhibits via NANC nerves (releasing NO and VIP) the internal sphincter, usually contracted thanks to a myogenic basal tone [42]. That is not usually enough to let defecation take part. In fact, it is necessary to reinforce this stimulus via afferent and efferent fibers conveyed by pelvic nerves. They increase the effects on peristalsis and relaxation of internal sphincter (parasympathetic reflex of defecation). But all these defecation reflexes are contrasted by another control mechanism, the voluntary one which acts upon the external sphincter and all the striated muscles involved in defecation. They can delay the stimulus of defecation, contracting the external sphincter, or let it take part, if there is a relaxation of this sphincter and of the levator ani [41].

NERVE SPARING RADICAL HYSTERECTOMY

The Techniques

Several studies have been published that relate the autonomic pelvic nerves to surgically important structures and describe NS-procedure. Direct injury of the pelvic autonomic nerves may occur at a number of different steps during RH: The superior hypogastric plexus at presacral and periaortic lymph node dissection; the hypogastric nerves at resection of the USLs; the proximal IHP at division of the USLs and CLs; and the distal IHP at division of the VVLs.

In order to solve this issue a new Class III RH with NS technique (NSRH) for cervical cancer has been proposed. Yabuki et al. [43] were the first group to elaborate the concept of NSRH and since then several feasibility studies on the technique have been published in Europe [23,44,45,46,47,48]. Recently, Raspagliesi et al. tested the feasibility of a particular new Class III NSRH with encouraging results [7,49].

There is a growing body of data about NSRH in cervical cancer [50]. However, there is not yet a consensus regarding which to part of uterine support ligaments a NS approach should be directed, due in part to an fragmentary knowledge of pelvic and urogenital neuroanatomy which derives from cadaver dissection or by personal operative experiences.

The principle of Raspagliesi technique [7] is to perform the resection uterine support ligaments based on a rationale approach which minimizes damage to the pelvic autonomic innervations without compromising oncological radicality. The class III RH was modified to spare the nerves at the level of the landmarks referred to below. These modifications were as follows:

A) During the first step of lymph node dissection, the sympathetic fibers running over the aorta were identified. The superior and medium hypogastric plexus are detached from the following structures: aorta bifurcation, presacral nodes, and left common iliac nodes (figure 3). The dissection continues cranially to detach the fibers from the paraortic lymph nodes up to the point at which the inferior mesenteric artery emerges. Then, the dissection continues caudally down to the origin of the two hypogastric nerves (figure 3). The USLs are divided into lateral and medial layers by blunt dissection, as described by Trimbos et al. [23]. As outlined, the lateral layer of the USL contains nerve fibers, and the medial is fibrous.

B) The CLs are dissected and cut close to the pelvic wall with the assistance of a hemoclip, according to Burghardt et al.'s technique. [16] All the vascular structures (venous, arterious, and lymphatic) that constitute the CL are isolated. After isolation, these structures are clamped with hemoclips. All the vessels are cut, and the loose connective tissue attached to the pelvic side wall are removed radically together with the CL. Unfortunately, during this step some fibers of the first group of parasympathetic fibers that run along the dorsomedial section of the CL are inevitably sacrificed.

C) The caudal part of the IHP runs along the lateral vaginal wall. The ureter tunnel is developed in the usual fashion and cut the anterior part of the VVL. After further dissection of the ureter, the fibers in the lateral vaginal wall are first identified and then cut the posterior part of the VVL.

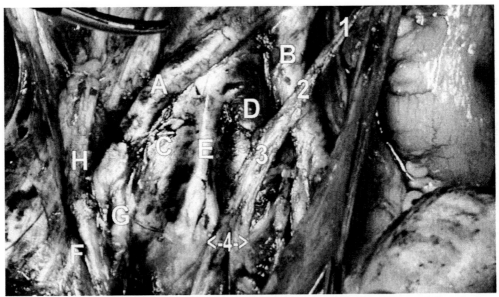

Figure 3: Sympathetic fibers from the twelfth thoracic and first two lumbar segments of the spinal cord run over left iliac vessels after lymph node dissection. The sympathetic trunk reaches superior hypogastric plexus (SHP) and traveling cross medium hypogastric plexus (MHP) giving off two hypogastric nerves. Frontal view of vessels and nerves. (1) sympathetic trunk; (2) SHP; (3) MHP; (4) hypogastric nerves; (A) right common iliac artery; (B) left common iliac artery; (C) right common iliac vein; (D) left common iliac vein; (E) sacral vein, (F) right external iliac artery; (G) right internal iliac artery; (H) right ureter.

D) After dissecting the VVL, nerve fibers (bladder branches) that run along the lateral vaginal wall are identified and the CL from the paracolpium are resected, detaching it from vaginal fornix. Then, the CLs are pulled up, maintaining slight tension on it to uncover the fibers that run from the IHP to the base of the bladder (Figure 4). The nerve fibers along the vaginal fornix for about 2 cm are gently moved down. Nerve fibers from the IHP run beside the lateral wall of the vagina to the bladder, and these will be preserved during this step in surgery, restricting the level of colpectomy to 2 cm below the cervix instead of resecting the cranial half of the vagina (figure 4). After this step the pelvic plexus is completely identifiable (figure 5).

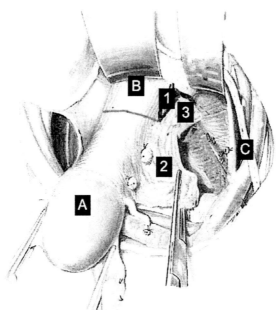

Figure 4: Nerve fibers run across right lateral wall of the vagina reaching the base of bladder. Right lateral view. A schematic representation of how, the cardinal ligament (CL) and vesico-vaginal ligament (VVL), is lifted from the vaginal wall clearing the fibers above the vagina highlighted in black. (1) nerve fibers; (2) CL and VVL; (3) paracolpium; (A) uterus; (B) vagina; (C) right pelvic wall with vessels and ureter.

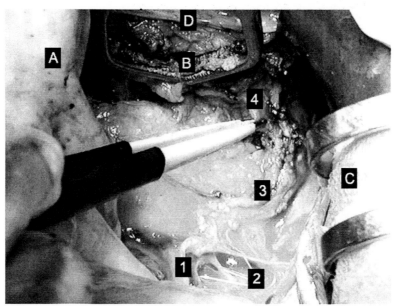

Figure 5: The hypogastric nerve merge with parasympathetic fibers forming inferior hypogastric plexus (IHP); from IHP nerve fibers run across lateral wall of the vagina, reaching the base of bladder. Lateral view of pelvic viscera. (1) hypogastric nerve; (2) parasympathetic nerve; (3) IHP; (4) terminal part of autonomic fibers. (A) rectum; (B) vagina; (C) right lateral pelvic wall; (D) bladder.

E) The hypogastric nerve and the initial part of the IHP are situated in the lateral part of the USL. During dissection of the USL and rectal pillars and after incision of the peritoneum of the Douglas pouch, the prerectal space is developed by blunt dissection. The USL between the prerectal and the pararectal spaces are identified. The medial USLs are separated from the lateral nervous fibers (Figure 6). The medial ligaments are resected, while the lateral parts are saved. This maneuver preserves the terminal part of the hypogastric nerve and the cranial part of the IHP (Figure 7).

Yabuki et al., [43] reported that surgical experience with carcinomas of the uterus has provided new insights into the surgical anatomy of a lamina, which separates the paravesical space from the pararectal space. It has been proved that each of the lamina consists of the CL and lateral ligaments and pelvic splanchnic nerves, descending in the following order: the CL and lateral ligaments, as a connective stalk, insert into the lateral walls of the uterus and rectum extending from the inner aspect of the pelvic wall. Clarification of this structural relationship led to the development of a new procedure for the dissection of the CL in RH, while still preserving the lateral ligament (neural part). This facilitated systematic dissection of the CLs and USLs with posterior manipulation, leading to a NS technique.

Hockel et al., [44] studied the topographic anatomy of the parametrial tissue with high-resolution magnetic resonance imaging and by dissection of fresh human cadavers. The perispinous adipose tissue contains the pelvic plexus, the pelvic splanchnic nerves, small blood vessels, and lymphatic tissue. Then, they performed a clinical feasibility study of the liposuction-assisted NS extended RH. Hockel stated that the NS removal of perispinous adipose tissue by liposuction is a feasible addition to wide en bloc parametrectomy in anatomically defined planes.

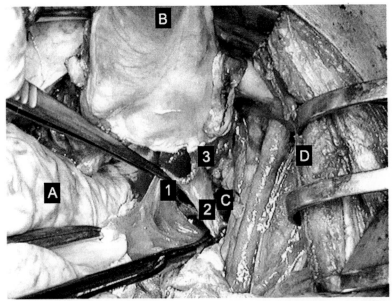

Figure 6: The hypogastric nerve traveling cross uterosacral ligament (USL). The medial USL are separated from the lateral nervous fibers. Right lateral view. (1) fibrous medial part of USL; (2) nervous lateral part of USL; (3) IHP: (A) rectum; (B) uterus; (C) pararectal space; (D) right lateral pelvic wall with vessels.

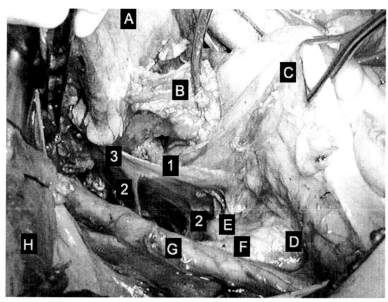

Figure 7: The hypogastric nerve merge with parasympathetic fibers forming inferior hypogastric plexus (IHP). Left lateral view of pelvic viscera. Nerve-sparing dissection of left uterosacral ligament (USL). This maneuver preserves the terminal part of the hypogastric nerve and the cranial part of the IHP. (1) hypogastric nerve; (2) parasympathetic nerve; (3) IHP; (A) uterus; (B) left USL resected; (C) rectum; (D) left common iliac artery; (E) left internal iliac artery; (F) left external iliac artery; (G) ureter; (H) left lateral pelvic wall.

More recently Hockel et al. [51] published on total mesometrial resection characterized by: a) the en bloc resection of the uterus, proximal vagina, and mesometrium as a developmentally defined entity; b) transection of the rectouterine dense subperitoneal connective tissue above the level of the exposed IHP; and c) extended pelvic/periaortic lymph node dissection preserving the superior hypogastric plexus.

Surgical procedure of total mesometrial resection is performed in up to 21 defined steps, 11 of which are carried out bilaterally: At the base of the mesosigma just caudal to the aortic bifurcation, the superior hypogastric plexus is identified and mobilized. Pararectal spaces are developed with the hypogastric nerves adhering medially to the mesorectum. This maneuver is carried out down to the level where the pelvic splanchnic nerves and the sacral splanchnic nerves join the hypogastric nerves to form the IHP but not further dorsally. The ureters are mobilized to the posterior side of the mesometrium which should be completely exposed. Anteriorly, paravesical spaces are developed with the umbilical arteries adhering medially to the bladder, down to the pubococcygeus and iliococcygeus muscles exposing the complete anterior side of the urogenital mesentery.

The umbilical artery together with the superior bladder mesentery is separated from the anterior mesometrium. The uterine arteries and veins are ligated at their origins. The peritoneum of the rectouterine pouch is incised and the anterior mesorectum is separated from the posterior vaginal wall down to the midvagina. Laterally, the mesorectum is separated from the dense subperitoneal connective tissue ('USLs') to the level of the IHP. The proximal IHP is mobilized from the lateral surface of the dense subperitoneal connective tissue which encases the rectum for 1—2 cm enabling the transection of the latter without nerve damage. Immediately above the superior margin of the IHP, the dense subperitoneal connective tissue ('rectouterine ligaments', 'USLs') is stepwise transected.

The operation proceeds in the anterior compartment. Mobilization of the mesometrium from its origin at the site of the already transacted uterine artery and vein(s) towards the uterus beyond the superior surface of the ureter. The vesicovaginal venous plexus together with the dense subperitoneal connective tissue above the prevesical segment of the ureter is ligated and divided. After mobilization and retraction of the superior hypogastric plexus, the presacral lymph node region is cleared exposing the medial sides of the internal iliac vein and the pelvic splanchnic nerves. The common iliac vessels can now be completely undermined. The right and left lumbar splanchnic nerves, the main roots of the superior hypogastric nerve plexus are preserved. Liposuction is applied within the inferior urogenital mesentery at the level of the IHP medial to the ischial spine to remove fatty tissue and small lymph nodes.

Possover et al. [48] investigated the parasympathetic innervations of the bladder in the CL in patients underwent laparoscopy-assisted radical vaginal hysterectomy class III. During laparoscopic dissection of the CL Possover showed that the middle rectal artery was identified as a landmark separating the vascular from the neural part of the CL.

In Possover' technique during pelvic lymphadenectomy, lymph nodes along the common and the external iliac vessels were dissected and removed, opening the lumbosacral and paravesical space. The obturator nerve, the sciatic nerve, and the lumbosacral trunk were exposed. The pararectal space was opened between the ureter medially and the internal iliac vessels laterally. Special attention was paid to preserve laterally the hypogastric fascia to avoid injury to the pelvic splanchnic nerves as well as sacral root.

The CL was completely freed of all lymphatic and fat tissue by blunt dissection and all vessels of the vascular part were identified, recognizing the border between the last vessels of the vascular part of the CL and the first branches of the pelvic splanchnic nerves. Thereafter, the neural part of the CL was freed of fat and lymphatic tissue anteriorly ("preneural lymph nodes"). After bipolar coagulation the vascular part of the CL was divided as lateral as possible at the pelvic side wall including the middle rectal vessels. The pelvic splanchnic nerves were completely exposed and preserved. Then, the operation was completed transvaginally.

Trimbos et al., [23] introduced elements of the Japanese NS techniques and carried out a feasibility study in Dutch patients. The following surgical steps facilitate the prevention of surgical damage to the pelvic autonomic nerves during RH, and are performed chronologically during the course of RH.

Step 1: Preserving the hypogastric nerve (and the proximal part of the IHP). This is a crucial first step that identifies the hypogastric nerve and the proximal (cranial) part of the IHP. It is performed during the dissection of the USLs and rectal pillars. The tissue between the prerectal space and the pararectal space consists of two parts: a firm medial part and a softer, looser lateral part. The firm medial part contains the USLs and the lateral part consists of the fibers of the hypogastric nerve and the proximal part of the IHP. This nerve tissue on one side and the ligamentous tissue on the other can be separated by blunt dissection. This sacrouterine dissection plane separates the medial ligamentous tissue (USL) and the lateral nerve fibers. The USL can then be safely clamped, cut, and ligated without damaging the hypogastric nerve or proximal part of the IHP.

Step 2: Preserving the pelvic splanchnic nerves and middle part of the IHP. This step is taken during the dissection of the parametrium. By dividing the parametrium, the paravesical and pararectal spaces are united. In a frontal section through the parametrium, two separate parts can be distinguished: an upper part containing vascular structures, fat, and loose connective tissue; and a lower part that feels tight on palpation and contains denser connective tissue and the nerve fibers of the middle part of the IHP. By dividing the parametrium with vascular clips, the course of the dissection line can be tailored to the individual anatomical situation. To avoid the IHP, the dissection follows the shape of the bow of a ship from a lateroventral to a mediodorsal position.

Step 3: Preserving the distal part of the IHP. The distal part of the IHP is situated in the posterior part of the VVL, lateral and caudal to the lower ureter. The anterior segment of the VVL is cut in the usual fashion, ensuring that the ureter tunnel is developed medially and ventrally to the ureter. By finger palpation, the lateral nerve part and the medial vascular part of the posterior sheath of the VVL can be distinguished. The vascular part can then be clamped and cut. By pulling the band in a lateral and caudal direction and by careful blunt dissection, the paravaginal tissue becomes separate from the nerve plexus and can be clamped and cut.

RESULTS OF NSRH

Raspagliesi et al. [7] reported on 23 cervical cancer patients treated by class III NSRH. One of the endpoint was to assess the impact of this technique on the incidence of early bladder dysfunctions. The mean operating time was 219 minutes (range: 150 - 270). The mean blood loss was 489 ml (range: 200-800). The average period of hospitalization was 10 days (range: 5-16). Two (9%) patients were discharged with self-catheterization and one of them recovered the ability to void her bladder spontaneously by the time of her first visit to the outpatient clinic. Raspagliesi concluded that the NSRH technique using the CUSA® is feasible, with promising results in terms of preventing early bladder dysfunction. The average time between surgery and the onset of spontaneous voiding was acceptable.

More recently the same group of investigators [52] retrospectively compared the safety of the NSRH procedure with that of other classes of RH in terms of incidence of early bladder dysfunctions and complications. One hundred and ten patients with cervical cancer were submitted to class II RH, class III NSRH and classical class III RH. The groups did not differ significantly in terms of GIII/IV morbidity. The class II RH and the class III NSRH groups presented a prompt recover of bladder function, significantly different from that of the class III RH group. The Class III NSRH is comparable to class II RH and superior to class III RH in terms of early bladder dysfunctions (Figure 8).

Yabuky et al. [43] reported about a new dissection method for the parametrium to demonstrate a reduction in the amount of blood loss for VVL dissection and to investigate the intrapelvic autonomic nerve pathway and its preservation by means of anatomic analysis. The amount of blood loss (mean +/- SD) during dissection of the VVL was ultimately 260.1+/- 114.8 ml. Postoperatively, the maximum capacity of the bladder was 393.9 +/- 40.4 ml, maximum detrusor pressure 6.3 +/- 4.1 cm H2O, mean compliance >10 ml/cm H2O, residual urine 23.8 +/- 9.4 ml, and maximum flow rate 25. +/- 8 2.2 ml/s, respectively. Yabuky concluded that the development of this new operative procedure has also contributed to a decrease in blood loss and preservation of bladder function.

Hockel et al. [44] developed the liposuction-assisted NS extended RH and applied it to seven consecutive patients with cervical or vaginal cancer. No intraoperative or postoperative complications occurred. Postoperative magnetic resonance imaging assured that perispinous adipose tissue was cleared in all cases. A metastatic lymph node was found in the perispinous adipose tissue removed by liposuction from one patient. Suprapubic cystostomies could be removed after a median period of 12 days. In conclusion Hockel stated that the NS removal of perispinous adipose tissue by liposuction is a feasible addition to wide en bloc parametrectomy in anatomically defined planes.

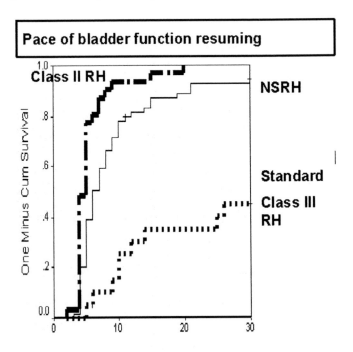

Event= Resuming the bladder function= ability to void spontaneously and post voiding residual <100cc

Figure 8: The pace of bladder function resuming along the immediate postoperative period is outlined. Class II RH and class III NSRH presented a prompt recover of bladder function, significantly different from that of the Class III RH without NS, in which a marked incidence of bladder dysfunction was reported.

Possover et al. [45] investigated the parasympathetic innervations of the bladder in the CL. During laparoscopic dissection of the CL, they used 7 x magnifications on 38 consecutive patients with cervical cancer stages IB1 to IIIA. The author performed laparoscopy-assisted radical vaginal hysterectomy class III. The results showed that the middle rectal artery was identified as a landmark separating the vascular from the neural part of the CL. The neural part was shown to contain the splanchnic pelvic nerves which anastomose with the pelvic plexus. Following preservation of these neural structures all patients were able to void their bladder spontaneously. Following NS technique, patients regained bladder function significantly quicker compared with a control group (n: 28) in which the neural part of the CLs had not been preserved: suprapubic drainage 11.2 days versus 21.4 days (P = 0.0007). Possover concluded that using the middle rectal artery as a landmark the neural part of the CL can be preserved, resulting in preservation of the motor function of the bladder.

Trimbos et al., [23] carried out a feasibility study of NS techniques in ten consecutive patients. Surgical preservation of the pelvic autonomic nerves in RH deserves consideration in the quest to improve both cure and quality of life in cervical cancer patients. In two of the 10 patients, identification of the autonomic nerve tissue was inadequate and the NS procedure was aborted. In the remaining eight patients, there were no technical problems. Nerve sparing caused virtually no blood loss, and the average extra operating time amounted to 20 min. The postoperative course in the 10 patients was uneventful. The suprapubic catheter was routinely removed after 5–7 days barring urine retention in excess of 100 ml. All patients left the hospital without catheters and with spontaneous voiding. The average admission time was 9 days (range 8–11 days). Five patients required treatment for bladder infection.

OPEN ISSUES AND FUTURE PROSPECTIVES

The issue of NSRH has attracted an increasing attention from the scientific community. Several groups of investigators emerged in the recent years proposing different approaches. The wide range of technical variation is the direct consequence of the scarce theoretical background concerning the surgical neuroanatomy and neurophysiology of the pelvis.

The actual knowledge on neuroanatomy results from the personal experience of pelvic surgeons and dissection of cadavers. A clear methodology to systematically study the surgical neuroanatomy has not been defined yet. Some authors have proposed the investigation of the neuroanatomy using immunohistochemistry to identify the nerve structures. However the experience is still incomplete [20].

Thus up to date there is still a lot to understand upon the mechanism regulating the pelvic organs function. Further studies are needed to clarify the pathways, neurotransmitters and neuromodulators involved in this process, as well as their inter relationship.

Despite the growing number of papers addressing the issue of NSRH no consensus has been reached on which parts of the uterine-supporting ligaments a preserving policy should be directed.

In the context of NS technique, the optimal dissection of CL has become one of the critical issues. Japanese authors [43] pioneered NS technique and they identified two parts of the CL, the vascular and the neural ones. They postulated that the neural part contained the pelvic splanchnic nerves. Possover and Hoeckel [45,44] proposed different techniques, focusing their NS approach in the CL. In particular, Hockel [44], described the preservation of the parasympathetic fibers by identifying them in the CL with liposuction; whilst Possover [45] reported on laparoscopy-assisted radical vaginal hysterectomy class III with NS. Both adopted the middle rectal artery as a landmark separating the vascular from the neural part of the CL. More recently, Trimbos et al [23] based on Japanese experiences used also the middle rectal artery as landmark to perform NS technique.

However, other authors have recently challenged the medial rectal artery as an actual reference point during the parametrial dissection [7,53]. While the above mentioned authors [23,43,44,45] stated that neural part of the CL contained the autonomic fibers, evidences emerged sustaining that the fibers runs along the medial aspect of CL [7].

Raspagliesi et al. [7] are of the opinion that the IHP is actually located in the medial aspect of CL or less frequently in lateral aspect of USL. In addition, as reported by Baader [26] the location of the IHP varies largely, the nerve fibers of the IHP were identified in four locations: USL, CL, and in a few cases pararectally and in the fold between the urinary bladder and the uterus, respectively. Thus, the so called neural part of the CL, according to these authors, is not likely to contain the autonomic fibers.

The best approach for dissecting the VVL has become another issue which warrants further investigation. Japanese authors state that the feasibility of the VVL dissection to spare the fibers has not yet been confirmed [53].

European authors stated that to spare nerves is necessary to preserve the deeper and /or more lateral portion of the VVL. Trimbos et al. [23] reported that by finger palpation, the lateral nerve part and the medial vascular part of the posterior sheath of the VVL can be distinguished.

On the other hand, Raspagliesi et al. [7] showed by direct intraoperative observation that nerve fibers from the hypogastric plexus run beside the lateral wall of the vagina to the bladder in the medial aspect of VVL.

In Raspagliesi technique after dissecting the VVL, nerve fibers that run along the lateral vaginal wall are identified and the CL from the paracolpium are resected, detaching it from vaginal fornix. These authors are of the opinion that the nerve fibers depart from the IHP and run beside the lateral wall of the vagina, in the medial aspect of VVL. According to them the preservation of such neural structures is feasible [7].

Another aspect to be considered is how to obtain an optimal balance between oncological radicality and neural structure sparing approach. Depending on how one conceives the nerve structures distribution inside the uterine supporting ligaments, the NS surgical approach could result in compromised local disease control. The lack of dissection of the most lateral part (including the neural part of the CL) is the major concern among the Japanese authors. Even Trimbos et al. [23] have described a technique, which involves a modified resection of the CLs. This may potentially compromise radicality.

On the other hand Raspagliesi et al. [7] proposed a NSRH technique which includes a complete resection of CL. They observed intraoperatively that the lateral part of the USL and the medial part of the CL contain nerve fibers. These fibers converge to form a uniform nerve plate medial to the vascular layer of the CL and deep into the peritoneum.

An understanding of the location of the autonomic pelvic network, including important landmarks, should help prevent iatrogenic injury through the adoption of surgical techniques that reduce postoperative autonomic dysfunction, without compromising the radicality.

Thus there is a lack of consensus in several of the technical aspects of NSRH. Besides these conflicting opinions another confounder factor should be considered among the studies. The majority of the investigations testing the NSRH are of feasibility nature. Thus the series are numerically limited, composed by patients with different stages and various presurgical treatments. Different methodologies to assess the results in terms of procedure related morbidity and local oncological control have been adopted, rendering the data among the different studies difficult to compare.

The surgeons variously use an ultrasonic surgical aspirator [7,43], liposuction [44], laparoscopy [45], sharp or blunt dissection [23] to clear the ligament from the nerves. Thus, another open issue is how to overcome the technically demanding characteristics of the various proposed approaches. This aspect hampers the wide application of the method which in turn could represent an obstacle to the conduction of controlled randomized studies.

Finally, the last point that deserves clarification is related to indications of NSRH. Further studies are warranted to identify the clinical situations in which the technique is applicable. The current data suggest that the procedure could be performed in disease stage Ib1 >2cm and Ib2-IIa after neoadjuvant chemotherapy.

In summary, progress in this field requires:

- More studies on neuroanatomy and neurophysiology;
- Standardization of the scientific methodology basing the clinical studies;
- Standardization of the methodology to assess the procedure related morbidity;
- Assessment of the impact on survival, local disease control and quality of life.

CONCLUSION

The successive technical modifications of RH allowed a substantial drop in the urinary fistula rate which was its main complication. Then, the attention was shifted to the strategies to minimize other important complications related to RH such as voiding, bowel and sexual dysfunctions. The NS technique has been shown to reduce the class III RH related postoperative visceral dysfunctions, improving quality of life.

NSRH does not seem to compromise radicality and could represent a consistent alternative to Class II RH in cervical cancer patients with disease stage Ib1 >2cm and Ib2-IIa after neoadjuvant chemotherapy.

Further studies clarifying the neuroanatomy and neurophysiology of autonomic nervous structures should be carried out, as well as a prospective randomized trial on NSRH to confirm the data not only with respect to morbidity, but also to the oncological outcome.

REFERENCES

[1]   Benedet JL, Odicino F, Maisonneuve P, Beller U, Creasman WT, Heintz AP, Ngan HY, Pecorelli S. Carcinoma of the cervix uteri. *Int J Gynaecol Obstet* 2003; 83 Suppl 1: 41-78.

[2]   Samlal RAK, van der Velden J, Ketting BW, González González D, Ten Kate FJW, Hart AAM, Lammes FB. Disease-free interval and recurrence pattern after the

Okabayashi variant of Wertheim's radical hysterectomy for stage Ib and IIa cervical carcinoma. *Int J Gynecol Cancer* 1996; 6: 120-7.

[3]   Trimbos JB, Adema B, Peters AA, Kenter GG, Snijders-Keilholz A. Morbidity and results of 100 radical hysterectomies performed in an oncology center. *Ned Tijdschr Geneeskd* 1992; 136: 323-7.

[4]   Lichtenegger W, Anderhuber F, Ralph G. Operative anatomy and technique of radical parametrial resection in the surgical treatment of cervical cancer. *Baillieres Clin Obstet Gynaecol* 1988; 2: 841-56.

[5]   Magrina JF, Goodrich MA, Weaver AL, Podratz KC. Modified radical hysterectomy: morbidity and mortality. *Gynecol Oncol* 1995; 59: 277-82.

[6]   Zullo MA, Manci N, Angioli R, Muzii L, Panici PB. Vesical dysfunctions after radical hysterectomy for cervical cancer: a critical review. *Crit Rev Oncol Hematol* 2003; 48: 287-93.

[7]   Raspagliesi F, Ditto A, Fontanelli R, Solima E, Hanozet F, Zanaboni F, Kusamura S. Nerve-sparing radical hysterectomy: a surgical technique for preserving the autonomic hypogastric nerve. *Gynecol Oncol* 2004; 93: 307-14.

[8]   Michalas S, Rodolakis A, Voulgaris Z, Vlachos G, Giannakoulis N, Diakomanolis E. Management of early-stage cervical carcinoma by modified (Type II) radical hysterectomy. *Gynecol Oncol* 2002; 85: 415– 22.

[9]   Magrina JF, Goodrich MA, Lidner TK, Weaver AL, Cornella JL, Podratz KC. Modified radical hysterectomy in the treatment of early squamous cervical cancer. *Gynecol Oncol* 1999; 72: 183– 6.

[10] Yang YC, Chang CL. Modified radical hysterectomy for early Ib cervical cancer. *Gynecol Oncol* 1999; 74: 241 –4.

[11] Girardi F, Lichtenegger W, Tamussino K, Haas J. The importance of parametrial lymph nodes in the treatment of cervical cancer. *Gynecol Oncol* 1989; 34: 206–11.

[12] Benedetti-Panici P, Maneschi F, Scambia G, Greggi S, Cutillo G, D'Andrea G, Rabitti C, Coronetta F, Capelli A, Mancuso S. Lymphatic spread of cervical cancer: an anatomical and pathological study based on 225 radical hysterectomies with systematic pelvic and aortic lymphadenectomy. *Gynecol Oncol* 1996; 62: 19-24.

[13] Benedetti-Panici P, Maneschi F, D'Andrea G, Cutillo G, Rabitti C, Congiu M, Coronetta F, Capelli A. Early cervical carcinoma: the natural history of lymph node involvement redefined on the basis of thorough parametrectomy and giant section study. *Cancer* 2000; 88: 2267–74.

[14] Landoni F, Maneo A, Cormio G, Perego P, Milani R, Caruso O, Mangioni C. Class II versus class III radical hysterectomy in stage IB–IIA cervical cancer: a prospective randomized study. *Gynecol Oncol* 2001; 80 : 3–12.

[15] Panici PB, Angioli R, Palaia I, Muzii L, Zullo MA, Manci N, Rabitti C. Tailoring the parametrectomy in stages IA2-IB1 cervical carcinoma: is it feasible and safe? *Gynecol Oncol* 2005; 96: 792-8.

[16] Burghardt E, Haas J, Girardi F. The significance of the parametrium in the operative treatment of cervical cancer. *Baillieres Clin Obstet Gynaecol* 1988; 2: 879-88.

[17]   Sartori E, Fallo L, La Face B, Bianchi UA, Pecorelli S. Extended radical hysterectomy in early-stage carcinoma of the uterine cervix: tailoring the radicality. *Int J Gynecol Cancer* 1995; 5: 143–7.

[18]   Kinney WK, Hodge DO, Egorshin EV, Ballard DJ, Podratz KC. Identification of a low-risk subset of patients with stage 1B invasive squamous cancer of the cervix possibly suited to less radical surgical treatment. *Gynecol Oncol* 1995; 57: 3– 6.

[19]   Meigs JV. *Radical hysterectomy with bilateral dissection of pelvic lymph nodes: surgical treatment of cancer of the cervix.* New York: Grune & Stratton, 1954.

[20]   Butler-Manuel SA, Buttery LD, A'Hern RP, Polak JM, Barton DP. Pelvic nerve plexus trauma at radical hysterectomy and simple hysterectomy: the nerve content of the uterine supporting ligaments. *Cancer* 2000; 89: 834-41.

[21]   Fritsch H. Topography of the pelvic autonomic nerves in human fetuses between 21-29 weeks of gestation. *Anat Embryol (Berl)* 1989; 180: 57-64.

[22]   Fraukenhauser F. *Dio nerven der Geba¨rmutter und ihre Endigung in den glatten Moskelfasern.* Jena: Mauke. p III, 1867.

[23]   Trimbos JB, Maas CP, Deruiter MC, Peters AA, Kenter GG. A nerve-sparing radical hysterectomy: guidelines and feasibility in Western patients. *Int J Gynecol Cancer* 2001; 11: 180-6.

[24]   Butler-Manuel SA, Buttery LD, A'Hern RP, Polak JM, Barton DP. Pelvic nerve plexus trauma at radical and simple hysterectomy: a quantitative study of nerve types in the uterine supporting ligaments. *J Soc Gynecol Investig* 2002; 9: 47-56.

[25]   Maas CP, Trimbos JB, DeRuiter MC, van de Velde CJ, Kenter GG. Nerve sparing radical hysterectomy: latest developments and historical perspective. *Crit Rev Oncol Hematol* 2003; 48: 271-9.

[26]   Baader B, Herrmann M. Topography of the Pelvic Autonomic Nervous System and Its Potential Impact on Surgical Intervention in the Pelvis. *Clinical Anatomy* 2003; 16: 119-30.

[27]   Williams, Warwick, *Gray's anatomy,* 36th ed. Jarrold and Sons, Norwich. Livingstone 1980, pp. 1406-1408

[28]   Guyton, Hall. *Fisiologia Medica.* II ed. EdiSES; 2002. p.373-376

[29]   Hegde SS, Eglen RM. Muscarinic receptor subtypes modulating smooth muscle contractility in the urinary bladder. *Life Sci* 1999; 64: 419-28.

[30]   Andersson KE, Hedlund P. Pharmacologic perspective on the physiology of the lower urinary tract. *Urology* 2002; 60 (5 Suppl 1): 13-20.

[31]   Ho MH, Bhatia NN, Khorram O. Physiologic role of nitric oxide and nitric oxide synthase in female lower urinary tract. *Curr Opin Obstet Gynecol* 2004; 16: 423-9.

[32]   Andersson KE, Arner A. Urinary bladder contraction and relaxation: physiology and pathophysiology. *Physiol Rev* 2004; 84: 935-86.

[33]   Giraldi A, Marson L, Nappi R, Pfaus J, Traish AM, Vardi Y, Goldstein I. Physiology of female sexual function: animal models. *J Sex Med* 2004; 1: 237-53.

[34]   McKenna KE. The neurophysiology of female sexual function. *World J Urol* 2002; 20: 93-100.

[35]   Giuliano F, Rampin O, Allard J. Neurophysiology and pharmacology of female genital sexual response. *J Sex Marital Ther* 2002; 28 Suppl 1 :101-21.

[36]   Guyton, Hall. *Fisiologia Medica*. II ed. EdiSES; 2002. pp. 965-6.

[37]   Wood JD, Alpers DH, Andrews PL. Fundamentals of neurogastroenterology. *Gut* 1999; 45 Suppl 2: II6-II16.

[38]   Wood JD. Neuropathophysiology of irritable bowel syndrome. *J Clin Gastroenterol* 2002; 35 Suppl 1: S11-22.

[39]   Jones MP, Dilley JB, Drossman D, Crowell MD. Brain-gut connections in functional GI disorders: anatomic and physiologic relationships. *Neurogastroenterol Motil* 2006; 18: 91-103.

[40]   Dinning PG, Szczesniak M, Cook IJ. Removal of tonic nitrergic inhibition is a potent stimulus for human proximal colonic propagating sequences. *Neurogastroenterol Motil* 2006; 18: 37-44.

[41]   Guyton, Hall. *Fisiologia Medica*. II ed. EdiSES; 2002. pp. 754-755

[42]   Rattan S. The internal anal sphincter: regulation of smooth muscle tone and relaxation. *Neurogastroenterol Motil* 2005; 17 Suppl 1 :50-9.

[43]   Yabuki Y, Asamoto A, Hoshiba T, Nishimoto H, Kitamura S. Dissection of the cardinal ligament in radical hysterectomy for cervical cancer with emphasis on the lateral ligament. *Am J Obstet Gynecol* 1991; 164: 7-14.

[44]   Hockel M, Konerding MA, Heussel CP. Liposuction-assisted nerve-sparing extended radical hysterectomy: Oncologic rationale, surgical anatomy, and feasibility study. *Am J Obstet Gynecol* 1998; 178: 971-6.

[45]   Possover M, Stober S, Plaul K, Schneider A. Identification and preservation of the motoric innervation of the bladder in radical hysterectomy type III. *Gynecol Oncol* 2000; 79: 154-7.

[46]   Querleu D, Narducci F, Poulard V, Lacaze S, Occelli B, Leblanc E, Cosson M. Modified radical vaginal hysterectomy with or without laparoscopic nerve-sparing dissection: a comparative study. *Gynecol Oncol* 2002; 85: 154-8.

[47]   Hockel M, Horn LC, Hentschel B, Hockel S, Naumann G. Total mesometrial resection: high resolution nerve-sparing radical hysterectomy based on developmentally defined surgical anatomy. *Int J Gynecol. Cancer* 2003; 13: 791-803.

[48]   Possover M. Technical modification of the nerve-sparing laparoscopy-assisted vaginal radical hysterectomy type 3 for better reproducibility of this procedure. *Gynecol Oncol* 2003; 90: 245-7.

[49]   Raspagliesi F, Ditto A, Kusamura S, Fontanelli R, Spatti G, Solima E, Zanaboni, F, Carcangiu ML: Nerve-sparing radical hysterectomy: a pilot study. *Tumori* 2003; 89: 497-501.

[50]   Sakuragi N, Todo Y, Kudo M, Yamamoto R, Sato T. A systematic nerve-sparing radical hysterectomy technique in invasive cervical cancer for preserving postsurgical bladder function. *Int J Gynecol Cancer* 2005; 15: 389-97.

[51]   Hockel M, Horn LC, Hentschel B, Hockel S, Naumann G. Total mesometrial resection: High resolution nerve-sparing radical hysterectomy based on developmentally defined surgical anatomy. *Int J Gynecol Cancer* 2003; 13: 791-803

[52]   Raspagliesi F, Ditto A, Fontanelli R, Zanaboni F, Solima E, Spatti G, Hanozet F, Vecchione F, Rossi G, Kusamura S. Type II versus Type III Nerve-sparing Radical

hysterectomy: Comparison of lower urinary tract dysfunctions. *Gynecol Oncol* 2006; 102: 256-62.

[53]   Kato T, Murakami G and Yabuki Y. A New Perspective on Nerve-sparing Radical Hysterectomy: Nerve Topography and Over-preservation of the Cardinal Ligament. *Jpn J Clin Oncol* 2003; 33: 589–91.

In: Trends in Cervical Cancer
Editor: Hector T. Varaj, pp. 125-148

ISBN: 1-60021-299-9
© 2007 Nova Science Publishers, Inc.

Chapter VI

ANTIBODIES IN SINGLE-CHAIN FORMAT AGAINST THE E7 ONCOPROTEIN: TOWARDS GENE-THERAPY OF THE HPV-ASSOCIATED CERVICAL CANCER?

Luisa Accardi[*]

Section of Molecular Pathogenesis, Dept. of Infectious, Parasitic and Immunomediated
Diseases, Istituto Superiore di Sanità, Rome, Italy

ABSTRACT

The recognized causal relation between the "high risk" human papillomavirus
(HPV) genotypes and the cervical neoplasia has allowed exploring new ways for
prevention and treatment of the HPV-associated tumors. One challenge of the non-
invasive cancer therapy is to generate tumor-specific strategies in order to achieve
targeted efficacy and to limit side effects. Most of the cervical carcinomas are caused by
the HPV genotype 16 (HPV16). The viral oncoproteins E6 and E7 are tumor-antigens
that play a crucial role in the virus-associated tumorigenicity by inhibiting apoptosis and
promoting cellular proliferation. They are considered as molecular targets for the
development of therapeutic strategies against the HPV-associated tumors. A main goal of
therapy is to impair the E6 and E7 oncogenic activity. Among the different strategies of
protein "knock out" used in gene-therapy, intracellular antibodies have emerged as
powerful tools. They offer the chance to interfere with the antigen function in a precise
intracellular compartment by a restricted and targeted expression. Recently, the phage
display technology has been used to select antibodies in single-chain format (scFv)
against the E7 oncoprotein of the high-risk HPV16. One of these scFvs has been
expressed in different compartments of HPV16-positive cells, showing a specific effect

---

[*] Correspondence concerning this article should be addressed to: Dr Luisa Accardi, Section of Molecular
Pathogenesis, Dept. of Infectious, Parasitic and Immunomediated Diseases, Istituto Superiore di Sanità, Viale
Regina Elena 299, 00161 Rome, Italy. accardi@iss.it

of proliferation inhibition when expressed in the nucleus and in the secretory compartment. The antiproliferative efficacy is, with high confidence, related to the antigen localization and to the scFv stability. The results obtained *in vitro* are encouraging and open the way to wide applications in gene therapy.

Keywords: human papillomavirus, E7 protein, intrabodies, single-chain variable fragment, antiproliferative effect, cervical cancer

INTRODUCTION

Cervical cancer is one of the leading causes of cancer mortality in women worldwide (zur Hausen 2002). Early diagnosis of cervical cancer still resides in regular screening. Once the tumor is claimed, surgery is the only therapeutic choice. After surgical removal, the potentially residual cancer cells can be managed with a variety of treatment options like radiotherapy and chemotherapy alone or, more effectively, in combination. These approaches are limited by the need of achieving therapeutically relevant drug concentrations in the tumor mass, usually accessible with difficulty, and by toxicity of the high drug dose required to maintain a state of remission while impeding the drug-resistance development. In this situation, to avoid the further worsening of the life quality of the patients, discontinuation of therapy is obliged (Vasir et al., 2005). Therefore, selectively providing therapeutic efficacy at the tumor site is a main challenge for improving cancer treatment and avoiding any significant adverse effect on the non-cancerous cells. This can be achieved either by targeted drug delivery or by use of reagents effective uniquely in the targeted tumor cells.

The comprehension of the tumor biology and of the causal relation between human papillomaviruses (HPV) and cervical neoplasia has allowed envisaging novel non-invasive therapies for both treatment of the existing cervical cancer and prevention of the disease in the long term (Durst et al., 1983). In particular, the identification of molecular mechanisms distinctive of cervical cancer can lead to development of strategies for correcting alterations of the cellular pathways involved and possibly reversing the malignant process.

The most important transforming effects of the carcinogenic HPVs, called "high-risk" genotypes (De Villiers et al., 1997), are ascribed to the actions of the E6 and E7 viral oncoproteins on the two cellular tumor-suppressors p53 and pRB, respectively; these combined actions, resulting in p53 degradation and pRB inactivation, lead to hampering of apoptosis, deregulation of cellular growth and ultimately to cell transformation. E6 and E7 are tumor specific antigens and their presence, limited to the HPV-infected cells, confers them an advantage over other cellular markers of malignancy. The quest for specificity can be then well addressed by targeting E6 and E7; in this case, the anti-tumor therapy could consist in a manipulation, rather than a direct killing, of the tumor cells. Moreover, the targeting of E6 and E7 is a valuable approach because the antitumoral effect might be obtained even in premalignant and in metastatic cells.

Among the methods to "knock out" the function of specific proteins, the "intracellular antibody" (intrabody) technology, mainly using recombinant antibodies in single-chain format (scFv), is gaining increasing importance (Visintin et al., 2004 a). The possibility of functionally neutralizing a protein in its intracellular environment even at the level of specific domains, represents an interesting alternative to the strategies of gene inactivation. ScFvs against the recombinant HPV16 E7 protein, selected from a phage-display library of human antibodies (Pini et al., 1998), were expressed in the different compartments of keratinocytes constitutively expressing the HPV16 E7. By this strategy, the cell proliferation was inhibited with success. These findings, together with those of other authors who obtained the restoring of apoptosis in HPV16-positive cells by anti-HPV16 E6 scFvs (Griffin et al., 2006), are encouraging, and suggest that advancements in the field could hopefully open the way to "gene therapy" of the HPV-associated cancers.

HPV INFECTION AND IMPLICATIONS FOR THERAPY

Since HPVs were recognized as etiological agents of the human cervical cancer, the study of their biology and immunology assumed increasing relevance in view of the important implications for therapy (zur Hausen, 2002). Just a low percentage of the HPV infections progress to cancer. Tumors generally arise several years after the initial infection and the oncogenesis process is partially linked to dependence of the viral replication on the host cell differentiation. The HPV has a DNA genome of about 8 Kb coding for 6 non structural or early (E1, E2, E4, E5, E6 and E7) and 2 structural or late (L1, L2) proteins. The late proteins form the viral capsid, and the early proteins play different roles that support the viral life cycle also by favoring cell proliferation. The virus infects primitive basal keratinocytes via micro abrasion of the mucosal epithelium. Initially it is in episomal form and the viral proteins are expressed at a low level. Then the infected keratinocyte enters the differentiating compartment of the epithelium and the virus forces the host cell towards S-phase entry in order to exploit the cell machinery for its replication. In this phase the expression of the viral L1, L2 and E4 proteins is up regulated. Virus assembly occurs in the terminally differentiated epithelium, and virus spreads from the exfoliating cells. In the cervical lesions, HPV is usually present in episomal form, but sometimes it is found integrated in the host cell genome. The integration event plays a central role in the development of cancer, with E6 and E7 being the main viral proteins implicated. During viral integration, the sequences encoding the E1 and E2 proteins are interrupted so that the expression of E6 and E7 is no more suppressed by E2. In the HPV-associated tumors, the oncoproteins are constitutively expressed at a level sufficient for cell immortalization and they are absolutely required for maintaining the transformed phenotype (zur Hausen, 2000; Munger & Howley, 2002).

There are many issues concerning integration that have still to be addressed, e. g. whether lesions with integrated HPV retain an elevated risk of cancer progression, the importance of the site of integration, and whether rates and sites of integration vary according to the different HPV types. Many studies revealing the presence of HPV DNA in cervical lesions have provided evidence for a strong association between cervical cancer and HPV infection persistence. Nevertheless, no clear consensus still exists on the distinction between transient and persistent infection; in fact HPV infections detectable over a certain interval of time can derive either from persistent HPV infection or from re-infection after early clearance (Wang & Hildesheim, 2003; Baseman & Koutsky, 2005).

Of note, neutralizing antibodies against the viral capsid proteins are able to prevent viral infection and spread in humans, but fail to hamper the development of tumor lesions when the infection is ongoing (Stanley, 2005). The intracellular localization of the E6 and E7 oncoproteins strongly suggests the importance of the cellular immune response in clearing the HPV lesions. As a matter of fact, T cell- mediated cellular immunity towards HPV16 E6 and E7 peptides has been found efficacious against the recurrence of cervical intraepithelial neoplasia, showing to be essential to clear virus-infected cells and to control the HPV-induced malignancies in humans (Lamikanra et al., 2001; Sarkar et al., 2005). Nevertheless, the natural existing anti-HPV cellular immunity seems to rise poorly or too late to eradicate the tumor, and another important role in tumorigenesis is certainly played by viral immunoevasion (O'Brien & Campo, 2003). In this view, most of the therapeutic interventions are tailored at triggering a vigorous immune response against the viral proteins and minimizing the risk for immune escape by eliminating the HPV-infected cells, thus avoiding persistent infection and development of lesions. These strategies include vaccine formulations based on virus-like particles and on proteins or their epitopes delivered by viral or non-viral systems, plasmid DNA immunizations and loaded dendritic cells (Govan, 2005; Santin et al., 2005).

The E6 and E7 proteins, as tumor-specific antigens, have been employed separately, together or in association to other viral proteins (L1, L2, E2, E5), to elicit a T-cell mediated immune response such to hamper or delay tumor arising or even to regress established tumors (Schiller & Lowy, 2001; Qian et al., 2006). Among the different methods of protein expression and delivering used to this aim, the plant system is particularly interesting because of its safety and adjuvant activity (Franconi et al., 2002; 2006). Some of these vaccine strategies have already been employed in clinical trials obtaining some success but further studies aimed at improving the clinical outcome in patients with early lesions are needed. Moreover, it must be underlined that cancer is more and more being considered a chronic disease that can be managed rather than eradicated. This consideration supports the need of new immunotherapy approaches able to control the neoplastic progression. Also in this perspective, approaches targeting E6 and E7 seem to be particularly appropriate.

E6 AND E7 PROTEINS IN TUMORS

Among the more than 100 HPV genotypes isolated so far (de Villiers, 1997), few are etiological agents of cervical cancer and also involved in other kinds of malignant tumors and are therefore identified as "high risk" genotypes (zur Hausen, 2000). The E6 and E7 proteins of the "high risk" genotypes are key factors in promoting and sustaining the neoplastic progression. Ongoing studies are constantly elucidating additional roles for these proteins. E6 and E7 interact with and inactivate several cellular proteins involved in the cell cycle control, alter their function and finally deregulate cell growth, thus leading to cell transformation (Mantovani & Banks, 2001; Zwerschke & Jansen-Durr, 2000). During these processes they cooperate with cellular oncogenes and modulate the expression and the subcellular localization of functional components of the NFkB signalling pathway (Mazurek et al., 2001; Havard et al., 2005).

E7 accumulates mainly in the nucleus, where it interacts with the p107 and p130 members of the pocket protein family pRb through its LYCYE motif (aa 22-26), and directly binds several transcription factors including members of the E2F family, thus contributing to the control of cell cycle progression (Dyson et al., 1989). The E7 binding causes the release of the E2Fs, and the consequent activation of genes encoding proteins that promote cell progression in phase S (Lavia & Jansen-Durr, 1999). Also, it has been recently reported that the HPV16 E7 is involved in the increase of phosphorylation level of the protein kinase B, that contributes to promoting cell transformation (Pim et al., 2005).

The E7 action is pleiotropic: the oncoprotein influences the transcriptional and non transcriptional cell-cycle control checkpoints, causes the expression of genes not involved in the cell cycle control, deregulates the cellular carbohydrate metabolism and modulates apoptosis. More than 18 cell proteins that bind E7 have been identified and others are still being uncovered. The E7 ability to associate the pocket proteins is considered a main cause of its oncogenicity, even though some E7 proteins of HPV genotypes different from HPV16 are unable to bind them but still able to deregulate the cell cycle (Caldeira et al., 2000). Moreover, some E7 activities are detectable *in vivo* even when pRb is inactivated in the same tissue (Balsitis et al., 2003). These considerations support the importance of targets other than pRb, at least for some HPV types, and suggest that mechanisms not involving the pocket proteins-binding can be implicated in the E7 oncogenicity (Munger et al., 2001; Balsitis et al., 2005).

One of the recently identified E7 targets is the promyelocytic leukaemia protein (PML). The loss of PML function leads to increased cell proliferation and one out of seven existing PML isoforms induces senescence in primary human fibroblasts, with increased levels of p53 and pRb and other tumor suppressor proteins. HPVs are among the DNA viruses that utilize the PML-associated nuclear bodies as replication centres; therefore it is not surprising that PML could be targeted by E7 to create a favourable cell environment for HPV replication (Bischof et al., 2005).

The E6 protein strongly contributes to malignant progression by both targeting cellular proteins involved in the host defence and overcoming the apoptosis and growth-arrest induced by E7. In particular, E6 induces degradation of the tumor suppressor protein p53 via the ubiquitin-proteasome pathway but it is also involved in p53-independent pathways (Thomas et al., 1999; Mantovani & Banks, 2001). The p53 degradation is mediated by the formation of a complex between E6 and the ubiquitin ligase E6AP, which mediates several additional E6 functions (Kelley et al., 2005). Furthermore, E6 is involved in the cell cycle entry in S-phase, necessary for viral DNA replication, and promotes pRb phosphorylation (Malanchi et al., 2002; 2004). All these and additional mechanisms, still under investigation, contribute to the accumulation of genetic mutations in the infected cells, and finally to malignant progression. However, the amount of E6 protein is low in the infected cell and the protein does not probably interact with all the targets at the same time but its interaction can change, depending on both the stage of cell differentiation and the specific cell compartment (Mantovani & Banks, 2001).

In summary, the tumor event can be considered as a result of the concerted action of the E6 and E7 oncoproteins, which cooperate to favor viral replication and to contrast the mechanisms of cell defence by direct or indirect interference with multiple cellular pathways.

THE "INTRABODY TECHNOLOGY"

The first applications of gene therapy were in the treatment of metabolism dysfunction diseases. The possibility of exploiting the molecular differences between normal and cancer cells has successively allowed targeting molecules involved in the carcinogenesis processes.

The main issues to address when dealing with cancer gene therapy are the identification of appropriate targets and the choice of the modality to interfere with them; the latter is strictly connected to the possibility of transferring and expressing the genes of interest in the target tumor cells (Bilbao et al., 2002).

The recombinant antibodies represent powerful alternatives to other methods of gene and protein inactivation based either on nucleic acids or on proteins, like antisense oligonucleotides, ribozymes, RNA interference, transdominant negative proteins, oligopeptides and suicide genes. In the last decades, the progress in biotechnology has allowed obtaining recombinant antibodies against antigens of interest by combining the building of antibodies from their genes with a specific selection.

The recombinant antibodies are available in different formats, among which the single-chain format (scFv) shows to be particularly versatile. The scFv molecule comprises only the variable heavy (VH) and variable light (VL) regions of an immunoglobulin G (IgG), linked by a polypeptide. Each variable region retains the three complementarity determining regions (CDR) forming the antigen-binding pocket. With its molecular weight of 27 KDa, the scFv represents the minimal molecule capable of antigen binding and still retaining sufficient stability (Holliger & Hudson, 2005). Of note, the small size confers to the scFv the advantage of a rapid tumor penetration with respect to larger antibody molecules, and the versatile structure allows tailoring the molecule by protein engineering whenever improvements in affinity and stability are needed.

The scFvs are derived from antibody libraries obtained by different methodologies. To amplify the immunoglobulin genes of interest, the RT-PCR is usually performed by specific primers either on the antibody germ-line genes or on the genes encoding specific monoclonal antibodies obtained by classical procedures following animal immunization. The immunoglobulin domains are then cloned into the appropriate plasmids to permit selection of scFvs with the desired binding specificity by recombinant systems. The "phage-display", the "ribosome display" and the "intracellular antibody capture" (IACT) are examples of powerful technologies that, bypassing *in vivo* immunization, allow obtaining human antibodies against virtually all the human proteins (Pini et al., 2004; Visintin et al., 1999; Hoogenboom, 2005). In Fig. 1 the structure of a scFv selected by phage-display technology and its comparison to that of an immunoglobulin G are shown.

The selected scFvs can be expressed by prokaryotic systems to be tested for their *in vitro* performance before being investigated as modulators of antigen function within the eukaryotic cells. The scFvs retaining the desired features of specificity and stability by *in vitro* tests, can be efficaciously employed as therapeutic agents (Kontermann, 2004). To this aim, they can be introduced into the target cells either by viral systems using retroviruses, adenoviruses and adeno-associated viruses, or by non-viral systems such as those employing liposomic and non-liposomic transfection and molecular conjugates (Mountain, 2000).

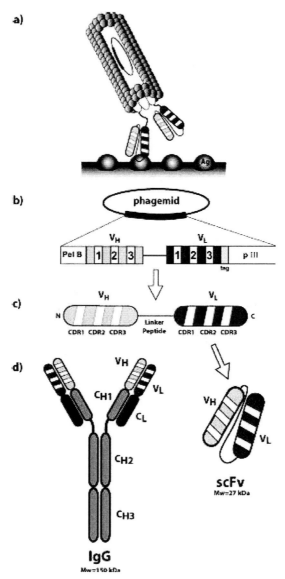

Figure 1. Selection of antibodies in single-chain format (scFv) by phage display. a) Phages from a library, retaining different binding specificities, are screened against the antigen (Ag) of interest. b) The phage DNA (phagemid) encodes the scFvs displayed on phage surface as pIII-fusions. Pel B sequence at the N-terminus allows secretion in the bacterial periplasm. A tag is present downstream the scFv coding sequence. c) The scFv is formed by a heavy (VH) and a light (VL) variable region linked by a flexible peptide. The complementarity-determining regions (CDR) form the antigen-binding site. d) The scFv format retains the antigen-binding capability in a smaller size with respect to an immunoglobuline G (IgG).

In order to configure the antibodies for utilization inside the cells, vector-deriving signal sequences able to direct the antibody fragments to subcellular compartments can be incorporated into the scFv sequence. The fusion of the antibody fragment to a nuclear localization signal or to a secretory sequence determines targeting to the nucleus and to the secretory pathway, respectively; when a SEKDEL sequence is incorporated downstream the scFv coding sequence in addition to the upstream secretory sequence, the antibody fragment is retained in the endoplasmic reticulum; in the absence of a signal sequence, the antibody fragment will remain in the cytoplasm (Persic et al., 1997a,b).

The proper *in vitro* activity of an antibody fragment does not ensure its intracellular activity, particularly in cell cytoplasm, which lacks the chaperone proteins necessary for the correct folding, thus representing a non-physiological environment for antibodies. Nevertheless, some antibodies are able to fold correctly in the cell cytoplasm even in the absence of disulphide bonds and have no tendency to aggregate, showing intrinsic properties of stability and solubility (Martineau et al., 1998). On the other hand, the antibodies retained in the endoplasmic reticulum by the SEKDEL signal sequence are able to acquire the proper tertiary structure by forming the necessary intra-chain disulphide bonds, and exhibit higher stability than their counterparts expressed in the reducing cytoplasm.

Recently, stability and solubility of an antibody fragment have been correlated to specific sequence requirements (Ewert et al., 2003a). Interesting studies have been carried out to determine the relation between sequence and structure of the immunoglobulin variable domains at atomic level, showing that the sites forming the "deep" structure of the immunoglobulin core have important implications in the overall molecular stability (Chothia et al., 1998).

It can also happen that scFvs randomly selected from a library do not retain the appropriate features of stability (Worn et al., 2000). To address this issue, different approaches can be utilized, including rational design of stable scFvs and *de novo* selection. Recently a "consensus" sequence for intracellular stable immunoglobulins has been identified by aligning the sequences of antibody fragments with recognized properties of stability (Visintin et al., 2002). Highly stable and soluble antibody frameworks identified either empirically or by comparison with the "consensus" can be used as acceptor backbones to "graft" known antigen specificities or even to construct randomised hypervariable loop libraries (Wirtz & Steipe, 1999; Tavladoraki et al., 1999; Desiderio et al., 2001; Worn & Plucktun, 2001; der Maur et al., 2002; Ewert et al. 2003b; Krauss et al., 2003). Alternatively, it is possible to directly select intracellular functional and stable binders by the IACT technology, which uses a two-hybrid in vivo system (Tse et al., 2002; Visintin et al., 1999; 2004b).

SCFV APPLICATIONS TO RESEARCH AND CLINICS

In virtue of their properties, the scFvs are versatile molecules useful in multiple and diversified antitumoral strategies. They can be manipulated at either genetic or protein level and conjugated to different kinds of molecules, like radioisotopes and toxins, to permit a number of applications including radioimmunotherapy, targeted destruction of specific cells, vehiculation of useful molecules like enzymes, and gene therapy (Onda et al., 2004; Marasco, 2005).

When the therapeutic molecules have to be administered systemically, one main goal is to achieve therapeutically relevant concentrations in the tumor mass. This is not an easy issue especially for solid tumors, which present a poor penetrability. In this regard it is interesting to note that the scFvs can easily penetrate the tumor mass because of their small size (Jang et al., 2003).

Another advantage of using scFvs can be represented by the existing possibility of expression inside the eukaryotic cells. Specific scFvs previously selected can be used as "intrabodies". By vectors carrying appropriate signals, they can be directed to the cell compartments where their target antigens are localized. This co localization allows an *in vivo* antigen-antibody interaction and can result in the phenotypic knock-out of the antigen due either to direct neutralizing effect or to delocalization of the target protein with indirect impairment of its function (Cattaneo & Biocca, 1997). Of note, low solubility in the cytoplasm and over expression of the scFvs can cause aggregation, but this event does not necessarily preclude their functioning, which can occur by alternative mechanisms like antigen-sequester and -inactivation in the aggresomes. The p21 ras is an example of antigen harbouring in the cytoplasm that was successfully targeted (Lener et al., 2000; Cardinale et al., 2001).

The use of intrabodies is particularly appropriate in pathologies caused by intracellular parasites, viruses and prions, or associated to the expression of proteins that can be targeted without affecting the cellular proteins. ScFvs against the vesicular stomatitis virus were capable of inhibiting viral transcription in infected cells (Cortay et al., 2006). ScFvs against the rotavirus NSP5 protein inhibited replication of the dsRNA and allowed disclosing the role of this protein (Vascotto et al., 2004). An anti-prion scFv targeted to the endoplasmic reticulum was able to retain the prion protein and to inhibit its translocation to the cell surface, thus affecting its maturation; these results have allowed studies on the molecular pathogenetic mechanisms of the prion disease (Cardinale et al., 2005). Anti-HIV-tat intrabodies have been evaluated for gene therapy of AIDS (Marasco et al., 1999). An anti-HIV-Vpr scFv able to inhibit the Vpr nuclear import was useful to study the role of this protein in HIV infection (Krichevsky et al., 2003). Recently, the selection of a secretory anti-HIV gp41 that successfully inhibited viral production by reducing viral assembly and expression has been reported (Liu et al., 2005).

Nevertheless, most applications of the scFvs to viral diseases are still limited to research studies and are not well fitting clinical purposes because of the difficulties of scFv delivery in the case of systemic infections (Lobato & Rabbitts, 2003). The scFvs expressed inside the cells are efficacious tools to target molecules involved in pathways associated with the carcinogenesis process, particularly the oncogenic proteins (Cochet et al., 1998; Caron de Fromentel et al., 1999). The choice of the molecular targets is of basic importance in determining success of the application. ScFvs have been used to counteract tumor angiogenesis, to modulate the immunologic response to cancer and to support conventional therapies like chemotherapy and radiation. An scFv targeting the vascular endothelial growth factor, which is known to stimulate endothelial cell proliferation and migration, was able to inhibit its activity *in vivo* in a murine system (Vitaliti et al., 2000). An scFv against the 5T4 oncofetal glycoprotein fused to the human IgG1 Fc domain was able to cause an antibody-dependent cell cytotoxic immune response against the tumoral cells (Myers et al., 2002). ScFvs have been used to enhance sensitivity of ovarian cancer and EBV-transformed lymphocytes to both chemotherapeutic agents and ionising radiation (Russell et al., 1999). A mutant form of the oncosuppressor p53 has been targeted to impair oncogenic transformation (Orgad et al., 2005). An antitumoral effect was also achieved in two different studies *in vitro*. The first study utilized an intracellular anti-c-Myb scFv to obtain antiproliferative effect in human leukaemia cells, whereas the second one succeeded in obtaining apoptosis by a scFv hampering the ErbB-2 translocation through the endoplasmic reticulum (Deshane et al., 1996; Kasono et al., 2000).

TARGETING CERVICAL CANCER BY INHIBITION OF E6 AND E7 PROTEIN FUNCTION

Since the very first association between HPV and cervical cancer, the viral proteins, and especially those encoded by the "high risk" genotypes, were main subjects of investigation.

On the basis of their strict implication in a plethora of processes underlying and promoting carcinogenesis, the HPV16 E6 and E7 proteins have been targeted with the aim of counteracting, at least in part, their oncogenic activity. The antisense methodologies have been largely explored to abrogate the E6 and E7 pleiotropic functions, e. g. by targeting their transcript or the HPV long control region, which contains the viral regulatory sequences, and have resulted rather efficacious (Venturini et al., 1999; Alvarez et al., 2003; Butz et al., 2003; Tang et al., 2006; Jang & Milner, 2005). However, E6 and E7 are expressed via a bicistronic mRNA, and the use of the siRNA methodology to block the protein expression does not allow to discriminate which is the contribution of each protein to the total effect. This goal can be accomplished by targeting the proteins directly, e.g. by using functional inhibitors like peptides, organic compounds (Beerheide et al., 2000; Liu et al., 2004) or antibody fragments. Moreover, approaches that directly target the oncoproteins allow dissecting their pleiotropic actions and then studying their function. Few years ago, the E7 down-regulation was obtained in HPV16-positive cells using anti-E7 scFvs targeted to the nucleolus and the endoplasmic reticulum (Wang-Johanning et al., 1998). Another interesting example of this approach is provided by an anti-HPV16 E6 recombinant antibody that, in cervical cancer cells *in vitro,* has shown to be able to hamper the association E6-p53 by binding the E6 zinc-finger domain, thus avoiding the degradation of the oncosuppressor. The efficacy of this antibody expressed in scFv, diabody and triabody format, and of specific peptides containing the ELLG E6-binding domain, was tested in different HPV-positive cell lines. The scFv format was able to inhibit the degradation of cellular substrates by E6, while the other formats were less efficacious, and the peptides were not at all (Griffin et al., 2006). Both the peptides and the scFvs gain easy access to the nucleus, where E6 is found; therefore the authors ascribe the failure of the peptides to their relatively low affinity for E6, and the success of the scFvs to their small size. These results support that the scFv format is adequate to control efficaciously proteins localized in the cell nucleus, like E6 and E7.

INTRABODIES IN SCFV FORMAT INHIBIT THE PROLIFERATION OF HPV-POSITIVE CELLS

The possibility to select specific scFvs and to express them by the "intrabody technology" opens new ways for counteracting the antigen function in the appropriate cellular sites. The use of this technology can be particularly appropriate to neutralize the action of the HPV16 oncoproteins, which are tumor-associated antigens of cervical cancer. The study reported in this chapter had the aim of counteracting the proliferative activity of the HPV16 E7 by specific scFvs. The selection was performed from the ETH-2 library of human recombinant antibodies provided by prof. D. Neri (Pini et al., 1998). The use of a synthetic library allows obtaining human antibodies with lower immunogenicity with respect to those derived from hybridomas, which require further processes of "humanization" to be useful for application in humans. The selected anti-E7 scFvs were expressed in and purified from *E. coli*. Sequence analysis showed they were belonging to three different groups, specifically scFv 32, 43 and 51. ScFv43 apparently showed to retain the highest reactivity against the antigen in different immunoassays *in vitro* whereas the affinity value of the three scFvs, as calculated by ELISA, was of the same order of magnitude, 10^6 M^{-1}. Of note, the scFvs characterization was performed *in vitro* even though the scFv molecular properties exhibited *in vitro* do not always mirror those exhibited in the intracellular environment. Biophysical properties of the scFvs such as solubility and stability can be decisive for the success in gene therapy application. In particular, stability is of outstanding importance, sometimes even more relevant than reactivity against the antigen, and should be considered when designing the most appropriate scFv for therapeutic applications (Willuda et al., 1999; Worn & Plucktun, 2001).

The scFv thermal stability ($T_{1/2}$) is considered as an appropriate indicator of stability in view of its relevance for extra cellular as well as for intracellular functioning of the antibody fragments. This parameter indicates the time at which the antigen-binding capability of a scFv, incubated at 37°C in the presence of human seroalbumin, halves with respect to that of the same scFv non-incubated. Interesting differences among the $T_{1/2}$ of the three antibodies were revealed. ScFv32 had a $T_{1/2}$ of few minutes, after which its E7-binding ability remained quite stable up to three days; scFv51 was rather stable all over the 72 h considered; scFv43 showed the lowest stability. The differences in thermal stability could have possible relevant implications for the *in vivo* use and might also be the cause of the different yields of purified products (Accardi, unpublished).

Considering that the major activity of E7 protein is to promote cellular proliferation, testing the anti-E7 scFv capability to interfere with cell proliferation was an important issue. This was accomplished in SiHa cells, an immortalized keratinocyte cell line harbouring the HPV16 genome and thus expressing the E7 oncoprotein. The coding sequences of scFv43, which had resulted the most reactive antibody fragment *in vitro*, were cloned into the eukaryotic vectors of the ScFvExpress series, containing targeting signals that allow expression in the nucleus and the secretory pathway, or not containing signals, for expression in the cytoplasm (Persic et al., 1997a,b). The recombinant vectors were used to transfect the SiHa cells. Immunofluorescence analysis showed the correct localization of the "intrabodies" in the cytoplasmic, nuclear and secretory compartments according to the targeting signals

(Fig. 2). When scFv43 was expressed in the cytoplasm, it accumulated in nodular structures. These aggregates have been described in numerous studies and are known as "aggresomes". They account for both the scFv insolubility and a production exceeding the cell degrading capacity (Kopito, 2000). The cell proliferation was estimated by the Bromodeoxy-Uridine (BrdU) assay, which reveals the actively DNA-synthesizing cells. The effect of the scFv43 expressed in each cellular compartment was tested by comparing DNA synthesis in transfected and not transfected cells. A significant effect of inhibition of the cell proliferation was observed when transfecting SiHa cells with the scFv43 targeting the nucleus and the secretory pathway; in contrast, no effect was detected when the antibody fragment was expressed in the cytoplasm (Accardi et al., 2005). The inefficacy of the cytoplasmic scFv43 might either be linked to its insolubility in the cytoplasm or depend on the E7 localization, which is predominantly nuclear. Of note, some authors showed that the scFvs could preserve their functionality in binding and inactivating the antigen even inside the "aggresomes" (Cardinale et al., 2001).

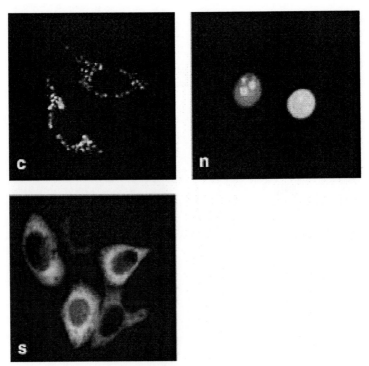

Figure 2. Immunofluorescence showing localization of the anti-HPV16 E7 scFvs in SiHa cells transiently transfected with the cytoplasmic (c), nuclear (n), and secretory (s) constructs. Detection is by an anti-tag monoclonal antibody (mAb) followed by a secondary fluorescein-labeled mAb.

The observed effects are highly specific because strictly related to the simultaneous presence of scFv43 and E7 protein, in fact no effect on proliferation was obtained neither when the HPV-negative cervical carcinoma C33A cells were transfected by the scFv43 nor when the HPV-positive SiHa cells were transfected by an irrelevant anti-β-galactosidase scFv (Martineau et al., 1998). The results are schematically reported in Fig. 3. The hypothesis on the scFv functioning is illustrated in Fig. 4.

The intracellular efficacy of scFv 32 and 51 is now under investigation. These scFvs show a rather low reactivity *in vitro* but, as above mentioned, not always the properties exhibited by the scFvs expressed in *E. coli* reflect those retained in the eukaryotic cells. For this reason, just a limited number of the scFvs selected against a specific antigen can be effectively employed *in vivo*. Of note, this is the first study reporting evidence of the intracellular efficacy of antibody fragments derived from the ETH-2 library.

Solubility in the cytoplasm is undoubtedly a relevant parameter for the scFv functioning in eukaryotic cells. Further studies on the solubility of the three scFvs are ongoing, and preliminary results indicate scFv51 as the most soluble among the antibody fragments (Accardi, unpublished).

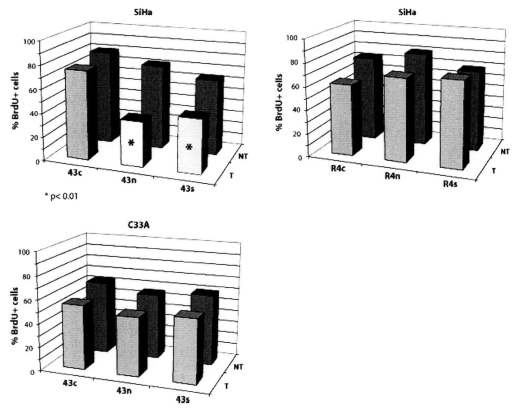

Figure 3. Cell proliferation analysis by Bromodeoxyuridine (BrdU) incorporation assay in a representative experiment. The assay was carried out 48 hr after the transfection of SiHa (HPV16-positive) and C33A (HPV-negative) cells with the recombinant cytoplasmic (c), nuclear (n) and secretory (s) constructs carrying the anti-HPV16 E7 scFv43 (43) or the irrelevant anti-β galactosidase scFv (R4) sequences. The percentage of BrdU-positive cells was determined for transfected (T) and non transfected (NT) cells. (*) statistically significant data.

Both stability and solubility ultimately depend on structural properties. Aminoacid sequences determine the capability of forming intra-chain disulphide bonds and therefore tertiary folding. Single residues may play a central role in maintaining the structure of the whole molecule (Chothia et al., 1998). As above mentioned, accurate folding is not possible in the reducing cytoplasmic environment but, in spite of that, some scFvs hold the intrinsic capability of correctly folding in the absence of disulphide bridges and are therefore stable even in the cytoplasm (Sibler et al., 2003; 2005). Many research studies are presently focussed on the direct selection of intrinsically stable scFvs, e.g. through systems in yeast like the above mentioned IACT (Visintin et al., 2004b).

All these considerations and results support the importance of sequence analysis to possibly identify variations responsible for the differences observed in stability and solubility of the three scFvs. To this aim, the deduced aminoacid sequences of the VH and VL region were aligned to the immunoglobulin sequences from the IMGT database. For construction, the VH regions of all the scFvs are deriving from the DP47 germ-line gene, whereas both the gene options available for the VL region are represented: DPL16 in scFv 32 and 51, and DPK22 in scFv43. By sequence analysis of the antibody scaffolds two potentially destabilizing variations were identified, the first one present in both the scFv 32 and 43 and the second one just in the latter. Studies are ongoing in our laboratory to validate the role of these variations on the scFv stability and to possibly design a mutational strategy aimed at improving intrabody efficacy as a consequence of improved stability.

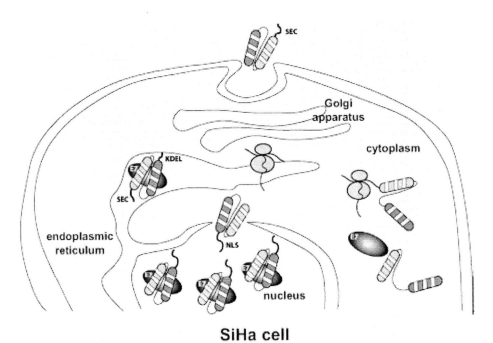

SiHa cell

Figure 4. Hypothesis of functioning of the anti-HPV16 E7 scFvs expressed in the cytoplasm, the nucleus and the secretory pathway of SiHa cells. The scFvs are targeted the nucleus by the nuclear localization signal (NLS), retained in the endoplasmic reticulum by the KDEL sequence, or secreted in virtue of the secretory leader (SEC). The scFvs localized in the nucleus and in the secretory compartment can block the E7 protein and inhibit its function. The scFvs expressed in the reducing cytoplasmic environment are not well-folded and fail to block E7.

METHODS FOR "INTRABODY" DELIVERING

One of the main issues of cancer gene therapy to address in the near future is the safe delivery of therapeutic molecules exclusively to the tumor site. Optimization of efficacy and avoiding of toxic side effects are imperative. In this context, the localized nature of a tumor target offers a guaranty of specificity, and bypasses the problem of the systemic administration of therapeutic molecules. In view of the causal link of the HPV-associated tumors to the expression of E6 and E7, a therapeutic strategy based on the knockout of these oncoproteins further warrants specificity.

The success of gene therapy largely depends on efficiency of the delivery systems in terms of level and duration of the therapeutic gene expression, although for most cancer gene therapies a short period of gene expression can give satisfactory results. Both virus-based and non-viral systems are objects of ongoing research (El-Aneed, 2004; Ohlfest et al., 2005).

Viral systems are biological systems that exploit vectors deriving from viruses, which naturally infect and transfer their genetic material into the host cells (Young et al., 2006). The main hindrance to the use viral vectors concerns safety and immunogenicity, besides their limited capability to carry transgenes. Several viral vectors have been constructed to eliminate viral toxicity while maintaining gene transfer capability. Viruses that have been managed to this aim include retroviruses, lentiviruses, adeno and adeno-associated viruses, herpes simplex viruses and poxviruses (Arafat et al., 2002; Anderson & Hope, 2005; Epstein et al., 2005; Essajee & Kaufman, 2004).

Retro, lentiviral and adenoviral vectors are major objects of investigation for cancer therapy applications. In both retro- and lentiviral systems, integration into the host genome occurs after viral transduction. Retroviruses infect actively dividing cells and, while this feature can be advantageous in protecting normal tissues, tumoral non-dividing cells can escape therapy. Their use resulted effective particularly in brain tumor of glial origin (Rainov & Ren, 2003). Lentiviruses are instead capable to infect non-proliferating cells but present major drawbacks for safety (Indraccolo et al., 2002). Adenoviral vectors do not permanently integrate into the host cell genome, require repetitive administration to be effective, and their efficacy is limited by the host immune response; they were responsible for the first death in clinical gene therapy trials (Raper et al., 2002). Nevertheless, for their oncolytic potential and the possibility to be "armed" with transgenes targeting multiple cellular pathways, transcriptionally regulated adenoviruses are now being developed and offer encouraging short-term opportunities to clinical applications (Ko et al., 2005).

Non-viral systems like peptides-, cationic polypeptides- or liposome-based gene transfer vehicles seem to be less efficient than viral vectors, albeit offering several advantages like no risk of infection or mutation, and large-scale production (Davis, 2002).

At present, nanobiotechnologies are emerging as a new interesting option for drug delivery in cancer and may be particularly helpful for the treatment of disseminated tumors. Different kinds of nanoparticles are investigated as nanobullets for cancer. Their application facilitates the delivery and overcomes the problems of insolubility linked to the administration of some drugs. Moreover, nanoparticles are versatile tools because they can be conjugated to or incorporated in other molecules, allowing combination of diagnosis with therapy. Polymer-based formulations can potentially allow modulations of both the level and the duration of gene expression, a property that can be advantageous depending on the tumor kind. Gene-delivery with nanoparticles usually requires direct intratumoral injection and it could also be possible to modify the nanoparticle surface to avoid its trapping by the reticuloendothelial system (Jain, 2005; Kommareddy et al., 2005; Vasir & Labhasetwar, 2005). Although promising, safety concerns still exist about the introduction of nanoparticles in the human body and many studies are required before their approval becomes possible (Gopalan et al., 2004).

Eventually, new kinds of molecules are now being developed that could be helpful for the application of scFvs to clinics: the "transbodies", antibodies able to translocate across the cell membrane thanks to fusion with a protein transduction domain. This approach exploits the ability of well-characterized peptides to translocate into living cells, thus providing a valuable tool to cross the permeable cell barrier (Joliot & Prochiantz, 2004; Heng & Cao, 2005).

CONCLUSION

Cervical cancer associated to high-risk papillomavirus infection is a serious problem of public health worldwide. The impending commercialization of a prophylactic anti-HPV vaccine is shifting the research efforts from prevention to tumor therapy (Mao et al., 2006). The delivery of antitumoral agents to the cervical cancer cells can represent a method alternative to surgery for the treatment of cancer lesions, especially at initial level. Cervical cancer mostly derives from the development of localized lesions caused by HPVs. The tumorigenic effect of HPVs is tightly linked to the pleiotropic action of the viral E6 and E7 proteins, that make these proteins appropriate targets for gene therapy. In the last decade, the "recombinant antibodies" technology has provided powerful tools for wide applications from sensitive diagnosis to tumor therapy, and many recombinant antibodies are already used successfully either in clinical trial or in therapy. Recently, progresses in biotechnology have offered the possibility to combine the "construction" of highly variable antibody libraries, with the selection of antibody fragments in a versatile format (scFvs), and specific for the antigen of interest. These molecules can be either targeted directly to the tumors or expressed in specific compartments of the tumoral cells. Recent studies have showed that scFvs against the "high risk" HPV16 E6 and E7 oncoproteins, selected by phage display, have succeeded in countering the activities of the proteins in inhibiting apoptosis and promoting proliferation, respectively. In a next future, it will be also possible to select scFvs targeting specific protein domains and functions, thus modulating the antitumoral activity. As a number of issues have still to be addressed to appropriately deliver these therapeutic agents, further research efforts are needed in this direction.

ACKNOWLEDGEMENTS

The author wishes to kindly acknowledge Dr M. G. Donà for her valuable contribution in performing the laboratory work, Dr C. Giorgi for criticism and suggestions, Mrs S. Tocchio for editorial assistance and Mr. W. Tranquilli for computer artwork.

REFERENCES

Accardi, L., Dona, M.G., Di Bonito, P. & Giorgi, C. (2005). Intracellular anti-E7 human antibodies in single-chain format inhibit proliferation of HPV16-positive cervical carcinoma cells. *Int. J. Cancer, 10*: 116(4): 564-570.

Alvarez-Salas, L.M., Benitez-Hess, M.L. & DiPaolo, J.A. (2003). Advances in the development of ribozymes and antisense oligodeoxynucleotides as antiviral agents for human papillomaviruses. *Antivir. Ther., 8(4)*: 265-278.

Anderson, J.L. & Hope, T.J. (2005). Intracellular trafficking of retroviral vectors: obstacles and advances. *Gene Ther., 12(23)*: 1667-1678.

Arafat, W.O., Gomez-Navarro, J., Buchsbaum, D.J., Xiang, J., Wang, M., Casado, E., Barker, S.D., Mahasreshti, P.J., Haisma, H.J., Barnes, M.N., Siegal, G.P., Alvarez, R.D., Hemminki, A., Nettelbeck, D.M. & Curiel, D.T. (2002). Effective single chain antibody (scFv) concentrations in vivo via adenoviral vector mediated expression of secretory scFv. *Gene Ther., 9(4)*: 256-262.

Balsitis, S.J., Sage, J., Duensing, S., Munger, K., Jacks, T. & Lambert, P.F. (2003). Recapitulation of the effects of the human papillomavirus type 16 E7 oncogene on mouse epithelium by somatic Rb deletion and detection of pRb-independent effects of E7 in vivo. *Mol. Cell Biol., 23(24)*: 9094-9103.

Balsitis, S., Dick, F., Lee, D., Farrell, L., Hyde, R.K., Griep, A.E., Dyson, N. & Lambert, P.F. (2005). Examination of the pRb-dependent and pRb-independent functions of E7 in vivo. *J. Virol., 79(17)*: 11392-11402.

Baseman, J.G. & Koutsky, L.A. (2005). The epidemiology of human papillomavirus infections. *J. Clin. Virol., 32*: S16-24.

Beerheide, W., Sim, M.M., Tan, Y.J., Bernard, H.U. & Ting, A.E. (2000). Inactivation of the human papillomavirus-16 E6 oncoprotein by organic disulfides. *Bioorg. Med. Chem., 8(11)*: 2549-2560.

Bilbao, G., Contreras, J.L. & Curiel, D.T. (2002). Genetically engineered intracellular single-chain antibodies in gene therapy. *Mol. Biotechnol., 22(2)*:191-211.

Biocca, S. & Cattaneo, A. (1995). Intracellular immunization: antibody targeting to sub cellular compartments. *Trends Cell Biol., 5(6)*: 248-252.

Bischof, O., Nacerddine, K. & Dejean, A. (2005). Human papillomavirus oncoprotein E7 targets the promyelocytic leukemia protein and circumvents cellular senescence via the Rb and p53 tumor suppressor pathways. *Mol. Cell Biol., 25(3)*: 1013-1024.

Butz, K., Ristriani, T., Hengstermann, A., Denk, C., Scheffner, M. & Hoppe-Seyler, F. (2003). siRNA targeting of the viral E6 oncogene efficiently kills human papillomavirus-positive cancer cells. *Oncogene, 22(38)*: 5938-5945.

Caldeira, S., de Villiers, E.M. & Tommasino, M. (2000). Human papillomavirus E7 proteins stimulate proliferation independently of their ability to associate with retinoblastoma protein. *Oncogene, 19(6)*: 821-826.

Cardinale, A., Filesi, I. & Biocca, S. (2001). Aggresome formation by anti-Ras intracellular scFv fragments. The fate of the antigen-antibody complex. *Eur. J. Biochem., 268(2)*: 268-277.

Cardinale, A., Filesi, I., Vetrugno, V., Pocchiari, M., Sy, M.S. & Biocca, S. (2005). Trapping prion protein in the endoplasmic reticulum impairs PrPC maturation and prevents PrPSc accumulation. *J. Biol. Chem., 280(1)*: 685-694.

Caron de Fromentel, C., Gruel, N., Venot, C., Debussche, L., Conseiller, E., Dureuil, C., Teillaud, J.L., Tocque, B. & Bracco, L. (1999). Restoration of transcriptional activity of p53 mutants in human tumor cells by intracellular expression of anti-p53 single chain Fv fragments. *Oncogene, 18(2)*: 551-557.

Cattaneo, A. & Biocca, S. (1997). *Intracellular antibodies: development and applications.* Springer Verlag,. pp 105-123.

Chothia, C., Gelfand, I. & Kister, A. (1998). Structural determinants in the sequences of immunoglobulin variable domain. *J. Mol. Biol., 278(2)*: 457-479.

Cochet, O., Kenigsberg, M., Delumeau, I., Virone-Oddos, A., Multon, M.C., Fridman, W.H., Schweighoffer, F., Teillaud, J.L. & Tocque, B. (1998). Intracellular expression of an antibody fragment-neutralizing p21 ras promotes tumor regression. *Cancer Res., 58(6)*: 1170-1176.

Cortay, J.C., Gerlier, D. & Iseni, F. (2006). Selection of single-chain antibodies that specifically interact with vesicular stomatitis virus (VSV) nucleocapsid and inhibit viral RNA synthesis. *J. Virol. Methods, 131(1)*: 16-20.

Davis, M.E. (2002) Non-viral gene delivery systems. *Curr. Opin. Biotechnol.*, 13(2):128-131.

Deshane, J., Grim, J., Loechel, S., Siegal, G.P., Alvarez, R.D. & Curiel, D.T. (1996). Intracellular antibody against erbB-2 mediates targeted tumor cell eradication by apoptosis. *Cancer Gene Ther., 3(2)*: 89-98.

de Villiers, E.M. (1997). Papillomavirus and HPV typing. *Clin. Dermatol., 15(2)*: 199-206.

der Maur, A.A., Zahnd C., Fischer F., Spinelli S., Honegger A., Cambillau C., Escher D., Pluckthun A. & Barberis A. (2002). Direct in vivo screening of intrabody libraries constructed on a highly stable single-chain framework. *J. Biol. Chem., 277(47)*: 45075-45085.

Desiderio, A., Franconi, R., Lopez, M., Villani, M.E., Viti, F., Chiaraluce, R., Consalvi, V., Neri, D. & Benvenuto, E. (2001). A semi-synthetic repertoire of intrinsically stable antibody fragments derived from a single-framework scaffold. *J. Mol. Biol., 310(3)*: 603-615.

Durst, M., Gissmann, L., Ikenberg, H. & zur Hausen, H. (1983). A papillomavirus DNA from a cervical carcinoma and its prevalence in cancer biopsy samples from different geographic regions. *Proc. Natl. Acad. Sci U.S.A., 80(12)*: 3812-3815.

Dyson, N., Howley, P.M., Munger, K. & Harlow, E. (1989). The human papilloma virus-16 E7 oncoprotein is able to bind to the retinoblastoma gene product. *Science, 243(4893)*: 934-937.

El-Aneed, A. (2004). An overview of current delivery systems in cancer gene therapy. *J. Control Release, 94(1)*: 1-14.

Epstein, A.L., Marconi, P., Argnani, R. & Manservigi, R. (2005). HSV-1-derived recombinant and amplicon vectors for gene transfer and gene therapy. *Curr. Gene Ther., 5(5)*: 445-458.

Essajee, S. & Kaufman, H.L. (2004) Poxvirus vaccines for cancer and HIV therapy. *Expert Opin Biol Ther. Apr, 4(4):* 575-588.

Ewert, S., Huber, T., Honegger, A. & Pluckthun, A. (2003a). Biophysical properties of human antibody variable domains. *J. Mol. Biol., 325(3)*: 531-553.

Ewert, S., Honegger, A. & Pluckthun, A. (2003b). Structure-based improvement of the biophysical properties of immunoglobulin VH domains with a generalizable approach. *Biochemistry, 42(6)*: 1517-1528.

Franconi, R., Di Bonito, P., Dibello, F., Accardi, L., Muller, A., Cirilli, A., Simeone, P., Dona, M.G., Venuti, A. & Giorgi, C. (2002). Plant-derived human papillomavirus 16 E7 oncoprotein induces immune response and specific tumor protection. *Cancer Res., 62(13)*: 3654-3658.

Franconi R, Massa S, Illiano E, Mullar A, Cirilli A, Accardi L, Di Bonito P, Giorgi C, Venuti A. (2006). Exploiting the plant secretory pathway to improve the anticancer activity of a plant-derived HPV16 E7 vaccine. *Int J Immunopathol Pharmacol. Jan-Mar, 19(1)*: 187-197.

Gopalan, B., Ito, I., Branch, C.D., Stephens, C., Roth, J.A. & Ramesh, R. (2004). Nanoparticle based systemic gene therapy for lung cancer: molecular mechanisms and strategies to suppress nanoparticle-mediated inflammatory response. *Technol. Cancer Res. Treat., 3(6)*: 647-657.

Govan, V.A. (2005). Strategies for human papillomavirus therapeutic vaccines and other therapies based on the e6 and e7 oncogenes. *Ann. N.Y. Acad. Sci., 1056*: 328-343.

Griffin, H., Elston, R., Jackson, D., Ansell, K., Coleman, M., Winter, G. & Doorbar, J. (2006). Inhibition of papillomavirus protein function in cervical cancer cells by intrabody targeting. *J. Mol. Biol., 355(3)*: 360-378.

Havard, L., Rahmouni, S., Boniver, J. & Delvenne, P. (2005). High levels of p105 (NFKB1) and p100 (NFKB2) proteins in HPV16-transformed keratinocytes: role of E6 and E7 oncoproteins. *Virology, 331(2)*: 357-366.

Heng, B.C. & Cao, T. (2005). Making cell-permeable antibodies (Transbody) through fusion of protein transduction domains (PTD) with single chain variable fragment (scFv) antibodies: potential advantages over antibodies expressed within the intracellular environment (Intrabody). *Med. Hypotheses, 64(6)*: 1105-1108.

Holliger, P. & Hudson, P.J. (2005). Engineered antibody fragments and the rise of single domains. *Nat. Biotechnol., 23(9)*: 1126-1136.

Hoogenboom, H.R. (2005). Selecting and screening recombinant antibody libraries. *Nat. Biotechnol., 23(9)*: 1105-1116.

Indraccolo, S., Habeler, W., Tisato, V., Stievano, L., Piovan, E., Tosello, V., Esposito, G., Wagner, R., Uberla, K., Chieco-Bianchi, L. & Amadori, A. (2002). Gene transfer in ovarian cancer cells: a comparison between retroviral and lentiviral vectors. *Cancer Res., 62(21)*: 6099-6107.

Jain, K.K. (2005). Nanotechnology-based drug delivery for cancer. *Technol Cancer Res. Treat., 4(4)*: 407-416.

Jang, S.H., Wientjes, M.G., Lu, D. & Au, J.L. (2003). Drug delivery and transport to solid tumors. *Pharm. Res., 20(9)*: 1337-1350.

Jiang, M. & Milner, J. (2005). Selective silencing of viral gene E6 and E7 expression in HPV-positive human cervical carcinoma cells using small interfering RNAs. *Methods Mol. Biol., 292*: 401-420.

Joliot, A. & Prochiantz, A. (2004). Transduction peptides: from technology to physiology. *Nat. Cell. Biol., 6(3)*: 189-196.

Kasono, K., Heike, Y., Xiang, J., Piche, A., Kim, H.G., Kim, M., Hagiwara, M., Nawrath, M., Moelling, K. & Curiel, D.T. (2000). Tetracycline-induced expression of an anti-c-Myb single-chain antibody and its inhibitory effect on proliferation of the human leukemia cell line K562. *Cancer Gene Ther., 7(1)*: 151-159.

Kelley, M.L., Keiger, K.E., Lee, C.J. & Huibregtse, J.M. (2005). The global transcriptional effects of the human papillomavirus E6 protein in cervical carcinoma cell lines are mediated by the E6AP ubiquitin ligase. *J. Virol., 79(6)*: 3737-3747.

Ko, D., Hawkins, L. &Yu, D.C. (2005). Development of transcriptionally regulated oncolytic adenoviruses. *Oncogene, 24(52)*: 7763-7774.

Kommareddy, S., Tiwari, S.B. & Amiji, M.M. (2005). Long-circulating polymeric nanovectors for tumor-selective gene delivery. *Technol. Cancer Res. Treat., 4(6)*: 615-625.

Kontermann, R.E. (2004). Intrabodies as therapeutic agents. *Methods, 34(2)*: 163-170.

Kopito, R.R. (2000). Aggresomes, inclusion bodies and protein aggregation. *Trends Cell Biol., 10(12)*: 524-530.

Krauss, J., Arndt, M.A., Martin, A.C., Liu, H. & Rybak, S.M. (2003). Specificity grafting of human antibody frameworks selected from a phage display library: generation of a highly stable humanized anti-CD22 single-chain Fv fragment. *Protein Eng., 16(10)*: 753-759.

Krichevsky, A., Graessmann, A., Nissim, A., Piller, S.C., Zakai, N. & Loyter, A. (2003). Antibody fragments selected by phage display against the nuclear localization signal of the HIV-1 Vpr protein inhibit nuclear import in permeabilized and intact cultured cells. *Virology, 305(1)*: 77-92.

Lamikanra, A., Pan, Z.K., Isaacs, S.N., Wu, T.C. & Paterson, Y. (2001). Regression of established human papillomavirus type 16 (HPV-16) immortalized tumors in vivo by vaccinia viruses expressing different forms of HPV-16 E7 correlates with enhanced CD8(+) T-cell responses that home to the tumor site. *J. Virol., 75(20)*: 9654-9664.

Lavia, P. & Jansen-Durr, P. (1999). E2F target genes and cell-cycle checkpoint control. *Bioessays, 21(3)*: 221-230.

Lener, M., Horn, I.R., Cardinale, A., Messina, S., Nielsen, U.B., Rybak, S.M., Hoogenboom, H.R., Cattaneo, A. & Biocca, S. (2000). Diverting a protein from its cellular location by intracellular antibodies. The case of p21Ras. *Eur J. Biochem., 267(4)*: 1196-1205.

Liu, F., Kumar, M., Ma, Q., Duval, M., Kuhrt, D., Junghans, R., Posner, M. & Cavacini, L. (2005). Human single-chain antibodies inhibit replication of human immunodeficiency virus type 1 (HIV-1). *AIDS Res. Hum. Retroviruses, 21(10)*: 876-881.

Liu, Y., Liu, Z., Androphy, E., Chen, J. & Baleja, J.D. (2004). Design and characterization of helical peptides that inhibit the E6 protein of papillomavirus. *Biochemistry, 43(23)*: 7421-7431.

Lobato, M.N. & Rabbitts, T.H. (2003). Intracellular antibodies and challenges facing their use as therapeutic agents. *Trends Mol. Med. 9(9)*: 390-396.

Malanchi, I., Caldeira, S., Krutzfeldt, M., Giarre, M., Alunni-Fabbroni, M. & Tommasino, M. (2002). Identification of a novel activity of human papillomavirus type 16 E6 protein in deregulating the G1/S transition. *Oncogene, 21(37)*: 5665-5672.

Malanchi, I., Accardi, R., Diehl, F., Smet, A., Androphy, E., Hoheisel, J. & Tommasino, M. (2004). Human papillomavirus type 16 E6 promotes retinoblastoma protein phosphorylation and cell cycle progression. *J. Virol., 78(24)*: 13769-13778.

Mantovani, F. & Banks, L. (2001). The human papillomavirus E6 protein and its contribution to malignant progression. *Oncogene, 20(54)*: 7874-7887.

Mao, C., Koutsky, L.A., Ault, K.A., Wheeler, C.M., Brown, D.R., Wiley, D.J., Alvarez, F.B., Bautista, O.M., Jansen, K.U. & Barr, E. (2006). Efficacy of human papillomavirus-16 vaccine to prevent cervical intraepithelial neoplasia: a randomized controlled trial. *Obstet. Gynecol., 107(1)*: 18-27.

Marasco, W.A., LaVecchio, J. & Winkler, A. (1999). Human anti-HIV-1 tat sFv intrabodies for gene therapy of advanced HIV-1-infection and AIDS. *J. Immunol. Methods, 231(1-2)*: 223-238.

Marasco, W.A. (2005). Therapeutic antibody gene transfer. Nat. Biotechnol., 23(5): 551-552.

Martineau, P., Jones, P. & Winter, G. (1998). Expression of an antibody fragment at high levels in the bacterial cytoplasm. *J. Mol. Biol., 280(1)*: 117-127.

Mazurek, S., Zwerschke, W., Jansen-Durr, P. & Eigenbrodt, E. (2001). Metabolic cooperation between different oncogenes during cell transformation: interaction between activated ras and HPV-16 E7. *Oncogene, 20(47)*: 6891-6898.

Mountain, A. (2000). Gene therapy: the first decade. *Trends Biotechnol., 18(3)*: 119-128.

Munger, K., Basile, J.R., Duensing, S., Eichten, A., Gonzalez, S.L., Grace, M. & Zacny, V.L. (2001). Biological activities and molecular targets of the human papillomavirus E7 oncoprotein. *Oncogene, 20(54)*: 7888-7898.

Munger, K. & Howley, P.M. (2002). Human papillomavirus immortalization and transformation functions. *Virus Res., 89(2)*: 213-228.

Myers, K.A., Ryan, M.G., Stern, P.L., Shaw, D.M., Embleton, M.J., Kingsman, S.M. & Carroll, M.W. (2002). Targeting immune effector molecules to human tumor cells through genetic delivery of 5T4-specific scFv fusion proteins. *Cancer Gene Ther., 9(11)*: 884-896.

O'Brien, P.M. & Campo, M.S. (2003). Papillomaviruses: a correlation between immune evasion and oncogenicity? *Trends Microbiol., 11(7)*: 300-305.

Ohlfest, J.R., Freese, A.B. & Largaespada, D.A. (2005). Nonviral vectors for cancer gene therapy: prospects for integrating vectors and combination therapies. *Curr. Gene Ther., 5(6)*: 629-641.

Onda, M., Wang, Q.C., Guo, H.F., Cheung, N.K. & Pastan, I. (2004). In vitro and in vivo cytotoxic activities of recombinant immunotoxin 8H9(Fv)-PE38 against breast cancer, osteosarcoma, and neuroblastoma. *Cancer Res., 64(4)*: 1419-1424.

Orgad, S., Goldfinger, N., Cohen, G., Rotter, V. & Solomon, B. (2005). Single chain antibody against the common epitope of mutant p53 restores wild-type activity to mutant p53 protein. *FEBS Lett., 579(25)*: 5609-5615.

Persic, L., Righi, M., Roberts, A., Hoogenboom, H.R., Cattaneo, A. & Bradbury, A. (1997a). Targeting vectors for intracellular immunisation. *Gene, 187(1)*: 1-8.

Persic, L., Roberts, A., Wilton, J., Cattaneo, A., Bradbury, A. & Hoogenboom, H.R. (1997b). An integrated vector system for the eukaryotic expression of antibodies or their fragments after selection from phage display libraries. *Gene, 187(1)*: 9-18.

Pim, D., Massimi, P., Dilworth, S.M. & Banks, L. (2005). Activation of the protein kinase B pathway by the HPV-16 E7 oncoprotein occurs through a mechanism involving interaction with PP2A. *Oncogene, 24(53)*: 7830-7838.

Pini, A., Giuliani, A., Ricci, C., Runci, Y. & Bracci, L. (2004). Strategies for the construction and use of peptide and antibody libraries displayed on phages. *Curr. Protein Pept. Sci., 5(6)*: 487-496.

Pini, A., Viti, F., Santucci, A., Carnemolla, B., Zardi, L., Neri, P. & Neri, D. (1998). Design and use of a phage display library. Human antibodies with subnanomolar affinity against a marker of angiogenesis eluted from a two-dimensional gel. *J. Biol. Chem., 273(34)*: 21769-21776.

Qian, J., Dong, Y., Pang, Y.Y., Ibrahim, R., Berzofsky, J.A., Schiller, J.T. & Khleif, S.N. (2006). Combined prophylactic and therapeutic cancer vaccine: Enhancing CTL responses to HPV16 E2 using a chimeric VLP in HLA-A2 mice. *Int. J. Cancer Jun 15, 118(12)*: 3022-3029.

Rainov, N.G. & Ren, H. (2003). Clinical trials with retrovirus mediated gene therapy--what have we learned? *J. Neurooncol., 65(3)*: 227-236.

Raper, S.E., Yudkoff, M., Chirmule, N., Gao, G.P., Nunes, F., Haskal, Z.J., Furth, E.E., Propert, K.J., Robinson, M.B., Magosin, S., Simoes, H., Speicher, L., Hughes, J., Tazelaar, J., Wivel, N.A., Wilson, J.M. & Batshaw, M.L. (2002). A pilot study of in vivo liver-directed gene transfer with an adenoral vector in partial ornithine transcarbamylase deficiency. *Hum. Gene Ther., 13(1)*: 163-175.

Russell, J.S., Lang, F.F., Huet, T., Janicot, M., Chada, S., Wilson, D.R. & Tofilon, P.J. (1999). Radiosensitization of human tumor cell lines induced by the adenovirus-mediated expression of an anti-Ras single-chain antibody fragment. *Cancer Res., 59(20)*: 5239-5244.

Santin, A.D., Bellone, S., Roman, J.J., Burnett, A., Cannon, M.J. & Pecorelli, S. (2005). Therapeutic vaccines for cervical cancer: dendritic cell-based immunotherapy. *Curr. Pharm. Des., 11(27)*: 3485-3500.

Sarkar, A.K., Tortolero-Luna, G., Follen, M. & Sastry, K.J. (2005). Inverse correlation of cellular immune responses specific to synthetic peptides from the E6 and E7 oncoproteins of HPV-16 with recurrence of cervical intraepithelial neoplasia in a cross-sectional study. *Gynecol. Oncol., 99*: S251-61.

Schiller, J.T. & Lowy, D.R. (2001). Papillomavirus-like particle vaccines. *J Natl Cancer Inst Monogr., (28)*: 50-54.

Sibler, A.P., Nordhammer, A., Masson, M., Martineau, P., Trave, G. & Weiss, E. (2003). Nucleocytoplasmic shuttling of antigen in mammalian cells conferred by a soluble versus insoluble single-chain antibody fragment equipped with import/export signals. *Exp. Cell Res., 286 (2)*: 276-287.

Sibler, A.P., Courtete, J., Muller, C.D., Zeder-Lutz, G. & Weiss, E. (2005). Extended half-life upon binding of destabilized intrabodies allows specific detection of antigen in mammalian cells. *FEBS J., 272(11)*: 2878-2891.

Stanley, M. (2003). Immune intervention in HPV infections: current progress and future developments. Expert Rev. Vaccines., 2(5): 615-617.

Stanley, M. (2005). Immune responses to human papillomavirus. *Vaccine, Sep 19.* [Epub ahead of print]

Tang, S., Tao, M., McCoy, J.P. & Zheng, Z.M. (2006). Short-term induction and long-term suppression of HPV16 oncogene silencing by RNA interference in cervical cancer cells. *Oncogene 25*: 2094-2104.

Tavladoraki, P., Girotti, A., Donini, M., Arias, F.J., Mancini, C., Morea, V., Chiaraluce, R., Consalvi, V. & Benvenuto, E. (1999). A single-chain antibody fragment is functionally expressed in the cytoplasm of both Escherichia coli and transgenic plants. *Eur. J. Biochem., 262(2)*: 617-624.

Thomas, M., Pim, D. & Banks, L. (1999). The role of the E6-p53 interaction in the molecular pathogenesis of HPV. *Oncogene, 18(53)*: 7690-7700.

Tse, E., Chung, G. & Rabbitts, T.H. (2002). Isolation of antigen-specific intracellular antibody fragments as single chain Fv for use in mammalian cells. *Methods Mol. Biol., 185*: 433-446.

Vascotto, F. Campagna, M., Visintin, M., Cattaneo, A. & Burrone, O.R. (2004). Effects of intrabodies specific for rotavirus NSP5 during the virus replicative cycle. *J. Gen. Virol., 85(Pt 11)*: 3285-3290.

Vasir, J.K. & Labhasetwar, V. (2005). Targeted drug delivery in cancer therapy. *Technol. Cancer Res. Treat., 4(4)*: 363-374.

Venturini, F., Braspenning, J., Homann, M., Gissmann, L. & Sczakiel, G., (1999). Kinetic selection of HPV 16 E6/E7-directed antisense nucleic acids: anti-proliferative effects on HPV 16-transformed cells. *Nucleic Acids Res., 27(7)*: 1585-1592.

Visintin, M., Tse, E., Axelson, H., Rabbitts, T.H. & Cattaneo, A. (1999). Selection of antibodies for intracellular function using a two-hybrid in vivo system. *Proc. Natl. Acad. Sci U.S.A., 96(21)*: 11723-11728.

Visintin, M., Settanni, G., Maritan, A., Graziosi, S., Marks, J.D. & Cattaneo, A. (2002). The intracellular antibody capture technology (IACT): towards a consensus sequence for intracellular antibodies. *J. Mol. Biol., 317(1)*: 73-83.

Visintin, M., Meli, G.A., Cannistraci, I. & Cattaneo, A. (2004a). Intracellular antibodies for proteomics. *J. Immunol. Methods., 290(1-2)*: 135-153.

Visintin, M., Quondam, M. & Cattaneo, A. (2004b). The intracellular antibody capture technology: towards the high-throughput selection of functional intracellular antibodies for target validation. *Methods, 34(2)*: 200-214.

Vitaliti, A., Wittmer, M., Steiner, R., Wyder, L., Neri, D. & Klemenz, R. (2000). Inhibition of tumor angiogenesis by a single-chain antibody directed against vascular endothelial growth factor. *Cancer Res., 60(16)*: 4311-4314.

Wang, S.S. & Hildesheim, A. (2003). Chapter 5: Viral and host factors in human papillomavirus persistence and progression. *J. Natl. Cancer Inst. Monogr., 31*: 35-40.

Wang-Johanning, F., Gillespie, G.Y., Grim, J., Rancourt, C., Alvarez, R.D., Siegal, G.P. & Curiel, D.T. (1998). Intracellular expression of a single-chain antibody directed against human papillomavirus type 16 E7 oncoprotein achieves targeted antineoplastic effects. *Cancer Res., 58(9)*: 1893-1900.

Willuda, J., Honegger, A., Waibel, R., Schubiger, P.A., Stahel, R., Zangemeister-Wittke, U. & Pluckthun, A. (1999). High thermal stability is essential for tumor targeting of antibody fragments: engineering of a humanized anti-epithelial glycoprotein-2 (epithelial cell adhesion molecule) single-chain Fv fragment. *Cancer Res., 59(22)*: 5758-5767.

Wirtz, P. & Steipe, B. (1999).Intrabody construction and expression III: engineering hyperstable V(H) domains. *Protein Sci., 8(11)*: 2245-2250.

Worn, A., Auf der Maur, A., Escher, D., Honegger, A., Barberis, A. & Pluckthun, A. (2000). Correlation between in vitro stability and in vivo performance of anti-GCN4 intrabodies as cytoplasmic inhibitors. *J. Biol. Chem., 275(4)*: 2795-2803.

Worn, A. & Pluckthun, A. (2001). Stability engineering of antibody single-chain Fv fragments. *J. Mol. Biol., 305(5)*: 989-1010.

Young, L.S., Searle, P.F., Onion, D. & Mautner, V. (2006). Viral gene therapy strategies: from basic science to clinical application. *J. Pathol., 208(2)*: 299-318.

zur Hausen, H. (2000). Papillomaviruses causing cancer: evasion from host-cell control in early events in carcinogenesis. *J. Natl. Cancer Inst., 92(9)*: 690-698.

zur Hausen, H. (2002). Papillomaviruses and cancer: from basic studies to clinical application. *Nat. Rev. Cancer, 2(5)*: 342-350.

Zwerschke, W. & Jansen-Durr, P. (2000). Cell transformation by the E7 oncoprotein of human papillomavirus type 16: interactions with nuclear and cytoplasmic target proteins. *Adv. Cancer Res., 78*: 1-29.

In: Trends in Cervical Cancer
Editor: Hector T. Varaj, pp. 149-165

ISBN: 1-60021-299-9
© 2007 Nova Science Publishers, Inc.

Chapter VII

PREDICTORS OF RADIATION RESPONSE IN CERVIX CANCER

L.T. Tan[*] and M. Zahra

Dept. of Oncology, Addenbrooke's NHS Trust, Cambridge, UK

ABSTRACT

Radiotherapy is the treatment of choice for locally advanced carcinoma of the cervix. Clinical trials have shown that the addition of concurrent platinum-based chemotherapy improves 3-year survival by 8-19%. Whilst the survival gains are impressive, the risk of serious late toxicity and its effect on long-term quality of life is a major concern. This is particularly important as a significant proportion of patients with advanced stage disease can be cured by radiotherapy alone. If techniques that have the potential to predict the response to radiotherapy could be identified, it may be possible to individualise treatment strategy in order to improve the therapeutic index of treatment. This could minimise morbidity in good prognosis patients (e.g. by omitting chemotherapy) whilst local control in poor prognosis patients could be maximised by intensification of treatment (e.g. by increasing the total dose, utilising alternative fractionation regimes, implementing novel sequencing of treatments, or by including additional modalities of treatment such as hypoxic cell sensitisers). For these predictive assays to be clinically useful, they would have to be reliable, reproducible and practical.

Several studies have attempted to identify potential predictive assays of radiation response in cervical cancer. Initial studies have investigated radiobiological predictors including cell proliferation kinetics, intrinsic tumour radiosensitivity and hypoxia. These assays assess the characteristics of the tumour and its microenvironment at the cellular level. Other studies have explored the potential of imaging techniques such as dynamic contrast enhanced magnetic resonance imaging, magnetic resonance spectroscopy and positron emission tomography, to predict radiation response. The early emphasis is on

---

[*] Correspondence concerning this article should be addressed to Dr L T Tan, Oncology Centre, Box 193, Cambridge University Hospitals NHS Foundation Trust, Hills Road, Cambridge CB2 2QQ, U.K Email: litee.tan@addenbrookes.nhs.uk

techniques for evaluating tumour vascular physiology and its effect on tumour oxygenation. More recently, new techniques and probes for studying other processes at the cellular and molecular levels have been developed, so-called molecular imaging. These techniques include immunohistochemistry assays as well as genomic and tissue microarray technology, and proteomics analyses.

This article reviews the published studies on predictive assays for cervix cancer and discusses their clinical relevance.

Keywords: cervical cancer, predictors, radiation response

INTRODUCTION

The ultimate goal of cancer treatment is the successful tailoring of treatment for individual patients in order to maximise cure while minimising morbidity. Good prognosis patients can be given less treatment to minimise unnecessary toxicity, whilst poor prognosis patients can be offered more intensive treatment to improve the chance of cure. For cervix cancer, the potential for individualisation of treatment is particularly promising as there is a wide range of treatment options available, including surgery, external beam radiotherapy, intracavitary and interstitial brachytherapy, cytotoxic chemotherapy and hypoxic cell sensitisers. There is therefore great scope for intensification of treatment e.g. by combining two or more modalities of treatment, introducing novel sequencing of treatments, increasing the radiation dose and utilising alternative fractionation regimes.

The clinicopathological factors known to influence prognosis in cervical cancer include disease stage, tumour volume, histological type, lymphatic spread, and vascular invasion. Of these, only stage, volume and lymphatic spread, are routinely used to guide treatment decision. Thus surgery and radiotherapy are equally effective treatments for early stage, small volume, node-negative disease. For bulky, advanced stage or node-positive disease, radiotherapy is the treatment of choice. The combination of surgery and radiotherapy appears to increase the risk of toxicity without improving cure rates [1]. In contrast, the addition of platinum-based chemotherapy to radiotherapy improves 3-year survival by 8-19% [2] and chemo-radiation is now the standard treatment for poor prognosis disease. Whilst the survival gains are impressive, the risk of increased serious late toxicity and its effect on long-term quality of life is a major concern. This is particularly important as a significant proportion of patients with poor prognosis disease are cured by radiotherapy alone. Improved techniques for predicting the response to radiotherapy are therefore necessary to facilitate individualisation and intensification of treatment strategy for poor prognosis disease.

The essential features of a clinically useful predictive tool were discussed in a recent review article by Simon [3]. He stated that such a tool should be therapeutically relevant and should offer additional predictive accuracy to that provided by standard prognostic factors. It must demonstrate reproducibility of measurements between centres, and between times and observers for the same centre. Its clinical usefulness should be independently validated in prospectively planned studies. For the purpose of treatment individualisation, the tool must also be practical, in terms of its ability to produce rapid results and the resources required for implementation.

The cellular factors that influence tumour response to radiotherapy include intrinsic radiosensitivity, proliferation, repair and apoptosis, and tumour vascularity and hypoxia. All these factors have been investigated as potential predictors of radiation response for clinical use. In general, the assays used to evaluate these factors can be divided into 4 groups:

- Radiobiological assays involving direct measurements of the various factors
- Immunohistochemical assays involving surrogate markers
- Molecular assays involving genomic and proteomic analyses and microarray technology
- Imaging assays involving magnetic resonance and positron emission tomography

This article reviews the published literature on those assays with clinical data and discusses their potential for treatment individualisation.

RADIOBIOLOGICAL ASSAYS

Radiosensitivity

The relationship between response to radiotherapy and cellular intrinsic radiosensitivity was first explored in the 1980s. The most widely used measure of intrinsic radiosensitivity is the surviving fraction after 2 Gray (SF2), following seminal work from the Institut Gustave-Roussy [4] indicating a good correlation between measured SF2 values of different tumour types and clinical experience of their radioresponsiveness. Thus measured SF2 values for radiosensitive tumours such as lymphomas and small cell carcinomas are 1.7-2.6 times smaller than for glioblastoma, a radioresistant tumour.

Much of the work evaluating SF2 as a predictive tool in cervix cancer has been undertaken by West and colleagues from the Patterson Institute for Cancer Research in Manchester. Using a soft agar clonogenic assay, they reported that the 5-year survival rate for tumours with SF2 values below the median was 81% compared to 51% for those with SF2 values above the median (p = 0.0002) [5]. The correlation between patient survival and decreasing tumour cell radiosensitivity remained significant when the SF2 values were divided into 4 quartiles (p = 0.0019). By independently processing multiple biopsies from 18 tumours, they found no significant heterogeneity in intra-tumour SF2 values (p = 0.30) [6]. However, other groups [7] suggest that intra-tumoural heterogeneity of cellular radiosensitivity may vary by as much as 3-fold which would be a major confounding factor to the use of pre-treatment measurements of radiosensitivity to predict clinical radioresponsiveness. Moreover, even in expert hands, successful colony growth was only in the region of 75%. The process is labour intensive and takes about 4 weeks to produce a result. Other assays of SF2 e.g. the cell adhesive matrix (CAM) assay and the tetrazolium (MTT) assay have similar shortcomings. Radiosensitivity assays in their present form are not useful as predictive tools for therapeutic individualisation in cervix cancer.

Cell Proliferation

It is well established that prolongation of overall treatment time in radical radiotherapy has an adverse effect on tumour control for certain tumour types. The hypothesis is that tumours undergo accelerated growth after 3-4 weeks of radiotherapy. This phenomenon is likely to be more pronounced in those tumours with short proliferation times and this is supported by clinical data which indicate that accelerated repopulation is particularly a problem in squamous cell tumours. An assay for measuring proliferation times could therefore be useful as a predictor for therapeutic individualisation in cervix cancer.

The most widely used technique for measuring proliferation rate involves *in vitro* or *in vivo* incorporation of bromodeoxyuridine followed by assessment of the labeling index (proportion of cells synthesizing DNA), DNA synthesis time and potential doubling time, using flow cytometry. Studies from different laboratories [8,9] have confirmed measurements of labelling index in cervix cancers ranging from around 1 to 40%. However, prospective studies [9] have failed to show a significant correlation between pretreatment proliferation parameters and tumour control. Interest in cell proliferation assays as a predictive tool in cervix cancer is currently limited.

Hypoxia

Tumour hypoxia is associated with decreased sensitivity to radiation. The mechanisms determining the degree of hypoxia in tumours include structural and functional abnormalities in tumour microvasculature, differences in diffusion distances and anaemia. Direct measurements of tumour oxygenation can be obtained by inserting polarographic needle electrodes into tumours. Using this method, several groups [10-13] have shown significant correlations between tumour oxygen pressure (pO2) and clinical outcome in cervix cancer. For example, Fyles *et al* [11] reported that progression-free survival for patients with hypoxic tumours was 37% at 3 years versus 67% in those patients with better oxygenated tumours (p = 0.004). However, the technique is invasive and requires the use of specialised equipment and skills. There is also significant intra-tumoural heterogeneity and multiple measurements are needed to adequately sample a tumour. The use of direct measurements of tumour oxygenation as a predictive tool in cervix cancer has not progressed beyond the research setting to date.

IMMUNOHISTOCHEMICAL (IHC) ASSAYS

In view of the problems with direct assays, interest has turned to the use of IHC markers as surrogate measures of the radiobiological factors influencing radiation response. A number of these markers have been identified and their potential as predictive assays is discussed below.

Hypoxia

Several IHC markers have been assessed as surrogate measures of hypoxia in cervix cancer. One of the more extensively studied markers is hypoxia inducible factor 1 alpha (HIF-1alpha), a nuclear protein which accumulates under hypoxic conditions and acts as a promoter for various genes involved in erythropoietin production, angiogenesis and glucose metabolism. HIF-1alpha expression can be assessed in formalin-fixed tumour biopsies, using a visual semi-quantitative scoring system. A number of studies [14,15] have shown significant but modest correlations between HIF-1alpha expression and polarographic oxygen measurements (r = 0.26-0.40). This correlation appears to be independent of tumour stage, grade, size and histology. Several studies [16-18] have shown correlations between increased HIF-1alpha expression and poor overall survival and distant metastasis in cervical cancer. However, other studies have shown either variable [15] or no correlation [14] between high HIF-1alpha expression and patient outcome. The value of HIF-1alpha as a predictor of outcome in cervix cancer requires further clarification.

Another intrinsic marker of tumour hypoxia that has aroused interest as a predictor of outcome in cervix cancer is carbonic anhydrase IX (CA IX). CA IX is a transmembrane glycoprotein involved in pH regulation whose production is regulated by several factors including HIF-1alpha. It is expressed in several tumour types including cervix cancer but is not normally expressed by non-malignant cells. Studies of the correlation of CA IX expression and polarographic oxygen measurements have produced contradictory results [19-21]. Similarly, the predictive value of CA IX in cervix cancer is unclear with one study [19] reporting an association with outcome whilst another [20] did not find any correlation. Based on current evidence, CA IX is unreliable as a predictor of outcome in cervix cancer. Other markers including thymidine phosphorylase [22] and glucose transporter Glut-1 [23] have also been studied as markers of hypoxia and correlated with outcome. The predictive value of these markers remains to be evaluated.

Vascularity

Angiogenesis is one of the compensatory mechanisms for hypoxia in tumours. The extent of this phenomenon can be assessed by scoring the microvessel density (MVD) in formalin-fixed, paraffin-embedded tumour biopsies stained with anti-factor VIII. In general, retrospective studies evaluating tumour vascularity in cervix cancer [24,25] have shown significant correlations with outcome after radiotherapy. For example, one study [24] showed that patients with low tumour MVD, indicating less tumour hypoxia, had a disease-free survival at 5 years of 65% compared to 40% for those with high MVD scores (p = 0.0036).

Tumour vascularity can also be assessed using a number of surrogate markers known to be involved in angiogenesis. Several groups [26-28] have shown that increased expression of cycloxygenase-2 (COX-2) is associated with poor outcome after radiotherapy in cervix cancer. For example, Kim *et al* [27] reported that the 5-year survival for COX-2 positive patients is 57% compared to 83% for COX-2 negative patients. COX-2 is an inhibitor of angiogenesis and its overexpression may impair the ability of the tumour to compensate for hypoxia. In contrast, high expression of vascular endothelial growth factor (VEGF) in cervical tumours has also been shown to be associated with poor overall and metastasis-free survival [29]. In this case, VEGF reflects the biological aggressiveness of the tumour rather than its ability to respond to hypoxia. Markers of angiogenesis are potentially promising as predictors of radiotherapy response and as targets for therapeutic intervention.

Repair and Apoptosis

The role of DNA repair pathways in determining radiation sensitivity has been evaluated in cervix cancer. Using IHC of formalin-fixed sections of tumour biopsies, one study [30] showed that patients whose tumours had a low expression of Ku70, a protein involved in the repair of DNA double-strand breaks, had significantly higher survival (p = 0.046). Another study [31] evaluating the related enzyme Ku80, also showed significantly better survival in Ku80-negative patients compared with those who were Ku80-positive (p = 0.04).

If the DNA damage induced by radiation is beyond repair, the cell proceeds to programmed cell death or apoptosis. Various methods have been used for quantifying apoptosis as a measure of radiation sensitivity. The most commonly used are morphological assays, which evaluate the histological features of apoptosis, or the TUNEL assay (terminal deoxynucleotidyl transferase-mediated dUTP nick end labelling), which detects DNA fragmentation. Several studies have evaluated the prognostic value of apoptosis in cervix cancer. Two retrospective studies [32,33] reported that a high apoptotic index (AI) in adenocarcinoma of the cervix correlated with better overall survival. For squamous cell carcinomas of the cervix, one retrospective study [34] reported that a high AI was associated with improved local control and survival but a prospective study [35] reported that a high AI prior to treatment correlated with poor local control and long term prognosis. The *in vivo* radiation-induced AI after 4 or 24 hours did not predict radiotherapy outcome. Other groups [36-38] have assessed the value of the oncoproteins, Bcl-2 (anti-apoptotic) and Bax (pro-apoptotic), as prognostic factors in cervix cancer with conflicting results. Further prospective studies are required to clarify the predictive role of assays of apoptosis in radiotherapy.

Cell Proliferation and Tumour Growth

There has been surprisingly little interest in the use of IHC markers of proliferation as predictive factors in cervical cancer. One study [39] suggested that tumours with increased proliferative activity, as indicated by high Ki67 antigen expression and argyrophilic nucleolar organiser region (AgNOR) counts, responded better to radiotherapy. Another study [40] did not find a correlation between growth fraction before radiotherapy and outcome although high growth fraction after 9 Gy of radiotherapy predicted good outcome. More work is required to evaluate the role of cell proliferation rates in determining outcome in cervical cancer.

Other Genetic Markers

The expression of multifunction genes involved in cell cycle control, DNA repair and genomic stability can also be assessed by IHC. The most widely studied of these is the tumour suppressor gene p53; its mutation and nuclear accumulation has been shown to be associated with tumour progression, resistance to radiation and unfavourable outcome in many tumours. In cervix cancer, p53 over-expression in adenocarcinomas treated with radiotherapy was associated with a 5 year disease free survival of 30% compared to 62% for p53 negative tumours [41]. Other groups have shown associations between poor prognosis and over expression of p63 [42], which functions as both an oncogene and a tumour suppressor gene, and the proto-oncogenes, epidermal growth factor receptor (EGFR/HER1) [42,43] and c-erbB-2 (HER2) [43,44]. Antibodies against several of these receptors have been developed e.g. cetuximab (anti-EGFR) and trastuzumab (anti-HER2) and IHC is used clinically to identify appropriate patients for treatment for other tumour types.

The large number of promising IHC markers identified has resulted in the development of high throughput histological studies based on tissue microarray technology. Tissue microarray involves the use of automated systems to analyse the expression of a particular marker in multiple samples simultaneously, using IHC, fluorescence in-situ hybridization, or RNA in-situ hybridization [45]. The technology is fast and cost efficient and has better standardization since the same batch of reagents can be used for a large number of samples from different sources.

MOLECULAR ASSAYS

Genetic Predictors

There has long been considerable interest in the genetic mechanisms underlying tumour genesis and growth but progress was limited by technical difficulties. The first efficient technique for genetic analysis is the polymerase chain reaction (PCR), first described in the 1980s, which allows amplification of specific DNA sequences in a matter of hours. PCR has been used to evaluate the presence of human papillomavirus (HPV) DNA as a prognostic indicator of response to radiotherapy in cervical cancers. Several studies [46-48] reported that HPV negative tumours had a poorer outcome after radiotherapy compared to HPV positive tumours. One hypothesis is that HPV infection leads to the inactivation of functional p53 [49]. Other studies have used PCR to evaluate the prognostic value of apoptotic genes [50,51] and DNA repair genes [52] on survival after radiotherapy in cervix cancer.

Traditional methods of genetic analysis can only examine a few genes at a time, and do not allow analysis of the complex interactions between different genes and their products. This has lead to the development of high throughput microarray gene expression profiling, which can monitor the expression of mRNA from thousands of genes simultaneously from large numbers of samples in parallel [53]. The technology requires high quality RNA usually from snap frozen tissues, and retrospective studies are limited as it is difficult to obtain RNA from formalin fixed tissues. The RNA can be obtained from malignant cells alone using micro-dissection techniques or from whole tumour sections, which should reflect the interactions between the tumour, its stroma and the immune system. Typical arrays will produce data on the expression of thousands of genes from a small number of samples requiring specialised data management and complex statistical analysis.

Two groups [54,55] have used molecular profiling in cervical cancer cell lines to identify signatures predictive of *in vitro* radiation response. Both groups identified a set of genes that statistically differentiated between radioresponsive and radioresistant tumours. Several of the genes identified were already known to influence the response to radiotherapy but there was almost no overlap between the two gene sets. Other studies [56,57] have reported gene sets that can classify patients with cervical cancers according to their radiation sensitivity and clinical outcome but again there was very little overlap in the gene sets identified by different groups.

The main limitation of molecular profiling studies to date is their small patient numbers, especially when compared to the number of genes interrogated by each microarray. There is considerable variation in the microarrays used, and in tissue preparation, probe hybridization and image analysis, resulting in poor intra and inter laboratory reproducibility. One review [53] has described high rates of tumour misclassification and frequent use of unstable molecular signatures in published studies. The magnitude of data sets generated can result in spurious correlations of no clinical significance being identified, especially when arbitrarily chosen cut-off levels are often used to identify differential gene expression. At present, the technology remains largely a research tool for generating hypothesis and any predictive molecular signatures identified will require validation in large, prospective clinical trials.

Protein Predictors

The emerging field of proteomics involves the large scale study of all the proteins expressed by a genome. Whilst the genome of a tumour is relatively constant, the protein complement or proteome differs from cell to cell and is constantly changing through its biochemical interactions with the genome and the environment. There is currently considerable interest in using the protein signatures resulting from cancer to guide diagnosis, prognosis, and response to therapy. At its most basic, this involves the measurement of a single protein in the serum. Various serum markers have been shown to correlate with outcome after radiotherapy in cervix cancer including squamous cell carcinoma antigen (SCC) [58-60], cancer antigen 125 (CA125) [60,61], the cytokeratin degradation product CYFRA 21.1 [62], vascular endothelial growth factor (VEGF) [63], N-acetylgalsctosamindase (NaGalase), which reflects immunological function [64], and tissue polypeptide antigen (TPA), which is a marker of proliferation [61]. Most of the studies are retrospective and none of the tumour markers has been incorporated into routine clinical use. A panel of protein markers that reflect the interplay of the underlying disease processes is more likely to be useful as predictor of treatment response.

Protein arrays, consisting of chip-based protein capture systems combined with mass spectroscopy, have been developed for high throughput analyses of protein signatures. The technology remains in its infancy and in cervix cancer, it has only been used in one study

[65] to differentiate between carcinoma and normal cervix. Protein arrays are more complicated to generate than DNA arrays and the protein antibody interactions are much more complex than DNA base pairing. The dynamic state and magnitude of the proteome pose a considerable challenge and advanced computational analyses are required to deal with the data generated.

IMAGING ASSAYS

Dynamic Contrast Magnetic Resonance (DCE-MRI)

In DCE-MRI, changes in signal intensity resulting from the rapid injection of a paramagnetic contrast agent are used to characterise tumour permeability and perfusion. A number of studies have shown significant correlations between DCE-MRI parameters and some parameters of tumour vascularity and oxygenation including MVD [66] and polarographic oxygen tension measurements [67]. Several studies [67-70] have shown that quantitative analysis of the DCE-MRI enhancement pattern, prior to or during radiotherapy, can predict response to treatment in cervix cancer. For example, Mayr *et al* [69] showed that tumours with high signal intensity, reflecting good tissue perfusion, prior to and early during therapy had a lower incidence of local recurrence (13% vs. 67%, p = 0.05). An increase in signal intensity early during therapy was the strongest predictor of subsequent local recurrence (0% vs. 78%, p = 0.002). Pixel-by-pixel analysis of the enhancement pattern showed a wide spectrum of heterogeneity in perfusion with the quantity of low-enhancement regions significantly predicting subsequent tumour recurrence (88% vs. 0%, p = 0.0004) [71]. DCE-MRI parameters have been shown to be independent of tumour volume [67,72] and a number of studies [67,73] have shown that the combined analysis of tumour volume and enhancement characteristics improved the prediction of local control following radiotherapy.

DCE-MRI is potentially a promising predictive tool for therapeutic individualisation in cervix cancer. It is a non-invasive technique that utilises a commonly available clinical resource and provides additional predictive information within a clinically useful time frame. Its potential for identifying regions that are more likely to be resistant to radiotherapy which could become relevant with technological advances that allow additional radiation dose to be directed to specific tumour subvolumes [74]. The advent of new contrast agents and more powerful 3 Tesla imagers, together with the development of common analytic platforms to allow better comparisons between different studies, may further enhance its potential as a predictive tool.

Positron Emission Tomography (PET)

Tumours are known to have an increased capacity for glycolysis, which allows cell growth in physiologically adverse conditions [75]. This physiological process is mediated by membrane glucose transporters and can be imaged by PET in conjunction with uptake of the glucose analogue, [18F]-2-fluoro-2-deoxy-D-glucose (FDG). FDG-PET has been shown to be useful for the assessment of initial stage, monitoring of treatment response and detection of recurrent disease and is used to guide patient management in a number of tumour sites e.g. lung cancer, lymphoma.

In cervix cancer, the role of FDG-PET in influencing primary management remains to be established. FDG-PET is more sensitive in detecting lymph node metastases than CT or MRI [76]. For patients with positive paraaortic nodes, this allows the option of dose escalation with intensity modulated radiotherapy [77] although the benefit of dose escalation for microscopic disease is uncertain [78]. For patients with locally advanced disease but negative lymph nodes on FDG-PET, a non-randomised prospective study [79] suggests that the addition of chemotherapy to radiotherapy confers no benefit (5-year overall survival: 85% with radiotherapy, 81% with chemoradiation (p = 0.91)). If this finding is validated, the risk of serious late toxicity in this group of patients could be reduced by the omission of chemotherapy. For early stage disease, FDG-PET has a low sensitivity for detecting lymph node metastases compared to standard surgical staging [80] and cannot be reliably used to guide patient management. Pre-treatment FDG uptake of the primary tumour [81] may also be predictive of survival and may potentially be used to influence patient management.

FDG-PET is therefore potentially useful as a tool for individualising therapy in cervix cancer. The emergence of new tracers, e.g. Cu-PTSM and Cu-ATSM for evaluating blood flow and hypoxia [82], should further enhance the potential of PET as a predictive tool in cervix cancer.

Magnetic Resonance Spectroscopy (MRS)

MRS involves the use of magnetic resonance to obtain chemical information about tissue metabolites [83]. Whilst conventional MRI detects the magnetic resonance of water for anatomical detail, MRS detects the resonance frequency of specific atoms, e.g. ^{31}P, ^{1}H or ^{13}C, to provide information on the structure of the chemical compound. At present, MRS is largely used as a research diagnostic tool to differentiate between normal and malignant tissues, including cervix cancer. Whilst there are no published reports on the role of MRS as a predictor of radiation response in cervical cancer, one report [84] has described a reduction of CH2-triglycerides after neo-adjuvant chemotherapy although there was no association with outcome in this small group of patients. The potential of MRS as a predictive tool for cervix cancer remains to be assessed.

Blood Oxygenation Level Dependent (BOLD) MRI

BOLD MRI assesses the distortion in the magnetic field resulting from the paramagnetic properties of deoxygenated haemoglobin, leading to a measurable effect on the T2 relaxation time. Most reports of BOLD MRI assess tumour oxygen status by comparing the differences in MRI images obtained when breathing air or carbogen. In this way, it is hoped that BOLD MRI could be used to identify tumours which are likely to benefit from the use of carbogen and other hypoxic sensitizers. However, animal studies [85] have failed to show a correlation between the BOLD signal and the absolute measured pO2. At present, the role of BOLD MRI in the management of cancer remains under evaluation.

CONCLUSION

The response to radiotherapy is a complex process influenced by innumerable biochemical, physiological and genetic factors interacting at the cellular and molecular level. Of the assays discussed in this article, it is likely that those that offer a global view of the cancer process would be the most useful as predictive assays for the individualisation of treatment rather than those that target single factors. The most promising assays appear to be microarray molecular profiling and DCE-MRI and PET imaging. The dynamics of protein profiling may be too volatile for clinical use. Much work is required to standardise and validate the tools being developed in order to realise the goal of individual tailoring of treatment to minimise treatment morbidity whilst maximising patient cure.

REFERENCES

[1]   Landoni F, Maneo A, Colombo A, Placa F, Milani R, Perego P, et al. Randomised study of radical surgery versus radiotherapy for stage Ib-IIa cervical cancer. *Lancet* 1997; 350(9077):535-40.

[2]   Green JA, Kirwan JM, Tierney JF, Symonds P, Fresco L, Collingwood M, et al. Survival and recurrence after concomitant chemotherapy and radiotherapy for cancer of the uterine cervix: a systematic review and meta-analysis. *Lancet* 2001; 358(9284):781-6.

[3]   Simon R. Roadmap for developing and validating therapeutically relevant genomic classifiers. *J Clin Oncol* 2005; 23(29):7332-41.

[4]   Malaise EP, Fertil B, Chavaudra N, Guichard M. Distribution of radiation sensitivities for human tumor cells of specific histological types: comparison of in vitro to in vivo data. *Int J Radiat Oncol Biol Phys* 1986; 12(4):617-24.

[5]   West CM, Davidson SE, Roberts SA, Hunter RD. The independence of intrinsic radiosensitivity as a prognostic factor for patient response to radiotherapy of carcinoma of the cervix. *Br J Cancer* 1997; 76(9):1184-90.

[6]   Davidson SE, West CM, Roberts SA, Hendry JH, Hunter RD. Radiosensitivity testing of primary cervical carcinoma: evaluation of intra- and inter-tumour heterogeneity. *Radiother Oncol* 1990; 18(4):349-56.

[7]   Britten RA, Evans AJ, Allalunis-Turner MJ, Franko AJ, Pearcey RG. Intratumoral heterogeneity as a confounding factor in clonogenic assays for tumour radioresponsiveness. *Radiother Oncol* 1996; 39(2):145-53.

[8]   Gasinska A, Urbanski K, Jakubowicz J, Klimek M, Biesaga B, Wilson GD. Tumour cell kinetics as a prognostic factor in squamous cell carcinoma of the cervix treated with radiotherapy. *Radiother Oncol* 1999; 50(1):77-84.

[9]   Tsang RW, Juvet S, Pintilie M, Hill RP, Wong CS, Milosevic M, et al. Pretreatment proliferation parameters do not add predictive power to clinical factors in cervical cancer treated with definitive radiation therapy. *Clin Cancer Res* 2003; 9(12):4387-95.

[10] Cooper RA, West CM, Logue JP, Davidson SE, Miller A, Roberts S, et al. Changes in oxygenation during radiotherapy in carcinoma of the cervix. *Int J Radiat Oncol Biol Phys* 1999; 45(1):119-26.

[11] Fyles A, Milosevic M, Hedley D, Pintilie M, Levin W, Manchul L, et al. Tumor hypoxia has independent predictor impact only in patients with node-negative cervix cancer. *J Clin Oncol* 2002; 20(3):680-7.

[12] Hockel M, Vorndran B, Schlenger K, Baussmann E, Knapstein PG. Tumor oxygenation: a new predictive parameter in locally advanced cancer of the uterine cervix. *Gynecol Oncol* 1993; 51(2):141-9.

[13] Lyng H, Sundfor K, Rofstad EK. Changes in tumor oxygen tension during radiotherapy of uterine cervical cancer: relationships to changes in vascular density, cell density, and frequency of mitosis and apoptosis. *Int J Radiat Oncol Biol Phys* 2000; 46(4):935-46.

[14] Haugland HK, Vukovic V, Pintilie M, Fyles AW, Milosevic M, Hill RP, et al. Expression of hypoxia-inducible factor-1alpha in cervical carcinomas: correlation with tumor oxygenation. *Int J Radiat Oncol Biol Phys* 2002; 53(4):854-61.

[15] Hutchison GJ, Valentine HR, Loncaster JA, Davidson SE, Hunter RD, Roberts SA, et al. Hypoxia-inducible factor 1alpha expression as an intrinsic marker of hypoxia: correlation with tumor oxygen, pimonidazole measurements, and outcome in locally advanced carcinoma of the cervix. *Clin Cancer Res* 2004; 10(24):8405-12.

[16] Bachtiary B, Schindl M, Potter R, Dreier B, Knocke TH, Hainfellner JA, et al. Overexpression of hypoxia-inducible factor 1alpha indicates diminished response to radiotherapy and unfavorable prognosis in patients receiving radical radiotherapy for cervical cancer. *Clin Cancer Res* 2003; 9(6):2234-40.

[17] Burri P, Djonov V, Aebersold DM, Lindel K, Studer U, Altermatt HJ, et al. Significant correlation of hypoxia-inducible factor-1alpha with treatment outcome in cervical cancer treated with radical radiotherapy. *Int J Radiat Oncol Biol Phys* 2003; 56(2):494-501.

[18] Ishikawa H, Sakurai H, Hasegawa M, Mitsuhashi N, Takahashi M, Masuda N, et al. Expression of hypoxic-inducible factor 1alpha predicts metastasis-free survival after radiation therapy alone in stage IIIB cervical squamous cell carcinoma. *Int J Radiat Oncol Biol Phys* 2004; 60(2):513-21.

[19] Loncaster JA, Harris AL, Davidson SE, Logue JP, Hunter RD, Wycoff CC, et al. Carbonic anhydrase (CA IX) expression, a potential new intrinsic marker of hypoxia: correlations with tumor oxygen measurements and prognosis in locally advanced carcinoma of the cervix. *Cancer Res* 2001; 61(17):6394-9.

[20] Hedley D, Pintilie M, Woo J, Morrison A, Birle D, Fyles A, et al. Carbonic anhydrase IX expression, hypoxia, and prognosis in patients with uterine cervical carcinomas. *Clin Cancer Res 2003*; 9(15):5666-74.

[21] *Mayer A, H*ockel M, Vaupel P. Carbonic anhydrase IX expression and tumor oxygenation status do not correlate at the microregional level in locally advanced cancers of the uterine cervix. *Clin Cancer Res* 2005; 11(20):7220-5.

[22] Kabuubi P, Loncaster JA, Davidson SE, Hunter RD, Kobylecki C, Stratford IJ, et al. No relationship between thymidine phosphorylase (TP, PD-ECGF) expression and hypoxia in carcinoma of the cervix. *Br J Cancer* 2006; 94(1):115-20.

[23] Airley R, Loncaster J, Davidson S, Bromley M, Roberts S, Patterson A, et al. Glucose transporter glut-1 expression correlates with tumor hypoxia and predicts metastasis-free survival in advanced carcinoma of the cervix. *Clin Cancer Res* 2001; 7(4):928-34.

[24] Cantu De Leon D, Lopez-Graniel C, Frias Mendivil M, Chanona Vilchis G, Gomez C, De La Garza Salazar J. Significance of microvascular density (MVD) in cervical cancer recurrence. *Int J Gynecol Cancer* 2003; 13(6):856-62.

[25] Cooper RA, West CM, Wilks DP, Logue JP, Davidson SE, Roberts SA, et al. Tumour vascularity is a significant prognostic factor for cervix carcinoma treated with radiotherapy: independence from tumour radiosensitivity. *Br J Cancer* 1999; 81(2):354-8.

[26] Pyo H, Kim YB, Cho NH, Suh CO, Park TK, Yun YS, et al. Coexpression of cyclooxygenase-2 and thymidine phosphorylase as a prognostic indicator in patients with FIGO stage IIB squamous cell carcinoma of uterine cervix treated with radiotherapy and concurrent chemotherapy. *Int J Radiat Oncol Biol Phys* 2005; 62(3):725-32.

[27] Kim YB, Kim GE, Pyo HR, Cho NH, Keum KC, Lee CG, et al. Differential cyclooxygenase-2 expression in squamous cell carcinoma and adenocarcinoma of the uterine cervix. *Int J Radiat Oncol Biol Phys* 2004; 60(3):822-9.

[28] Chen HH, Su WC, Chou CY, Guo HR, Ho SY, Que J, et al. Increased expression of nitric oxide synthase and cyclooxygenase-2 is associated with poor survival in cervical cancer treated with radiotherapy. *Int J Radiat Oncol Biol Phys* 2005; 63(4):1093-100.

[29] Loncaster JA, Cooper RA, Logue JP, Davidson SE, Hunter RD, West CM. Vascular endothelial growth factor (VEGF) expression is a prognostic factor for radiotherapy outcome in advanced carcinoma of the cervix. *Br J Cancer* 2000; 83(5):620-5.

[30] Wilson CR, Davidson SE, Margison GP, Jackson SP, Hendry JH, West CM. Expression of Ku70 correlates with survival in carcinoma of the cervix. *Br J Cancer* 2000; 83(12):1702-6.

[31] Harima Y, Sawada S, Miyazaki Y, Kin K, Ishihara H, Imamura M, et al. Expression of Ku80 in cervical cancer correlates with response to radiotherapy and survival. *Am J Clin Oncol* 2003; 26(4):e80-5.

[32] Sheridan MT, Cooper RA, West CM. A high ratio of apoptosis to proliferation correlates with improved survival after radiotherapy for cervical adenocarcinoma. Int J Radiat Oncol *Biol Phys* 1999; 44(3):507-12.

[33] Wheeler JA, Stephens LC, Tornos C, Eifel PJ, Ang KK, Milas L, et al. ASTRO Research Fellowship: apoptosis as a predictor of tumor response to radiation in stage IB cervical carcinoma. American Society for Therapeutic Radiology and Oncology. *Int J Radiat Oncol Biol Phys* 1995; 32(5):1487-93.

[34] Chung EJ, Seong J, Yang WI, Park TK, Kim JW, Suh CO, et al. Spontaneous apoptosis as a predictor of radiotherapy in patients with stage IIB squamous cell carcinoma of the uterine cervix. *Acta Oncol* 1999; 38(4):449-54.

[35] Kim JY, Cho HY, Lee KC, Hwang YJ, Lee MH, Roberts SA, et al. Tumor apoptosis in cervical cancer: its role as a prognostic factor in 42 radiotherapy patients. *Int J Cancer* 2001; 96(5):305-12.

[36] Green MM, Hutchison GJ, Valentine HR, Fitzmaurice RJ, Davidson SE, Hunter RD, et al. Expression of the proapoptotic protein Bid is an adverse prognostic factor for radiotherapy outcome in carcinoma of the cervix. *Br J Cancer* 2005; 92(3):449-58.

[37] Jain D, Srinivasan R, Patel FD, Kumari Gupta S. Evaluation of p53 and Bcl-2 expression as prognostic markers in invasive cervical carcinoma stage IIb/III patients treated by radiotherapy. *Gynecol Oncol* 2003; 88(1):22-8.

[38] Wootipoom V, Lekhyananda N, Phungrassami T, Boonyaphiphat P, Thongsuksai P. Prognostic significance of Bax, Bcl-2, and p53 expressions in cervical squamous cell carcinoma treated by radiotherapy. *Gynecol Oncol* 2004; 94(3):636-42.

[39] Pillai MR, Jayaprakash PG, Nair MK. Tumour-proliferative fraction and growth factor expression as markers of tumour response to radiotherapy in cancer of the uterine cervix. *J Cancer Res Clin Oncol* 1998; 124(8):456-61.

[40] Oka K, Suzuki Y, Nakano T. High growth fraction at 9 grays of radiotherapy is associated with a good prognosis for patients with cervical squamous cell carcinoma. *Cancer* 2000; 89(7):1526-31.

[41] Suzuki Y, Nakano T, Kato S, Ohno T, Tsujii H, Oka K. Immunohistochemical study of cell cycle-associated proteins in adenocarcinoma of the uterine cervix treated with radiotherapy alone: P53 status has a strong impact on prognosis. *Int J Radiat Oncol Biol Phys* 2004; 60(1):231-6.

[42] Cho NH, Kim YB, Park TK, Kim GE, Park K, Song KJ. P63 and EGFR as prognostic predictors in stage IIB radiation-treated cervical squamous cell carcinoma. *Gynecol Oncol* 2003; 91(2):346-53.

[43] Lee CM, Shrieve DC, Zempolich KA, Lee RJ, Hammond E, Handrahan DL, et al. Correlation between human epidermal growth factor receptor family (EGFR, HER2, HER3, HER4), phosphorylated Akt (P-Akt), and clinical outcomes after radiation therapy in carcinoma of the cervix. *Gynecol Oncol* 2005; 99(2):415-21.

[44] Nishioka T, West CM, Gupta N, Wilks DP, Hendry JH, Davidson SE, et al. Prognostic significance of c-erbB-2 protein expression in carcinoma of the cervix treated with radiotherapy. *J Cancer Res Clin Oncol* 1999; 125(2):96-100.

[45] Simon R, Sauter G. Tissue microarrays for miniaturized high-throughput molecular profiling of tumors. *Exp Hematol* 2002; 30(12):1365-72.

[46] Harima Y, Sawada S, Nagata K, Sougawa M, Ohnishi T. Human papilloma virus (HPV) DNA associated with prognosis of cervical cancer after radiotherapy. *Int J Radiat Oncol Biol Phys* 2002; 52(5):1345-51.

[47] Ishikawa H, Mitsuhashi N, Sakurai H, Maebayashi K, Niibe H. The effects of p53 status and human papillomavirus infection on the clinical outcome of patients with stage IIIB cervical carcinoma treated with radiation therapy alone. *Cancer* 2001; 91(1):80-9.

[48] Lindel K, Burri P, Studer HU, Altermatt HJ, Greiner RH, Gruber G. Human papillomavirus status in advanced cervical cancer: predictive and prognostic significance for curative radiation treatment. *Int J Gynecol Cancer* 2005; 15(2):278-84.

[49] Thomas M, Massimi P, Banks L. HPV-18 E6 inhibits p53 DNA binding activity regardless of the oligomeric state of p53 or the exact p53 recognition sequence. *Oncogene* 1996; 13(3):471-80.

[50] Harima Y, Harima K, Shikata N, Oka A, Ohnishi T, Tanaka Y. Bax and Bcl-2 expressions predict response to radiotherapy in human cervical cancer. *J Cancer Res Clin Oncol* 1998; 124(9):503-10.

[51] Liu SS, Leung RC, Chan KY, Chiu PM, Cheung AN, Tam KF, et al. p73 expression is associated with the cellular radiosensitivity in cervical cancer after radiotherapy. *Clin Cancer Res* 2004; 10(10):3309-16.

[52] Santucci MA, Barbieri E, Frezza G, Perrone A, Iacurti E, Galuppi A, et al. Radiation-induced gadd45 expression correlates with clinical response to radiotherapy of cervical carcinoma. *Int J Radiat Oncol Biol Phys* 2000; 46(2):411-6.

[53] Ramaswamy S, Golub TR. DNA microarrays in clinical oncology. *J Clin Oncol* 2002; 20(7):1932-41.

[54] Achary MP, Jaggernauth W, Gross E, Alfieri A, Klinger HP, Vikram B. Cell lines from the same cervical carcinoma but with different radiosensitivities exhibit different cDNA microarray patterns of gene expression. *Cytogenet Cell Genet* 2000; 91(1-4):39-43.

[55] Tewari D, Monk BJ, Al-Ghazi MS, Parker R, Heck JD, Burger RA, et al. Gene expression profiling of in vitro radiation resistance in cervical carcinoma: a feasibility study. *Gynecol Oncol* 2005; 99(1):84-91.

[56] Kitahara O, Katagiri T, Tsunoda T, Harima Y, Nakamura Y. Classification of sensitivity or resistance of cervical cancers to ionizing radiation according to expression profiles of 62 genes selected by cDNA microarray analysis. *Neoplasia* 2002; 4(4):295-303.

[57] Harima Y, Togashi A, Horikoshi K, Imamura M, Sougawa M, Sawada S, et al. Prediction of outcome of advanced cervical cancer to thermoradiotherapy according to expression profiles of 35 genes selected by cDNA microarray analysis. *Int J Radiat Oncol Biol Phys* 2004; 60(1):237-48.

[58] Hong JH, Tsai CS, Chang JT, Wang CC, Lai CH, Lee SP, et al. The prognostic significance of pre- and posttreatment SCC levels in patients with squamous cell carcinoma of the cervix treated by radiotherapy. *Int J Radiat Oncol Biol Phys* 1998; 41(4):823-30.

[59] Ohno T, Nakayama Y, Nakamoto S, Kato S, Imai R, Nonaka T, et al. Measurement of serum squamous cell carcinoma antigen levels as a predictor of radiation response in patients with carcinoma of the uterine cervix. *Cancer* 2003; 97(12):3114-20.

[60] Takeda M, Sakuragi N, Okamoto K, Todo Y, Minobe S, Nomura E, et al. Preoperative serum SCC, CA125, and CA19-9 levels and lymph node status in squamous cell carcinoma of the uterine cervix. *Acta Obstet Gynecol Scand* 2002; 81(5):451-7.

[61] Sproston AR, Roberts SA, Davidson SE, Hunter RD, West CM. Serum tumour markers in carcinoma of the uterine cervix and outcome following radiotherapy. *Br J Cancer* 1995; 72(6):1536-40.

[62] Gadducci A, Cosio S, Carpi A, Nicolini A, Genazzani AR. Serum tumor markers in the management of ovarian, endometrial and cervical cancer. *Biomed Pharmacother* 2004; 58(1):24-38.

[63] Mitsuhashi A, Suzuka K, Yamazawa K, Matsui H, Seki K, Sekiya S. Serum vascular endothelial growth factor (VEGF) and VEGF-C levels as tumor markers in patients with cervical carcinoma. *Cancer* 2005; 103(4):724-30.

[64] Reddi AL, Sankaranarayanan K, Arulraj HS, Devaraj N, Devaraj H. Serum alpha-N-acetylgalactosaminidase is associated with diagnosis/prognosis of patients with squamous cell carcinoma of the uterine cervix. *Cancer Lett* 2000; 158(1):61-4.

[65] Wong YF, Cheung TH, Lo KW, Wang VW, Chan CS, Ng TB, et al. Protein profiling of cervical cancer by protein-biochips: proteomic scoring to discriminate cervical cancer from normal cervix. *Cancer Lett* 2004; 211(2):227-34.

[66] Hawighorst H, Knapstein PG, Weikel W, Knopp MV, Zuna I, Knof A, et al. Angiogenesis of uterine cervical carcinoma: characterization by pharmacokinetic magnetic resonance parameters and histological microvessel density with correlation to lymphatic involvement. *Cancer Res* 1997; 57(21):4777-86.

[67] Loncaster JA, Carrington BM, Sykes JR, Jones AP, Todd SM, Cooper R, et al. Prediction of radiotherapy outcome using dynamic contrast enhanced MRI of carcinoma of the cervix. *Int J Radiat Oncol Biol Phys* 2002; 54(3):759-67.

[68] Hawighorst H, Knapstein PG, Knopp MV, Weikel W, Brix G, Zuna I, et al. Uterine cervical carcinoma: comparison of standard and pharmacokinetic analysis of time-intensity curves for assessment of tumor angiogenesis and patient survival. *Cancer Res* 1998; 58(16):3598-602.

[69] Mayr NA, Yuh WT, Magnotta VA, Ehrhardt JC, Wheeler JA, Sorosky JI, et al. Tumor perfusion studies using fast magnetic resonance imaging technique in advanced cervical cancer: a new noninvasive predictive assay. *Int J Radiat Oncol Biol Phys* 1996; 36(3):623-33.

[70] Yamashita Y, Baba T, Baba Y, Nishimura R, Ikeda S, Takahashi M, et al. Dynamic contrast-enhanced MR imaging of uterine cervical cancer: pharmacokinetic analysis with histopathologic correlation and its importance in predicting the outcome of radiation therapy. *Radiology* 2000; 216(3):803-9.

[71] Mayr NA, Yuh WT, Arnholt JC, Ehrhardt JC, Sorosky JI, Magnotta VA, et al. Pixel analysis of MR perfusion imaging in predicting radiation therapy outcome in cervical cancer. *J Magn Reson Imaging* 2000; 12(6):1027-33.

[72] Gong QY, Brunt JN, Romaniuk CS, Oakley JP, Tan LT, Roberts N, et al. Contrast enhanced dynamic MRI of cervical carcinoma during radiotherapy: early prediction of tumour regression rate. *Br J Radiol* 1999; 72(864):1177-84.

[73] Mayr NA, Yuh WT, Zheng J, Ehrhardt JC, Magnotta VA, Sorosky JI, et al. Prediction of tumor control in patients with cervical cancer: analysis of combined volume and dynamic enhancement pattern by MR imaging. *AJR Am J Roentgenol* 1998; 170(1):177-82.

[74] Bentzen SM. Theragnostic imaging for radiation oncology: dose-painting by numbers. *Lancet Oncol* 2005; 6(2):112-7.

[75] Harris AL. Hypoxia--a key regulatory factor in tumour growth. *Nat Rev Cancer* 2002; 2(1):38-47.

[76]   Grigsby PW, Siegel BA, Dehdashti F. Lymph node staging by positron emission tomography in patients with carcinoma of the cervix. *J Clin Oncol* 2001; 19(17):3745-9.

[77]   Esthappan J, Mutic S, Malyapa RS, Grigsby PW, Zoberi I, Dehdashti F, et al. Treatment planning guidelines regarding the use of CT/PET-guided IMRT for cervical carcinoma with positive paraaortic lymph nodes. *Int J Radiat Oncol Biol Phys* 2004; 58(4):1289-97.

[78]   Grigsby PW, Singh AK, Siegel BA, Dehdashti F, Rader J, Zoberi I. Lymph node control in cervical cancer. *Int J Radiat Oncol Biol Phys* 2004; 59(3):706-12.

[79]   Grigsby PW, Mutch DG, Rader J, Herzog TJ, Zoberi I, Siegel BA, et al. Lack of benefit of concurrent chemotherapy in patients with cervical cancer and negative lymph nodes by FDG-PET. *Int J Radiat Oncol Biol Phys* 2005; 61(2):444-9.

[80]   Wright JD, Dehdashti F, Herzog TJ, Mutch DG, Huettner PC, Rader JS, et al. Preoperative lymph node staging of early-stage cervical carcinoma by [18F]-fluoro-2-deoxy-D-glucose-positron emission tomography. *Cancer* 2005; 104(11):2484-91.

[81]   Xue F, Lin LL, Dehdashti F, Miller TR, Siegel BA, Grigsby PW. F-18 fluorodeoxyglucose uptake in primary cervical cancer as an indicator of prognosis after radiation therapy. *Gynecol Oncol* 2006; 101(1):147-51.

[82]   Rust TC, Kadrmas DJ. Rapid dual-tracer PTSM+ATSM PET imaging of tumour blood flow and hypoxia: a simulation study. *Phys Med Biol* 2006; 51(1):61-75.

[83]   Shah N, Sattar A, Benanti M, Hollander S, Cheuck L. Magnetic resonance spectroscopy as an imaging tool for cancer: a review of the literature. *J Am Osteopath Assoc* 2006; 106(1):23-7.

[84]   deSouza NM, Soutter WP, Rustin G, Mahon MM, Jones B, Dina R, et al. Use of neoadjuvant chemotherapy prior to radical hysterectomy in cervical cancer: monitoring tumour shrinkage and molecular profile on magnetic resonance and assessment of 3-year outcome. *Br J Cancer* 2004; 90(12):2326-31.

[85]   Baudelet C, Gallez B. How does blood oxygen level-dependent (BOLD) contrast correlate with oxygen partial pressure (pO2) inside tumors? *Magn Reson Med* 2002; 48(6):980-6.

In: Trends in Cervical Cancer
Editor: Hector T. Varaj, pp. 167-184
ISBN: 1-60021-299-9
© 2007 Nova Science Publishers, Inc.

Chapter VIII

Lymphatic Mapping and Sentinel Lymph Node Biopsy in Early-Stage Cervical Cancer

Antonio Maffuz[1] and Sergio A. Rodríguez-Cuevas[2]

[1]Gynecologic Oncology Department, Hospital de Oncología, Centro Médico Nacional Siglo XXI (CMN-SXXI), Instituto Mexicano del Seguro Social (IMSS), Mexico City, Mexico;
[2]Honorary Research Surgeon, Hospital de Oncología, CMN-XXI, IMSS, Mexico City, Mexico.

ABSTRACT

The concept for sentinel lymph node is one of the most significant and interesting achievements in surgical oncology in the last 10 years. The sentinel lymph node (SLN) is defined as the first draining lymph node of an anatomical region, so that a histologically negative SLN would predict the absence of tumor metastases in the other non-sentinel lymph nodes. The detection of SLN is currently a standard component of the surgical treatment of malignant melanoma, breast cancer and is a promising staging technique for patients with vulvar cancer. In cervical cancer SLN mapping is more recent and only a few studies have been published so far, those preliminary studies indicated that is a feasible technique. SLN are currently detected by the application of two techniques, blue dye and radioactive tracer technetium-99-m. The combination of the two techniques increases its sensitivity.

Lymph node status is a major prognostic factor for patients with cervical carcinoma and is a decision criterion for adjuvant therapy. Radical hysterectomy with pelvic and with or without paraaortic lymphadenectomy is the most commonly performed definitive surgical procedure for patients with early cervical cancer. In patients with early stage cervical cancer, pelvic node metastases are expected in 10-15% of the cases. This means that in the most favorable group of patients, the majority who undergo lymphadenectomy derive no benefit from the procedure yet must endure the associated increase in the risk of lymphocyst and lymphedema. Furthermore, in case of lymph node metastases, patients with cervical cancer could be treated with primary chemoradiotherapy without radical surgery.

SLN identification in early stage cervical cancer is feasible, and extends our knowledge on the pathways of lymphatic spread of cervical cancer. The use combination technique with of technetium-99-m-labeled nanocolloid and blue dye achieved in the majority of trials near than 100% detection rate, and a predictive negative value of 100%. This method currently allows a more precise examination of the most critical nodes through serial sections and immunohistochemistry. The results obtained at this moment with the use of lymphatic mapping and SLN biopsy in cervical cancer must be confirmed in multicentric and controlled trials before it could be considered a standard of care.

BACKGROUND

The concept of the sentinel lymph node comprises one of the most significant and interesting achievements in surgical oncology in the last 10 years. The sentinel lymph node (SLN) is defined as the first draining lymph node of an anatomic region. When nodal metastases occur, SLN will be initially involved, so that a histologically negative SLN would predict the absence of tumor metastases in the remaining non-sentinel lymph nodes of the corresponding lymphatic chain. Likewise, if the sentinel node is positive the risk exists that other nodes in the area may be involved [1,2].

Clark, at the end of 19th century, was the first to apply the Halstedian concept of radical surgery to cervical cancer management. In the first radical hysterectomy he performed, regional lymph nodes were removed at the same time as the uterus as were the structures joining it to the nodes: the parametria. Since that time, the concept of systematic lymphadenectomy has prevailed for decades [3]. New surgical strategies in cancer management have been continuously sought. Anatomists have established that lymph node drainage is predictable yet not uniform; thus, identification of SLN as the indicator of a cervical metastatic disease would be useful to improve detection of cancer cell spread and to reduce the morbidity and mortality related with the procedure of its detection.

Lymphatic mapping technique involves injection of a chromatic (vital) dye or of a radioisotope suspension, or both, into primary tumor-adjacent tissue. The material is taken up by regional lymphatics and collects in a SLN. Sometimes there are two or more unilateral or bilateral lymphatic channels originating in the region of the primary tumor and running to two or more different lymph nodes on each side. In some cases, a SLN could be a false negative, meaning that a SLN identified in a basin is histologically negative but a tumor is present in other lymph node(s) from that basin.

The term sentinel lymph node was coined in 1960 by Gould for carcinoma of the parotid gland [4]. This term and the lymphatic mapping technique was used first by Ramón Cabañas in 1977, who suggested that penile cancer initially drains into a particular lymph node in the groin that is defined by its constant anatomic position [5]. In the late 1980s, Donald L. Morton proposed and utilized the concept of lymphatic mapping and sentinel lymph node biopsy for patients with cutaneous melanoma [6]. SLN detection is currently a standard component of surgical treatment for malignant melanoma and breast cancer, and is a promising staging technique for patients with vulvar cancer and other neoplasms such as squamous cell carcinoma of head and neck, prostate, gastric and colorectal cancer. In cervical cancer lymphatic mapping with SLN identification is more recent, the first report described by Echt in 1999 [7].

The physiology of lymphatic drainage from the cervix has been variously described and is not well established. Some authors noted the existence of a first-level lymph node drainage station where the probability of detecting SLNs is greater; contrariwise, other authors suggested that lymph node metastasis from early stage cervical cancer is a random event because any pelvic node site may be the first stage for metastases [8]. Lymphatic mapping procedures are well tolerated overall and add only a small amount of extra time to the planned surgical procedure.

JUSTIFICATION

Several prognostic factors, including disease stage, tumor size, and nodal status, have been clearly identified in patients with cervical carcinoma. In patients with early-stage disease (defined as International Federation of Gynecology Obstetrics [FIGO] stages IA, IB1, and non-bulky IIA), prognostic factors have been discussed and clarified more recently.

A Gynecologic Oncology Group (GOG) study was conducted in 1990 on prognostic factors for FIGO stage IB cervical carcinoma treated with primary radical hysterectomy. The study concluded that clinical size, tumor invasion depth, and capillary lymphatic space status were independent prognostic factors [9]. Other more recent studies have clearly shown three independent prognostic factors: stromal invasion depth; nodal status, and lymphovascular space status [10].

Clinical staging of patients with cervical cancer according to FIGO becomes increasingly inaccurate with the advancing stage: the failure rate rises from 25% in FIGO stages I and II to 65–90% in FIGO stage IIIb. Prognosis of patients with cervical cancer is determined not only by tumor size as reflected by FIGO stage, but also and most importantly by the metastasizing potential reflected by lymph node status and lymphovascular space. Lymph node metastasis—either regional or distant—is considered the most important prognostic factor. Thus, clinically based FIGO classification, which does not take into account lymph node status, may lead to patient undertreatment. Alternatively, patients may be assigned to primary chemoradiation for suspected nodal disease and are shown to be tumor-free following histopathologic evaluation [11,12].

Surgical staging is the ideal method to determine the extent of the disease histopathologically. SLN identification became a less invasive alternative for patients with invasive cervical cancer.

Early-stage cervical cancer is a good candidate disease for lymphatic mapping for several reasons:

a) Lymph node status is a major prognostic factor for patients with cervical carcinoma, it is a decision criterion for adjuvant therapy, and unfortunately the clinical FIGO staging system for cervical cancer does not include assessment of lymph node involvement. Positive lymph node location cannot be determined on the basis of clinical factors.

b) Incidence of positive nodes in early surgical stages that in theory possesses a benefit with lymphadenectomy is approximately 6% for stage IA2, 15% for stage IB1, and 26% for non-bulky stage IIA. This means that the majority of patients who undergo lymphadenectomy derive no benefit from the procedure but must endure the associated increase in surgical complications such as increase in operative time, blood loss, risk of lymphocyst, and lymphedema.

c) Complete lymphadenectomy may be unnecessary in patients with nodal involvement; this subgroup of patients could be treated by radiation or chemoradiation therapy alone.

d) Cervix is a central structure with complex anatomic lymphatic drainage; thus, extensive bilateral lymphadenectomy is necessary to assess nodal involvement.

e) Conventional imaging techniques (lymphangiography, computed tomography [CT], and magnetic resonance imaging [MRI]) notoriously fail to identify lymph node metastases accurately.

Therefore, the indication for lymphatic mapping (LM) and sentinel lymph node biopsy (SLNB) in cervical cancer is to identify patients with metastasic lymph nodes to avoid complete lymphadenectomy or radical hysterectomy for the latter and to treat these with radiation alone or with chemoradiation therapy. Morbidity for combined surgery and radiotherapy is higher than for either of these alone, and combined treatment does not assure better survival. Patients with unaffected SLN will benefit from radical hysterectomy. Patients with positive pelvic SLN must be submitted to careful para-aortic node evaluation, because if these are metastatic extended radiation fields are necessary [13–16].

TECHNIQUE

a) Preoperative Lymphoscintigraphy

Pre-operative lymphoscintigraphy are performed by injection of 200 µCi of filtered technicium-99 radiocolloid into the cervix. This was divided into four injections around the tumor, or at 12, 3, 6 and 9 o'clock positions around the cervix for midline tumors. The majority of patients reported mild to moderate pain with the injection, but also reported that the pain passed quickly. Injections were performed with a 25- or 27-gauge needle with constant gentle pressure in an attempt to prevent spillage into the vagina. In the majority of cases, the first lymphoscintigrams were obtained within 30 minutes of radionuclide injection. Lymphoscintigrams were repeated as necessary for up to 3 additional hours to identify sentinel nodes. Anterior/posterior and lateral views were obtained with markers placed on bony landmarks such as pubic symphysis and anterior superior iliac crests. In some cases, transmission scans were obtained to demonstrate the outline of the body at the discretion of the nuclear medicine specialist. (Figure 1)

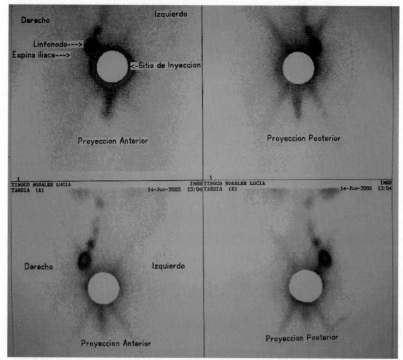

Figure 1. Pre-operative lymphoscintigram; an SLN is visible in the right pelvis (right- quadrant anterior view and left-quadrant posterior view).

Technetium-99 (Tc-99m) half-life is approximately 6 hours. For this reason, if pre-operative lymphoscintigraphy was performed >18 hours (three half-lives) prior to surgery the radionuclide injection was repeated on the morning of the procedure 1–6 hours before surgery. No side effects have been reported from the Tc-99m injection to date [17,18].

b) Intraoperative Lymphatic Mapping

On the day of surgery and after induction of general anesthesia, patients are placed in low lithotomy position and examined. Routine preparation and draping are performed. Skin-incision or the laparoscopic approach is performed and the abdomen is explored. At this point, a speculum is placed in the vagina and 2–4 mL of isosulfan blue dye (Lymphazurin 1%, U.S. Surgical Co., Norwalk, CT) or patent blue dye (bleu patenté V, France Guebert, F-95943 ROISSY CdG Cedex) or methylene blue (sterile methylene blue 1%) are injected into the cervix in four quadrants (at 12, 3, 6, and 9 o'clock) as previously described, and at 0.5–1.0 cm in depth. (Figure 2) A needle extender or spinal needle are used with gentle pressure to minimize spillage of the blue dye, and when possible direct tumoral injection are avoided. Before, during, or after blue dye injection and depending on surgeon preference, incisions are made in the pelvic peritoneum to expose the retroperitoneum, and avascular, paravesical, and pararectal spaces are gently developed. Grossly involved lymph nodes should be confirmed by frozen section prior to continuing the procedure. Up to 10 minutes must be allowed for nodal dye uptake. The retroperitoneum is then visually inspected and scanned with the hand-held gamma counter to locate sentinel nodes. Both pelvic and para-aortic regions are surveyed. The probe is collimated and angled laterally to the greatest degree possible to reduce detection of residual radioactivity from the primary cervical tumor. Preoperative lymphoscintigram should be available in the operating room to help guide the search for sentinel nodes.

Adverse reactions with blue dye injection are infrequent. The majority of patients have blue-green urine discoloration during the first 24–48 post-operative hours. The remaining two side effects include transient oxygen desaturation (measured by pulse oxymetry) in the majority of cases without clinical consequence, and anaphylactic reaction, which varies from self-limited blue urticaria to severe anaphylactoid reaction. The reported rate of severe anaphylactic reaction with blue dye in large series of breast cancer and melanoma falls within the range of 1–2% and appears to be dose-related, the majority of reactions occuring when 4 cc or more of dye is injected. In view of the rarity of severe allergic reactions, routine pre-operative skin-prick testing is not advocated at present. However, because a negative history of blue dye allergy does not totally preclude the possibility of an allergic reaction some authors suggest premedication with both H_1 and H_2 antihistamines to all patients prior to blue dye injection to prevent severe allergic reactions [19–22].

Last, there is controversy surrounding the issue of massaging the lesion after dye injection because of the potential risk of driving tumor cells into the lymphatics. This is currently under discussion with regard to breast cancer, but there is no consensus and the concern cannot be addressed with data available at present. Concerning breast cancer, it is felt that if this were true in a few patients it would probably not have clinical significance. Nevertheless, it may be more prudent to simply conduct regular pelvic examination after dye injection without massaging the cervix too vigorously and without a massage of several minutes, as frequently performed in breast cancer [23].

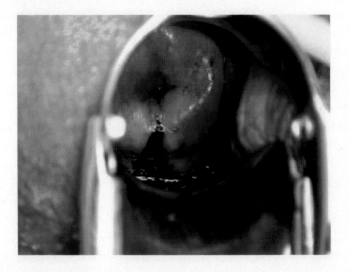

Figure 2. Blue dye cervical injection.

c) Sentinel Lymph Node Identification

Any blue or hot nodes are considered SLNs. Gamma probe-identified radioactive lymph nodes were removed and radioactivity was measured *ex vivo*. If counts are at least 10-fold above background radiation levels, the node is considered sentinel. Sentinel nodes are label as blue, hot (radioactive), or blue/hot. Radioactive counts and location of each sentinel node are recorded. (Figure 3)

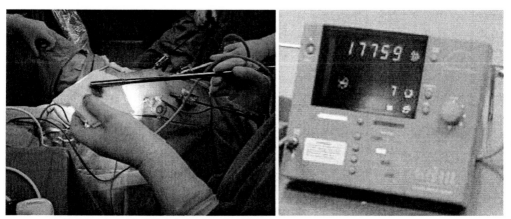

Figure 3. Radioactivity measured *ex vivo* by laparoscopic gamma probe.

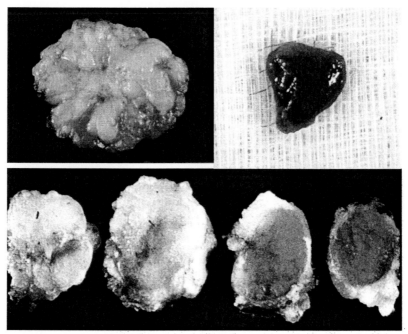

Figure 4. Blue stained sentinel lymph node.

d) Pathologic Processing

SLN are visually inspected by the pathologist. Two procedures are performed: imprint cytology or frozen section analysis, this variable among different hospitals. The sensitivity of each method will be discussed later. In the imprint cytology method, sentinel node(s) were sent fresh to the Pathology Department and were cut into several sections 2–3-mm-thick sections. Lymph node(s) are only bisected when they measure <0.5 cm or less in diameter. Imprints are made of the cut surfaces of each section obtained. The imprints are then stained with hematoxylin & eosin (H&E). Results are reported as positive or negative. The remaining sentinel lymph node tissue sections are fixed in formaldehyde and processed into paraffin blocks, with sections are taken of each.

The frozen section method is performed in the customary manner, If the initial section is negative, five 40 μm-wide interval sections are obtained for H&E staining and unstained slides are prepared for cytokeratin immunohistochemical analysis. (Figure 4)

Considerations for the Technique

Over the course of experience in lymphatic mapping in patients with cervical cancer, several observations in the technique have been described. First, timing for opening the retroperitoneum after dye injection is important. There is a 5–10-minute window during which the dye passes through the cervical lymphatics into the parametrial tissues and ultimately into the pelvic sidewall. Some authors found it most feasible to incise the retroperitoneum and initiate opening retroperitoneal spaces prior to dye injection. This allows adequate visualization of node-bearing tissues without significant disruption of parametrial and sidewall lymphatics. After dye uptake is noted in lymphatic node-bearing tissues, thorough dissection of pelvic spaces and attempts at SLN identification should proceed.

Second, retention of dye within the cervical stroma was occasionally problematic, requiring exploration of several different injection techniques. In patients with prior conization, it is easy to overestimate the amount of remaining stroma and to cause intraperitoneal or rectal deposition. Care must also be taken to control needle-penetration depth in these patients. Patients with large exophytic tumors presented greater difficulty, often requiring lateral retractors or angled needles to facilitate dye injection. Alternatively, a Potocky needle (used for paracervical nerve block) may facilitate infusion. Overall, some authors found that a 25-gauge needle attached to a needle extender with a 5-cc syringe produced best results for dye injection.

Failure to identify SLNs may be due to limited dye or radioisotope uptake from excessive vaginal or peritoneal spillage, disruption of lymphatic channels during initial dissection, or poor operative exposure of lymphatic tissues. It is also possible that cancer-related occlusion of cervical stromal lymphatic channels could limit dye uptake. The latter limitation could also explain low frequency of bilateral SLN identification and the difficulty among patients with large tumors [11,17,18].

Surgical Approach

In cervical cancer, lymphatic mapping can be conducted by laparotomic or laparoscopic approach. It would appear perfectly logical to perform lymphatic mapping laparoscopically now that a laparoscopic gamma probe is available. The advantages are several and obvious: first, the laparoscopic surgical approach allows a more delicate and bloodless dissection of the retroperitoneum; second, laparoscope permits magnification of the image, which facilitates visualization of blue lymphatic vessels, and third, if positive nodes are identified the surgeon has the opportunity to end the procedure, thus avoiding radical hysterectomy, and to offer patients chemoradiation with minimal delay and reduced morbidity compared with laparotomy.

Validation and Learning Curve

The benefit of SLN biopsy appears clear, but the technique is a new one, long-term consequences are not fully defined, and medicolegal risks are unknown. Institutions beginning to perform this procedure should do so under a formalized review protocol in which selection and technique are carefully specified, patients are fully informed, backup pelvic/para-aortic lymph node dissection is carried out to validate the early experience, and careful audits of individual and institutional results (short- and long-term) are maintained. A success rate of 90–95% in finding SLN and no more than 5–10% false negative results would appear to be reasonable targets for validation trials.

Some trials in breast cancer have found that success in localizing SLN continues to improve over the surgeon's first cases, and more than one half of false negative results occurred in the first cases of each surgeon. The majority of authorities recommend that each surgeon initially perform 20 or 30 SLN procedures in breast cancer; with backup axillary lymph node dissection, fewer validated cases may be necessary.

SLN may be identified by either radioisotope or blue dye methods, and while each technique in itself enjoys the vocal support of a few investigators in breast cancer an emerging international consensus supports the use of both methods in combination. McMasters et al. demonstrated that false negatives occur one half as often with a combined technique as with single-agent SLN mapping technique. Although experience in melanoma, breast cancer, and also in cervical cancer has shown that the combined technique for SLN detection is superior to the blue dye technique only, some authors continue to use the blue dye technique only because of greater convenience, rapidity, and in their opinion technical adequacy in the cervical cancer field. Contrariwise, the combined technique is more expensive, requires greater patient healthcare coordination, and leads to identification of an elevated mean number of SLN in multiple sites [24,25].

Initial studies with SLN detection utilizing lymphazurin dye, isosulfan blue dye, patent blue, or technetium-99m colloidal albumin in patients with cervical cancer showed sensitivity, negative predictive value, and 100% accuracy. Subsequent studies only partly confirmed the high validity of this concept in patients with cervical cancer. SLN localization varies and the detection rate proves highest using a combination of radioactively labeled albumin with blue dye. The value of detection of circulating tumor cells or micrometastases in SLN by immunohistochemical or molecular-biological methods is not clear. Additional studies in cervical cancer should be carried out to establish the number of procedures with backup pelvic/para-aortic lymph node dissection for validating the technique.

Rate of SLN detection in cervical cancer can be influenced by the following various factors:

a) Type of marker used. Initially, only dyeing agents were used, thus rendering a lower detection rate (between 15 and 100%, average 76%). Use of radioisotopes infers that detection rates >80% can be obtained. The combination of both techniques yields the best results (detection rates between 80 and 100%, mean 93%)

b) Amount of marker injected. More detection errors were found when a smaller amount of dyeing substance was injected. Optimal amount of dyeing substance or radioisotope is probably 4 mL.

c) Injection site and puncture number. The majority of authors performed four intracervical punctures. Puncture at the fundus of the vagina is associated with a higher detection error rate.

d) Time elapsed between administration of the dyeing substance and detection. Some authors recommended a time lapse of >20 minutes when using patent blue; nonetheless, when employing isosulfan blue an average lapse for identification of 7 minutes was reported.

e) Previous conization does not appear to influence identification rates.

The procedure's learning curve must include all members of the healthcare team involved, i.e., the gynecologic oncologist, the nuclear physician, and the pathologist [25–29].

In Tables 1–3, we summarized the majority of studies published in the English-language literature regarding lymphatic mapping and SLN identification with the three different methods, demonstrating the combined technique as the most accurate.

Table 1. Summary of published literature by blue-dye-only method.

Author, year	No. of cases	Detection rate by patient %	False negative /all positives	NPV (%)
Echt, 1999 [7]	13	15.4	0/2	*
Medl, 2000 [23]	3	100	0/3	*
O'Boyle, 2000 [14]	20	60	0/3	100
Malur, 2001 [30]	9	55.5	1/2	75
Plante, 2003 [31]	70	87.1	0/12	100
Dargent, 2003 [17]	70	100	0/19	100
Holub, 2004 [32]	7	100	0/1	100
Di Stefano, 2005 [24]	50	90	1/10	97.2
TOTAL	*242*	*76*	*2/52*	*95.36*

*Not calculable. NPV = Negative Predictive Value.

Table 2. Summary of published literature by radiocolloid tracer only.

Author, year	No. of cases	Detection rate by patient %	False negative /all positives	NPV (%)
Kamprath, 2000 [33]	18	88.8	0/1	100
Malur, 2001 [30]	21	76.2	0/0	100
Lantzsch, 2001 [34]	14	92.8	0/1	100
Van Dam, 2003 [35]	25	84	0/5	100
Li, 2004 [36]	28	96.4	0/6	100
Angioli, 2005 [37]	37	70.3	0/6	100
Silva, 2005 [38]	56	92.8	3/17	100
TOTAL	*199*	*85.9*	*3/36*	*100*

NPV = Negative Predictive Value.

Table 3. Summary of published literature by blue dye and radiocolloid tracer.

Author, year	No. of cases	Detection rate by patient (%)	False negative /all positives	NPV (%)
Verheijen, 2000 [39]	10	80	0/1	100
Malur, 2001 [30]	20	90	0/4	100
Levenback, 2002 [13]	39	100	1/8	96.9
Rhim, 2002 [40]	26	100	1/6	95.2
Hubalewska, 2003 [41]	37	100	0/5	100
Lambaudie, 2003 [42]	12	91.7	0/2	100
Chung, 2003 [43]	2	100	0/5	100
Plante, 2003 [31]	29	93.1	0/4	100
Lelievre, 2004 [44]	8	75	0/0	100
Martínez-Palones, 2004 [18]	25	100	0/3	100
Barranger, 2004 [45]	36	94.4	0/8	100
Nikura, 2004 [46]	20	90	0/2	100
Pijpers, 2004 [47]	34	100	1/12	95.7
Gil-Moreno, 2005 [48]	12	100	0/0	100
Maffuz, 2005 [49]	10	90	0/0	100
TOTAL	*344*	*93.61*	*3/56*	*99.18*

NPV = Negative Predictive Value.

Sentinel Lymph Node Localization

The average number of pelvic and para-aortic sentinel nodes in patients with cervical cancer is 2.7 and 1.6, respectively. The most common site for SLN identification can vary among different studies. Dargent and colleagues in 35 patients submitted to lymphatic mapping with blue dye technique found that the majority of SLNs are located in the so-called Leveuf et Godard area, meaning lateral to the inferior vesical artery, ventral to the origin of the uterine artery, and medial or caudal to the external iliac vein. In the series reported by Di

Stefano in 50 patients, the most common SLN sites comprised the external iliac and obturator areas, with an overall detection of 93%. In the report written by Levenback, the interiliac and obturator areas were the most frequent SLN localizations. One of the largest series by Plante, which included 70 patients, found that external iliac, obturator, and bifurcation were the most common SLN identification sites [13,17,24,50].

Positive Nodes

SLN detection rate in patients with macroscopically suspicious nodes is low in comparison with patients with normally appearing lymph nodes. The difficulty in identifying macroscopic nodes may be explained by the fact that lymphatic vessels may be blocked by tumor cells, thus preventing migration of the injected dye/technetium, or may be due to blockage of the lymph node capsule by tumor cell emboli, again preventing the dye/technetium from entering the node. However, the objective of the lymphatic mapping and SLN technique clearly is not to identify macroscopically involved lymph nodes, which are readily visible at surgery, but to identify the potential SLN involved due to sub-clinical micrometastases [24].

Pathologic Evaluation

The issue of SLN intraoperative pathologic evaluation remains under debate concerning all tumor sites for which SLN mapping is performed. There is currently no standardized protocol for SLN evaluation. Two histopathologic procedures are performed: imprint cytology, or frozen section analysis. In a recent paper, the results of imprint cytology were very poor (overall sensitivity, 8%) and appeared to be worse than those obtained in breast cancer or melanoma. In this interesting series of 36 patients (eight of whom had nodal spread), the rate of micrometastases was particularly high (four of eight) and six of eight patients had positive nodes located exclusively in sentinel nodes. Perhaps these poor results could be correlated with the high rate of micrometastases. Frozen section analysis of cervical-cancer pelvic nodes was evaluated in three series with a sensitivity that varied from 68–92%. Nevertheless, none of the papers addressed the results of frozen section analysis in cervical-cancer sentinel nodes. Ideal SLN management approaches during surgical management should be evaluated in further studies [51–53].

Another important point is to know whether standard microscopic examination is sufficient or whether biological marker determination should be performed on the SLN (immunohistochemistry [IHC] or reverse transcriptase-polymerase chain reaction of cytokeratin). A recent major paper by Van Trappen et al. in 2001 demonstrated that 44% of negative nodes (using standard microscopic examination) had high cytokeratin 19 expression (detected using reverse transcriptase-polymerase chain reaction) [53]. The cytokeratin 19 expression level was found correlated with survival. Two recent conflicting papers examined the implications of this paper with respect to the concept of SLN. In the paper by Marchiolé et al. that reported on 29 patients who underwent SLN biopsy for early-stage cervical cancer, routine pathologic examination and IHC staining were performed on sentinel and non-sentinel nodes. Three patients had micrometastases in non-sentinel lymph node, whereas the sentinel node biopsy was negative. The authors concluded that given the high rate of false negative results, SLN biopsy is not accurate. Notwithstanding this, 1 month later Barranger et al. reported satisfactory results with a similar methodology (no false negative results). How can this difference be explained? In the paper by Marchiolé, SLN were detecting using patent blue dye, whereas in the series reported by Barranger the combined detection procedure was employed. This essential difference could probably explain the conflicting results. To date, there is no guideline as to whether IHC should be routinely performed on sentinel nodes in cervical cancer [51,55].

Micrometastases

One of the main contributions of SLN biopsy is its capacity to identify metastases of <2mm. Extensive experience of SLN in breast cancer has led to a modification in criteria for metastatic staging. According to the American Joint Commission on Cancer/International Union Against Cancer (AJCC/UICC) staging system, micrometastases have been defined with a lower limit and are designated pN1mi for metastases >0.2 mm but not <2.0 mm. A new category of metastases of ≤0.2 mm has been designated as isolated tumor cells and these are classified as pN0. At present, research is focused on prognosis and clinical implementation in patients with micrometastases and isolated tumor cells in gynecologic cancer. Until additional findings are obtained, patients with micrometastases and isolated tumor cells should be considered as N+. Imprint cytology possesses low sensitivity for detecting micrometastases in SLN [54,56].

False Negative Rate

The true false negative, defined as a case in which SLN is negative but other non-sentinel nodes are found to be positive, comprises solely a few cases in the results published in English literature with regard to SLN mapping in cervical cancer, for an overall rate of <1%. In one case, it is not clear whether the positive non-sentinel node was on the same side as the negative SLN, or on the contralateral side. Additionally, the SLN was evaluated using the standard H&E method and not with serial sections and IHC. In another case, the false negative SLN was actually found on frozen section and not on final pathology. Accuracy in frozen section SLN analysis is actually an interesting concept because from a clinical point of view, this is the information on which we would eventually rely to determine whether more complete lymph node dissection is required (if the SLN is positive) or not (if the SLN is negative).

However, parametrial nodes are the most frequent cause of false negatives, located as they are near the cervix where blue coloration is intense and radioactivity is high, rendering them particularly difficult to identify [13,24,30,40,47].

CONCLUSIONS

Lymphatic mapping is a promising strategy for intra-operative assessment of nodal status in a variety of solid tumor types. Sentinel lymphadenectomy techniques have been applied successfully in treating patients with breast cancer and melanoma and may decrease morbidity by allowing omission of complete lymphadenectomy in some patients. Successful implementation of these techniques is dependent on operator skill as well as on tumor-specific factors such as tumor size, predictability of regional lymphatic drainage pattern, and accessibility of lymphatic basins. In this chapter, we explored and described the feasibility of lymphatic mapping in patients with early-stage cervical cancer in their attempts in undergoing radical hysterectomy and pelvic lymphadenectomy.

Lymph node status is a major prognostic factor for patients with cervical carcinoma and is a decision criterion for adjuvant therapy. Radical hysterectomy with pelvic or para-aortic lymphadenectomy is the most commonly performed definitive surgical procedure for patients with early cervical cancer. In patients with early-stage cervical cancer, pelvic node metastases are expected in 10–15% of cases. This means that in the most favorable group of patients, the majority who undergo lymphadenectomy derive no benefit from the procedure, yet must endure the associated increase in risk for lymphocyst and lymphedema. Furthermore, in the case of lymph node metastases patients with cervical cancer could be treated with primary chemoradiotherapy without radical surgery.

In their classic article, Plentl and Friedman [8] describe a predictable pattern of lymphatic drainage with step-wise progression from cervical stroma and serosal lymphatics to successive nodal groups in the parametria, pelvic lymphatics, pararectal lymphatics, and para-aortic lymphatics, although significant variations exist and have been demonstrated in the different lymphatic mapping studies.

Among the different series, the percentage of false negative SLN lies between 3 and 11%. Possible causes might include massive lymphatic chain infiltration and the presence of positive parametrial nodes, which are difficult to distinguish from isotopic activity of the cervix and which are not very accessible for dissection. The majority of series show a high negative predictive value (between 75 and 100%, mean 97%). SLN identification in early-stage cervical cancer is feasible and furthers our knowledge concerning the lymphatic spread pathways of cervical cancer. Several lymphatic mapping studies have been performed on patients with cervical cancer; previous experience with blue dye alone was disappointing, with a low SLN detection rate. The use of a combination technique with technetium-99-m-labeled nanocolloid and blue dye achieved a nearly 100% detection rate in the majority of trials, and a predictive negative value of 100%. This method currently allows more precise examination of the most critical nodes by means of serial sections and immunohistochemistry. The results obtained at present with the application of lymphatic mapping and SLN biopsy in cervical cancer must be confirmed in multicenter and controlled trials before being considered a standard of care.

Detection of SLN or the practice of lymphoscintigraphy at present does not modify the posterior therapeutic procedure and presents no additional morbidity. In the future, novel imaging technologies such as positron emission tomography (PET) would be compared with this pre- or intra-operative detection of sentinel lymph nodes to detect, prior to treatment, the possibility of pelvic spread of cervical cancer. On the other hand, SLN identification enables the pathologist to analyze the node with greater precision or to submit these nodes to immunostaining against cytokeratin or molecular quantification reverse transcriptase PCR for identification of micrometastases.

REFERENCES

[1]   Nieweg OE, Tanis PJ, Kroon BBR. The definition of a sentinel lymph node. *Ann Surg Oncol* 2001;8(6):538-541.

[2]   Cody HS III. Clinical aspects of sentinel lymph node biopsy. *Breast Cancer Res* 2001;3:104-108.

[3]   Clark JG. A more radical method of performing hysterectomy for cancer of the uterus. *Bull Johns Hopkins Hosp 6*, 1896.

[4]   Gould EA, Winship T, Philbin PH, et al. Observations on a "sentinel node" in cancer of the parotid. *Cancer* 1960;13:77-78.

[5]   Cabañas RM. An approach for the treatment of penile cancer. *Cancer* 1977;39:456-466.

[6]   Morton DL, Wen D, Wong JH, et al. Technical details of intraoperative lymphatic mapping for early stage melanoma. *Arch Surg* 1992;127:392-399.

[7]   Echt ML, Finan MA, Hoffman MS, et al. Detection of sentinel lymph nodes with lymphazurin in cervical, uterine and vulvar malignancies. *South Med J* 1999;92(2):204-208.

[8]   Plentl A, Friedman E. Lymphatic system of the female genitalia. In: Plentl AFE (ed), *Lymphatics of the Cervix Uteri*. Vol. 2. Philadelphia, PA: Saunders;1971.

[9]   Delgado G, Bundy B, Zaino R, et al. Prospective surgical-pathological study of disease-free interval in patients with stage IB squamous cell carcinoma of the cervix: a Gynecologic Oncology Group study. *Gynecol Oncol* 1990;38:352-357.

[10]   Grisaru DA, Covens A, Franssen E, et al. Histopathologic score predicts recurrence free survival after radical surgery in patients with stage IA2-IB1-2 cervical carcinoma. *Cancer* 2003;97:1904-1908.

[11]   Morice P, Castaigne D. Advances in the surgical management of invasive cervical cancer. *Curr Opin Obstet Gynecol* 2005;17:5-12.

[12]   Ho CM, Chien TY, Huang SH, et al. Multivariate analysis of the prognostic factors and outcomes in early cervical cancer patients undergoing radical trachelectomy. *Gynecol Oncol* 2004;93:458-464.

[13]   Levenback C, Coleman RL, Thomas W, et al. Lymphatic mapping and sentinel lymph node identification in patients with cervix cancer undergoing radical hysterectomy and pelvic lymphadenectomy. *J Clin Oncol* 2002;20:688-693.

[14]   O'Boyle JD, Coleman RL, Bernstein SG, et al. Intraoperative lymphatic mapping in cervix cancer patients undergoing radical hysterectomy: a pilot study. *Gynecol Oncol* 2000;79:238-243.

[15]   Schneider A, Hertel H. Surgical and radiographic staging in patients with cervical cancer. *Curr Opin Obstet Gynecol* 2004;16:11-18.

[16]   Torné A, Puig-Tintoré LM. The use of sentinel lymph nodes in gynaecological malignancies. *Curr Opin Obstet Gynecol* 2004;16:57-64.

[17]   Dargent D, Enria R. Laparoscopic assessment of the sentinel lymph nodes in early cervical cancer. Technique- preliminary results and future developments. *Crit Rev Oncol Hematol* 2003;48(3):305-310.

[18] Martínez-Palones JM, Gil-Moreno A, Pérez-Benavente MA, et al. Intraoperative sentinel node identification in early stage cervical cancer using a combination of radiolabeled albumin injection and isosulfan blue dye injection. *Gynecol Oncol* 2004;92(3):845-850.

[19] Leong SP, Donegan E, Heffernon W, et al. Adverse reactions to isosulfan blue during selective sentinel lymph node dissection in melanoma. *Ann Surg Oncol* 2000;7(5):361-366.

[20] Montgomery LL, Thorne AC, Van Zee, et al. Isosulfan blue dye reactions during sentinel lymph node mapping for breast cancer. *Anesth Analg* 2002;95(2):385-388.

[21] Sadiq TS, Burns WW 3rd, Taber DJ, et al. Blue urticaria: a previously unreported adverse event associated with isosulfan blue. *Arch Surg* 2001;136(12):1433-1435.

[22] Cimmino VM, Brown AC, Szocik JF, et al. Allergic reactions to isosulfan blue during sentinel node biopsy- a common event. *Surgery* 2001;130(3):439-442.

[23] Medl M, Peters-Engl C, Schutz P, et al. First report of lymphatic mapping with isosulfan blue dye and sentinel node biopsy in cervical cancer. *Anticancer Res* 2000;20(2B):1133-1134.

[24] Di Stefano AB, Acquaviva G, Garozzo G, et al. Lymph node mapping and sentinel node detection in patients with cervical carcinoma: a 2-year experience. *Gynecol Oncol* 2005;99(3):671-679.

[25] McMasters KM, Tuttle TM, Carlson DJ, et al. Sentinel lymph node biopsy for breast cancer: a suitable alternative to routine axillary dissection in multi-institutional practice when optimal technique is used. *J Clin Oncol* 2000;18:2560-2566.

[26] Barranger E, Cortéz A, Commo F, et al. Histopathological validation of the sentinel node concept in cervical cancer. *Ann Oncol* 2004;15:870-874.

[27] Metcalf KS, Johnson N, Calvert S, et al. Site specific lymph node metastasis in carcinoma of the cervix: is there a sentinel node? *Int J Gynecol Cancer* 2000;10:411-416.

[28] Schwartz GF, Guiliano AE, Veronesi U & the Consensus Conference Committee. Proceedings of the Consensus Conference on the role of sentinel lymph node biopsy in carcinoma of the breast. April 19-22, 2001, Philadelphia, Pennsylvania. *Hum Pathol* 2002;33:579-589.

[29] Morice P, Sabourin JC, Pautier P, et al. Indications and results of extemporaneous examination of pelvic lymph nodes in the surgical strategy of stage Ib or II cancers of the cervix uteri. *Ann Chirurg* 1999;53:583-586.

[30] Malur S, Krause N, Köhler C, Schneider A. Sentinel lymph node detection in patients with cervical cancer. *Gynecol Oncol* 2001;80(2):254-257.

[31] Plante M, Renaud MC, Têtu B, et al. Laparoscopic sentinel node mapping in early-stage cervical cancer. *Gynecol Oncol* 2003;91(3):494-503.

[32] Holub Z, Jabor A, Lukac J, Kliment L. Laparoscopic detection of sentinel lymph nodes using blue dye in women with cervical cancer and endometrial cancer. *Med Sci Monit* 2004;10(10):CR587-CR591.

[33] Kamprath S, Possover M, Schneider A. Laparoscopic sentinel lymph node dissection in patients with cervical cancer. *Am J Obstet Gynecol* 2000;182(6):1648. (Abstract).

[34] Lantzsch T, Wolters M, Grimm J, et al. Sentinel node procedure in Ib cervical cancer: a preliminary series. *Br J Cancer* 2001;85(6):791-794.

[35] Van Dam PA, Hauspy J, Vanderheyden T, et al. Intraoperative sentinel node identification with Technetium-99m-labeled nanocolloid in patients with cancer of the uterine cervix: a feasibility study. *Int J Gynecol Cancer* 2003;13(2)182-186.

[36] Li B, Zhang WH, Liu L, et al. Sentinel lymph node identification in patients with early stage cervical cancer undergoing radical hysterectomy and pelvic lymphadenectomy. *Chin Med J* 2004;117(6):867-870.

[37] Angioli R, Palaia I, Cipriani C, et al. Role of sentinel lymph node biopsy procedure in cervical cancer: a critical point of view. *Gynecol Oncol* 2005;96(2):504-509.

[38] Silva BL, Silva-Filho AL, Traiman P, et al. Sentinel node detection in cervical cancer with ^{99m}Tc-phytate. *Gynecol Oncol* 2005;97(2):588-595.

[39] Verheijen RH, Pijpers R, Van Diest PJ, et al. Sentinel node detection in cervical cancer. *Obstet Gynecol* 2000;96(1):135-138.

[40] Rhim CC, Park JS, Bae SN, Namkoong SE. Sentinel node biopsy as an indicator for pelvic nodes dissection in early stage cervical cancer. *J Korean Med Sci* 2002;17(4):507-511.

[41] Hubalewska A, Sowa-Staszczak A, Huszno B, et al. Use of Tc99m-nanocolloid for sentinel nodes identification in cervical cancer. *Nucl Med Rev Cent East Eur* 2003;6(2):127-130.

[42] Lambaudie E, Collinet P, Narducci F, et al. Laparoscopic identification of sentinel lymph nodes in early stage cervical cancer: prospective study using a combination of patent blue dye injection and technetium radiocolloid injection. *Gynecol Oncol* 2003;89(1):84-87.

[43] Chung YA, Kim SH, Sohn HS, et al. Usefulness of lymphoscintigraphy and intraoperative gamma probe detection in the identification of sentinel nodes in cervical cancer. *Eur J Nucl Med Mol Imaging* 2003;30(7):1014-1017.

[44] Lelievre L, Camatte S, Le Frere-belda MA, et al. Sentinel lymph node biopsy in cervix and corpus uterine cancers. *Int J Gynecol Cancer* 2004;14(2):271-278.

[45] Barranger E, Cortéz A, Grahek D, et al. Laparoscopic sentinel node procedures for cervical cancer: impact of neoadjuvant chemoradiotherapy. *Ann Surg Oncol* 2004;11(4):445-452.

[46] Niikura H, Okamura C, Akahira J, et al. Sentinel lymph node detection in early cervical cancer with combination 99mTc phytate and patent blue. *Gynecol Oncol* 2004;94(2):528-532.

[47] Pijpers R, Buist MR, van Lingen et al. The sentinel node in cervical cancer: scintigraphy and laparoscopic gamma probe-guided biopsy. *Eur J Nucl Med Mol Imaging* 2004;31(11):1479-1486.

[48] Gil-Moreno A, Díaz-Feijoo B, Roca I, et al. Total laparoscopic radical hysterectomy with intraoperative sentinel node identification in patients with early invasive cervical cancer. *Gynecol Oncol* 2005;96(1):187-193.

[49] Maffuz A, Cortés G, Escudero P, et al. Mapeo ganglionar y biopsia de ganglio centinela en cáncer cervicouterino. *GAMO* 2005;4(5):S112.

[50] Leveuf J, Godard H. Les lymphatiques de l'uterus. *Rev Chir* 1923; 219-248.

[51] Barranger E, Cortéz A, Uzan S, et al. Value of intraoperative imprint cytology of sentinel node in patients with cervical cancer. *Gynecol Oncol* 2004;94:175-180.

[52] Bjornsson BL, Nelson BE, Reale FR, Rose PG. Accuracy of frozen section for lymph node metastases in patients undergoing radical radical hysterectomy for carcinoma of the cervix. *Gynecol Oncol* 1993;51:50-53.

[53] Scholz HS, Lax SF, Benedicic C, et al. Accuracy of frozen section examination of pelvic lymph nodes in patients with FIGO stage Ib1 to IIb cervical cancer. *Gynecol Oncol* 2003;90:605-609.

[54] Van Trappen PO, Gyselman VG, Lowe DG, et al. Molecular quantification and mapping of lymph-node micrometastases in cervical cancer. *Lancet* 2001;357:15-20.

[55] Marchiolé P, Buenerd A, Scoazec JY, et al. Sentinel lymph node biopsy is not accurate in predicting lymph node status for patients with cervical carcinoma. *Cancer* 2004;100:2154-2159.

[56] *American Joint Committee on Cancer (AJCC) Cancer Staging Manual.* 6th ed. Philadelphia, PA: Lippincott-Raven;2002.

In: Trends in Cervical Cancer
Editor: Hector T. Varaj, pp. 185-205

ISBN: 1-60021-299-9
© 2007 Nova Science Publishers, Inc.

Chapter IX

DOCETAXEL LABELED WITH RADIONUCLIDE SHOWS HIGH EFFICIENCY AGAINST CERVICAL CANCER CELL LINES IN VITRO

Emil Rudolf[*] and Miroslav Červinka

Department of Medical Biology and Genetics, Charles University in Prague, Faculty of
Medicine in Hradec Králové, 500 38 Hradec Králové, Czech Republic.

ABSTRACT

Advanced carcinoma of the uterine cervix is conventionally treated with radiotherapy. Moreover, several lines of evidence show that chemotherapy administered concurrently with radiotherapy often overcomes developed resistance of cancer cells, thereby improving therapeutical efficiency of this treatment modality. Besides traditionally used cytostatics such as cisplatin or fluorouracil, taxanes represent a relatively new group of agents in this field, showing cytostatic activity against some advanced forms of cervical carcinoma. In addition, recently, it has been experimentally demonstrated that paclitaxel and docetaxel act as radiosensitizing agents, promisingly enhancing the cytotoxic effect of radiation in the treatment of cervical cancer. In this study, we present a new treatment modality in which chemotherapeutic agent (docetaxel) was labeled with radionuclide iodine 131 which is an emittor of β- and γ-radiation and its cytotoxic potential was evaluated and compared with non-labeled docetaxel on the HeLa Hep2 cell lines (chemosensitive and resistant) during 48 hours. Unlike non-labeled docetaxel which induced apoptosis in sensitive HeLa Hep-2 cell line only, the radiolabeled docetaxel was significantly more toxic in both cell lines, inducing cell cycle arrest, DNA damage and subsequent p53-dependent apoptosis as early as 12 hours after the beginning of the treatment. Our results thus show that ^{131}I-docetaxel holds a

---

[*] Correspondence concerning this article should be addressed to Dr. Emil Rudolf, Ph.D. Department of Medical Biology and Genetics, Charles University in Prague, Faculty of Medicine in Hradec Králové, Šimkova 870, 500 38 Hradec Králové, Czech Republic. Tel: +420 495816393; Fax: +420 495816495; email: rudolf@lfhk.cuni.cz.

promising therapeutic potential whose mechanism as well as efficacy might be worth of further investigation both *in vitro* as well as *in vivo*.

Keywords: Cervical cancer, Docetaxel, Radiolabeled docetaxel, p53, Apoptosis, Chemosensitivity.

1. INTRODUCTION

Cervical carcinoma is one of the most common malignancies among women in the world. Its prevalence and incidence are linked to human papillomavirus (HPV) infection which remains high in many world countries despite continuing educational and screening efforts [1,2]. The standart treatment modalities for newly diagnosed cases of cervical carcinoma include surgery and radiotherapy [3,4] which may lead to a significant clinical improvement. On the other hand, recurrent and advanced cervical carcinoma continue to be therapeutical problem and management of these cases is rather difficult, including some traditional as well as new treatment strategies such as fractionation therapy schedules or hyperthermia; however, always with varying clinical outcomes [5]. Chemotherapy whose use in cervical cancer has traditionally been restricted to palliation nowadays emerges as a potentially beneficial approach, in particular when combined with other local modalities (radiation or surgery) [6,7,8].

Generally, chemotherapy may (A) precede local treatment (neoadjuvant) or (B) it may be indicated after radical local treatment (adjuvant) or (C) it is administered concurrently with radiation. Each of these approaches holds some advantages and disadvantages but based on the results of many in vitro and in vivo studies it is the concominant approach which seems to be most promising [8,9]. Several lines of evidence show that chemotherapy administered concurrently with radiotherapy increases combined cytotoxicity of radiation and antineoplastic drugs towards malignant cell populations and overcomes inherent or developed resistance of cancer cells, thereby improving therapeutical efficiency [10,11]. Traditionally used cytostatics in the treatment of cervical cancer comprise cisplatin, fluorouracil, ifosfamide, epirubicin, bleomycin or etoposide [12].

Taxanes (paclitaxel and its synthetic analogue docetaxel) represent a relatively new group of agents in this field, showing cytostatic activity against some advanced forms of cervical carcinoma [13]. Taxanes bind to heterodimers subunit of microtubules and through increased tubulin polymerization prevent microtubular depolymerization. This stabilizing effect promotes cell cycle arrest and leads to an induction of many intracellular pathways and genes [14]. Ultimately, taxanes may induce cell death – apoptosis by p53-mediated pathway. In addition, by acting via microtubules taxanes have a profound effect on mitosis and mitosis-associated cell death – mitotic catastrophe [15]. Recently, it has also been experimentally demonstrated that paclitaxel and docetaxel act as radiosensitizing agents, promisingly enhancing the cytotoxic effect of radiation in the treatment of cervical cancer [16,17].

In this study, we wanted to study a new treatment approach in which chemotherapeutic agent (docetaxel) was labeled with radionuclide iodine 131 which is an emittor of β- and γ-radiation and its cytotoxic potential was evaluated and compared with non-labeled docetaxel on the HeLa Hep2 cell lines (chemosensitive and resistant) during 48 hours. Unlike non-labeled docetaxel which induced apoptosis in sensitive HeLa Hep-2 cell line only, radiolabeled docetaxel was significantly more toxic in both cell lines, inducing cell cycle arrest, DNA damage and subsequent p53-dependent apoptosis as early as 12h after the beginning of the treatment in both cell lines. Our results thus show that radiolabeled taxane docetaxel combines DNA-damaging as well as microtubule-inhibiting properties which show a synergistic effect and may overcome an acquired or inherent chemoresitance of malignant cervical cells. This modality therefore holds a promising therapeutic potential whose mechanism as well as efficacy might be worth of further investigation both in vitro as well as in vivo.

2. MATERIALS AND METHODS

Cell Line

Human cervical cell line HeLa Hep2 (EATCC, No. 86030501, Porton Down, United Kingdom) was cultivated as stationary monolayer in plastic tissue-culture dishes (Nunclon, Roskilde, Denmark). Cells were grown in Dulbecco's modified Eagle's medium – DMEM (Gibco, Prague, Czech Republic), supplemented with 10% bovine serum (Gibco, Prague, Czech Republic), 100 U/ml penicillin, and 100 µg/ml streptomycin. Cells were passaged every third day using 0.25% trypsin and their mycoplasma-free status was frequently checked.

In order to generate chemoresistant cells (HeLa Hep2R), HeLa Hep2 cells were seeded in cultivation flasks and upon reaching 80% confluency, 0.5 nM paclitaxel (Taxol® pro inj., Bristol-Myers Squibb, New York, U.S.A.) was added. Surviving cells were pooled and allowed to grow to 80% confluency again. Cells were kept in the presence of steadily increasing concentrations of paclitaxel for a period of 6 months until they were able to tolerate the concentrations several fold higher than was the starting one.

Tested Chemical

Docetaxel (Taxotere® inj.) was obtained from Rhône-Poulenc Rorer (Antony, France). The stock solution (100 µM) was prepared by dissolving it in DMSO. The final tested concentrations (1 nM, 5nM, 10, nM, 100 nM, 500 nM and 1 000 nM) were obtained by diluting stock in DMEM. Radiolabeling of docetaxel with iodine 131 radionuclide (^{131}I) was performed by Nuclear Research Institute (Řež u Prahy, Czech Republic). Radiochemical purity of labeled docetaxel measured by thin layer chromatography was determined as exceeding 95%.

Nonactive lipiodol oil solution (ethiodized poppy seed oil) was obtained from LIPIODOL® Ultra-Fluid (BYK, Konstanz, Germany). One ml of lipiodol with dissolved ^{131}I-docetaxel (10 mg) was added dropwise to the 4 ml solution containing Poloxamer 188

(Synperonic PE/F 68, ICI Surfactants, Cleveland, England), Polysorbat 20 (Tween 20, ICI Surfactants, Cleveland, England), and water and ultrasonicated with 40 W input in pulses lasting 2 seconds with 0.5 second pauses for 2 minutes. The radioactivity of the emulsion was determined at 20 MBq/ml. The emulsion of lipiodol with dissolved ^{131}I-docetaxel was diluted with DMEM to yield a range of tested concentrations (1 nM, 5nM, 10, nM, 100 nM, 500 nm and 1 000 nM).

Cytotoxicity Assay

Cytotoxicity of non-labeled docetaxel and ^{131}I-docetaxel on both HeLa Hep-2 cell lines was carried out by WST-1 colorimetric assay (Boehringer Mannheim-Roche, Prague, Czech Republic), which is based on the cleavage of the tetrazolium salt to colored formazan by mitochondrial dehydrogenases as well as other cytoplasmic enzymes in viable cells. HeLa Hep2 and HeLa Hep2R cells at a concentration 6,000 cells/well in 200 μl of DMEM containing 10% bovine serum were seeded in 96-well microtiter plates, with the first column of wells without cells (blank). The cells were incubated 24 hours at 37°C and in 5% CO_2. After incubation, the medium was replaced with a medium containing tested emulsions and cultivated for 48 hours at 37°C and 5% CO_2. After this period, 100 μl of WST-1 was added. The cells were further incubated for 2 hours. The absorbance was recorded at 450 nm with 650 nm of reference wavelength by a multiplate reader TECAN SpectraFluor Plus (TECAN Austria GmbH, Grödig, Austria). In all cases, the absorbance of the tested substance in medium alone was recorded to determine whether it interfered with the assay.

Time - Lapse Video Microscopy

Studied cell lines HeLa Hep2 and HeLa Hep2R were grown in DMEM under standard laboratory conditions (37°C, 5 % CO_2). After 24 hours of cultivation, the standard medium was replaced with a medium containing non-labeled docetaxel or ^{131}I-docetaxel. The culture flasks were left in an incubator for 20 minutes and then transferred to a 37 °C heated chamber where all recordings were carried out. Cells were examined using an inverted microscope Olympus IX-70 (Olympus Corporation, Tokio, Japan) equipped with a long-working-distance condenser, and a 20x phase contrast lens. For time-lapse recording, the microscope was mounted with a Mitsubishi CCD-100 E camera (Mitsubishi Corporation, Tokyo, Japan) and connected to a Mitsubishi video recorder HS-S5600 (Mitsubishi Corporation, Tokyo, Japan). The recording was performed in a 480 mode, with a slowing factor 160. Recording continued for 48 hours, with a subsequent image analysis of digitised files using Adobe Premiere.

Flow Cytometry

HeLa Hep2 and HeLa Hep2R cells were seeded into cultivation flasks, cultivated upon standard laboratory conditions (see above) and at the end of each treatment interval were harvested using 0.25% trypsin. After rinsing with cold PBS (5 minutes), cells were fixed in 5 ml of 70% cold ethanol (2 hours, 4°C), rinsed with PBS and resuspended in 0.5 ml propidium iodide (PI – Sigma, Prague, Czech Republic). Following the inclubation with PI (15 minutes, dark, room temperature – RT), the fluorescence emission of examined cells was measured with a flow cytometer (Coulter Electronic, Hialeah, U.S.A.) with subsequent cell cycle analysis.

Measurement of DNA Damage – Comet Assay

DNA single-strand breaks in treated cells were determined by alkali single-cell gel electrophoresis (comet assay). This assay is based on analysis of labile DNA damage sites where DNA forms characteristic tails – comets. Control and treated HeLa Hep2 and HeLa Hep2R cells were at particular time intervals harvested by 0.25% trypsin, centrifuged for 5minutes at 1,500 rpm at 4°C, suspended in 0.6% agarose and mounted to microscopic slides. Next, cells were lysed in cooled lysis buffer (2.5 M NaCl, 100 mM EDTA, 10 mM Trizma, 1% Triton X-100 and 10% DMSO) for 1.5 hours at 4°C. After rinsing in TRIS, cells were allowed to unwind DNA in alkali buffer for 30 minutes. Electrophoresis was performed at 25 V and 300 mA for 30 minutes. After neutralizing slides and draining them, cells were stained by 100 µl ethidium bromide (Sigma-Aldrich, Prague, Czech Republic). One hundred cells from three independent samples were scored for tail migration intensity.

Immunocytochemistry

Treated and control HeLa Hep2 and HeLa Hep2R cell lines were seeded into cytospin chambers and cultivated overnight in an incubator at 5% CO_2 at 37°C. After exposure to non-labeled docetaxel and ^{131}I-docetaxel at 12, 24, 36 and 48h they were centrifuged (50 x g, 5minutes, 4°C), fixed with 1 ml of 2% paraformaldehyde (20 minutes, 25°C), rinsed with PBS with 1% Triton X (PBS-T) and then treated to skimmed milk for 30 minutes at 25°C. The cells were then incubated with mouse anti-phospho p53 (1:200, Sigma-Aldrich, Prague, Czech Republic) or anti-caspase 3 (1:150, DAKO, Glostrup, U.S.A.) at 4°C for 1 hour. After washing with cold PBS (5 minutes, 25°C), Alexa Fluor 488 or 546-labeled goat anti-mouse IgG (Genetica, Prague, Czech Republic) was added for additional 1 hour (25°C). Next, the specimens were rinsed three times with cold PBS, optionally post-labeled with DAPI (Sigma-Aldrich, Prague, Czech Republic - 10 µg/ml) and mounted into SlowFade® medium (Molecular Probes, Inc., Eugene, U.S.A.). The localization and status of protein p53 and caspase-3 were examined under a fluorescence microscope Nikon Eclipse E 400 (Nikon Corporation, Kanagawa, Japan) equipped with the digital color matrix camera COOL 1300 (VDS, Vosskůhler, Germany), using TRITC, FITC and DAPI specific filters. Photographs were taken using the software LUCIA DI Image Analysis System LIM (Laboratory Imaging Ltd., Prague, Czech Republic) and analyzed. For the purpose of analysis, at least 2,000 cells were scored at 200 and 600x magnifications.

Statistics

Statistical analysis was carried out with a statistical program GraphPad Prism, using one-way Anova test with Dunnet's post test for multiple comparisons. Results were compared with control samples, and means were considered significant if P<0.05.

3. RESULTS

Cytotoxicity of ^{131}I-Docetaxel and Docetaxel

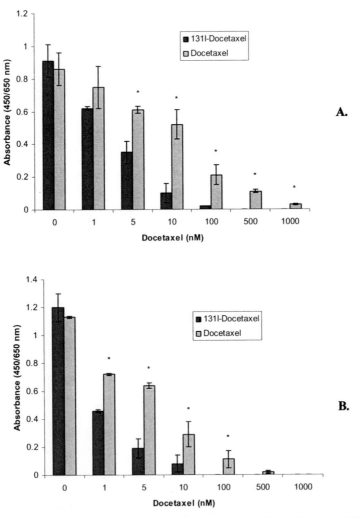

Figure 1. Viability and proliferation of chemosensitive human cervical carcinoma cell line HeLa Hep2 treated with non-labeled and radiolabeled docetaxel (0- 1000 nM) during 48 hours as measured by WST-1 cleavage assay, (A) 24 hours (B) 48 hours. Values represent means ± SD of at least three experiments *P<0.05 with one way-Anova test and Dunnett's post test for multiple comparisons.

To determine the cytotoxicity of ^{131}I-docetaxel and non-labeled docetaxel to human cervical carcinoma cell lines (normal and chemoresistant to paclitaxel), HeLa Hep2 and HeLa Hep2R cells were treated with a range of concentrations of both docetaxels during 48 hours and metabolic activity of exposed cells was measured by WST-1 assay. Fig. 1 shows that in the interval of 24 hours both docetaxels produced concentration-dependent inhibition of cellular metabolism which was visible already with the lowest employed concentration (1 nM). In addition, ^{131}I-docetaxel proved to be much more toxic than docetaxel alone at all the used concentrations. These results were even more apparent during 48 hours lasting treatment (Fig. 2).

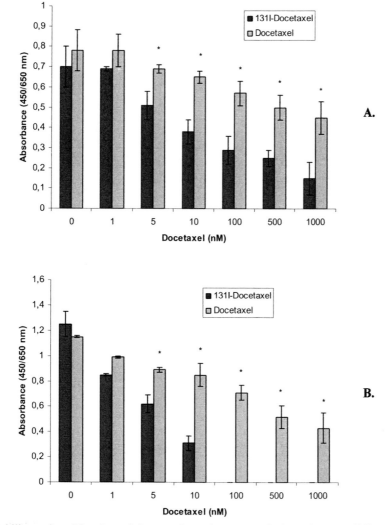

Figure 2. Viability and proliferation of chemoresistant human cervical carcinoma cell line HeLa Hep2R treated with non-labeled and radiolabeled docetaxel (0- 1000 nM) during 48 hours as measured by WST-1 cleavage assay, (A) 24 hours (B) 48 hours. Values represent means ± SD of at least three experiments *P<0.05 with one way-Anova test and Dunnett's post test for multiple comparisons.

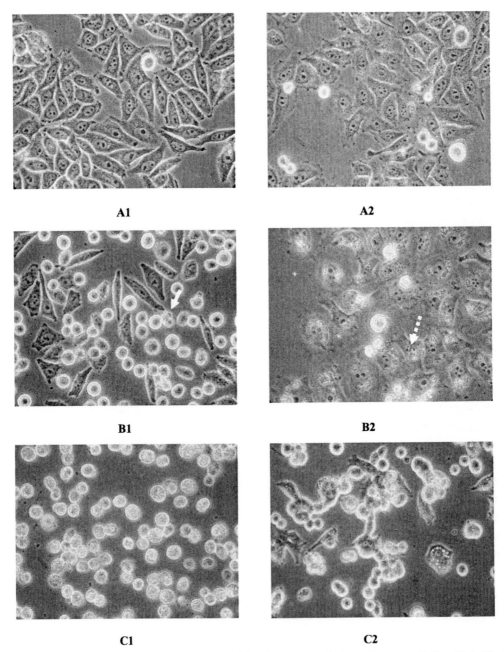

A1   A2

B1   B2

C1   C2

Figure 3. Morphology of (A1-C1) chemosensitive human cervical carcinoma cell line HeLaHep2 treated with 100 nM docetaxel during 24 hours and (A2-C3) chemoresistant human cervical carcinoma cell line HeLa Hep2R treated with 10 nM radiolabeled docetaxel during 24 hours. After 12 hours, chemosensitive cells became rounded and started blebbing (white arrow). In the same time interval (12 hours), chemoresistant cells developed vacuoles in the cytoplasm in the absence of typical blebbing (dashed white arrow).

When the same treatment regimen was used in Hela Hep2R cell line, cytotoxic effects of non-labeled docetaxel were relatively poor – the highest treatment concentration (1000 nM) reduced metabolic activity of exposed cells by only 30% during 24 hours treatment and 60% during 48 hours treatment, respectively. On the other hand, ^{131}I-docetaxel inhibited cell growth and metabolism more potently – 50% inhibition was achieved after 10 nM concentration during 24 hours and 5 nM during 48 hours, respectively.

Morphology of Cells Exposed to ^{131}I-Docetaxel and Docetaxel

To characterise morphology of HeLa Hep2 and HeLa Hep2R cells exposed to both ^{131}I-docetaxel and non-labeed docetaxel, time-lapse videomicroscopy as well as sequential recording were used. In sensitive HeLa Hep2 cells, both ^{131}I-docetaxel and docetaxel produced a similar concentration-dependent sequence of morphological alterations starting with an increased transparency of nucleoli, detachment from substratum followed by cell rounding. The cells often showed surface blebbing which lasted several hours before they shrank and remained motionless (Fig. 3A2). While these changes occurred mostly at low and medium concentrations (up to 100 nM in docetaxel and between 1 and 5 nM in ^{131}I-docetaxel) during 48 hours, the use of higher concentrations resulted in accelerated cells' demise where some morphologies were reduced or altogether missing (cell blebbing), with the entire course of cell death completed by 24 hours. In HeLa Hep2R cells the timing and dynamics of morphological changes was essentially different. In docetaxel-treated cultures, almost no avisible changes were recorded during 24 hours of treatment at all the employed concentrations. During 36 hours and at the highest concentrations (500 and 1000 nM) some cells exhibited the coarsening of the cytoplasm and started to lose their adherence. By 48 hours, approximately 25% of cells developed vacuoles in the cytoplasm and started shrinking without any other distinct membrane changes.

In comparison to docetaxel treated cells, the effect of ^{131}I-docetaxel on chemoresistant cervical cells was more pronounced albeit different from normal cervical cultures. With exception of the lowest dose (1 nM), all other concentrations induced relatively rapid cytoplasmic vacuolization, loss of adherence and irregular cells shrinkage (Fig. 3C2). Upon the highest employed concentrations (500 nM and 1000 nM), the process culminated in a massive relase of cytoplasmic content and the fragmentation of cells which was again not observed at medium and lower concentrations.

Distribution of Cell Cycle

Analysis of cell cycle and proapoptotic effects of both chemosensitive and chemoresistant cervical carcinoma cell lines treated with ^{131}I-docetaxel and non-labeled docetaxel was carried out by flow cytometry. The distribution of chemosensitive cells with respect to phases of the cell cycle after 36 hours of treatment is shown in Fig. 4A. It is evident that in comparison to docetaxel which induced cells into G2/M phase, the effect of ^{131}I-docetaxel was less significant. In addition, the time course of G2/M synchronization shows that the maximum effect of both employed docetaxels was reached at 36 hours of treatment (Fig. 4B). Apoptotic peak was detected in cells treated for 36 hours with both docetaxels too.

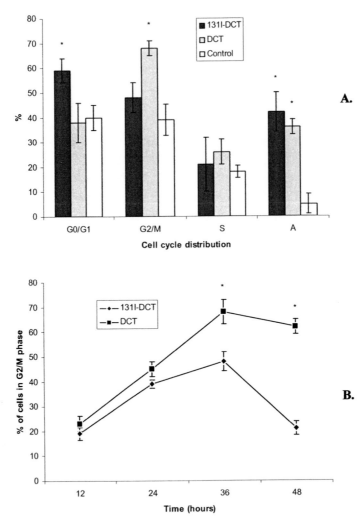

Figure 4. Cell cycle distribution in chemosensitive human cervical carcinoma cell line HeLa Hep2 treated with non-labeled and radiolabeled docetaxel (0- 1000 nM) during 48 hours as measured by flow cytometry, (A) general distribution of the cell cycle phases at 36 hours of the treatment (B) time course of G_2/M arrest in docetaxels treated cells during 48 hours. Values represent means ± SD of at least three experiments *P<0.05 with one way-Anova test and Dunnett's post test for multiple comparisons.

As displayed in Fig. 5A and B, in comparison to ^{131}I-docetaxel, the percentage of G2/M cells treated with docetaxel was significantly lower at all the followed time intervals, with its maximum (23%) reached between 24 and 36 hours of treatment. Furthermore, only insignificant apoptotic peak was observed in docetaxel-treated HeLa Hep2R cells.

DNA Damage

DNA damage in chemosensitive HeLa Hep2 cells after treatment with radiolabeled and non-labeled docetaxel during 24 hours was estimated by means of single cell electrophoresis – comet assay. As shown in Fig. 6A, ^{131}I-docetaxel induced dose-dependent DNA damage which was at all the employed concentrations significantly higher than in non-labeled docetaxel. The extent of DNA damage after the treatment with non-labeled docetaxel was at the lowest concentrations (1 nM and 5 nM) insignificant but starting with 10 nM it exhibited almost exponential increase.

In chemoresistant HeLa Hep2R cells, the DNA-damaging effect of non-labeled docetaxel was only minor at all the employed concentrations. On the other hand, ^{131}I-docetaxel induced dose-dependent DNA alterations in exposed cells in a manner similar to its effects in chemosensitive HeLa Hep2 cells (Fig. 6B).

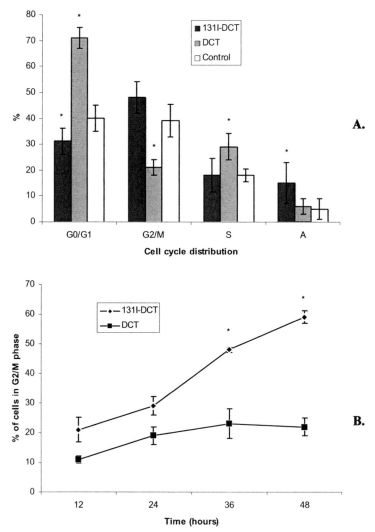

Figure 5. Cell cycle distribution in chemoresistant human cervical carcinoma cell line HeLa Hep2R treated with non-labeled and radiolabeled docetaxel (0- 1000 nM) during 48 hours as measured by flow cytometry, (A) general distribution of the cell cycle phases at 36 hours of the treatment (B) time course of G_2/M arrest in docetaxels treated cells during 48 hours. Values represent means ± SD of at least three experiments *P<0.05 with one way-Anova test and Dunnett's post test for multiple comparisons.

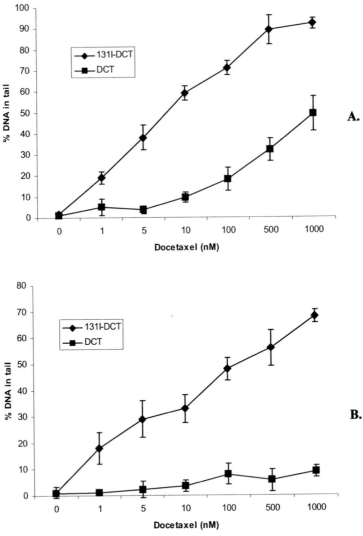

Figure 6. DNA damage in human cervical carcinoma cell lines treated with non-labeled and radiolabeled docetaxel (0- 1000 nM) during 24 hours as measured by comet assay, (A) chemosensitive HeLa Hep2 cells (B) chemoresistant HeLa Hep2R. Values represent means ± SD of at least three experiments. All the concentrations of radiolabeled docetaxel produced statistically more significant response than non-labeled docetaxel.

Immunocytochemical Detection of Cell Death

To determine whether ^{131}I-docetaxel and non-labeled docetaxel induced cell death involved p53 signalling and subsequent activation of apoptosis-specific caspase-3, we detected the presence of the phosphorylated p53 (after 12 hours of treatment) and the active caspase-3 (after 24 hours of treatment) in both model cell lines. Non-labeled docetaxel stimulated p53 phosphorylation in dose-dependent manner in chemosensitive HeLA Hep2 cells. In chemoresistant cells HeLa Hep2R, p53phosphorylation reached significant levels only at high employed docetaxel concentrations (100 nM and higher) (Fig. 7B). ^{131}I-docetaxel induced a massive dose-dependent p53 phosphorylation in chemosensitive cells, with the maximum response being observed at 100 nM concentration. Further concentrations (500 and 1000 nM) had an opposite effect on p53 status in HeLa Hep2 cells (Fig. 7). In case of chemoresistant cells, p53 phosphorylation after treatment with ^{131}I-docetaxel was increased; however, there was no difference between lower treatment concentrations (1 – 10 nM). The maximum effect was recorded at 100 nM concentration after which a dose-dependent decline in p53 phosphorylation was noticed.

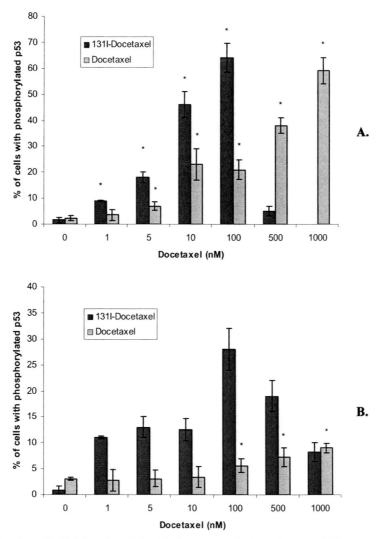

Figure 7. Activation of p53 (phosphorylation) in human cervical carcinoma cell lines treated with non-labeled and radiolabeled docetaxel (0- 1000 nM) during 12 hours as determined by immunohistochemistry, (A) chemosensitive HeLa Hep2 cells (B) chemoresistant HeLa Hep2R cells. Values represent means ± SD of at least three experiments. *P<0.05 with one way-Anova test and Dunnett's post test for multiple comparisons. In HeLa Hep2R cells all concentrations of radiolabeled docetaxel produced a significant increase in p53 phosphorylation as compared with control.

Activation of caspase-3, one of the major apoptosis executioner enzymes, is regarded as a hallmark of this type of cell death. In chemosensitive cervical cancer cells, exposure to radiolabeled docetaxel or non-labeled docetaxel led to a significant activation of caspase-3 already at the lowest treatment concentrations (Fig. 8A). While the maximum effect after non-labeled docetaxel was reached at the highest concentrations (1000 nM), dose-response curve of ^{131}I-docetaxel was shifted to the left. Similar results were recorded in chemoresistant cervical carcinoma cells too (Fig. 8B).

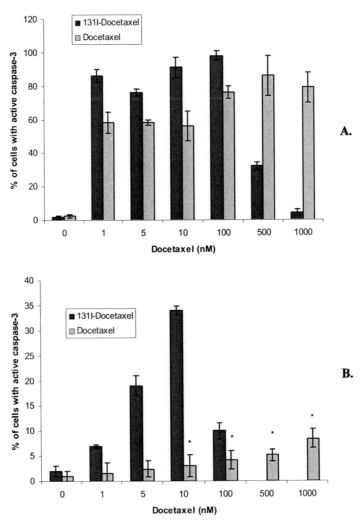

Figure 8. Activation of caspase-3 in human cervical carcinoma cell lines treated with non-labeled and radiolabeled docetaxel (0- 1000 nM) during 24 hours as determined by immunohistochemistry, (A) chemosensitive HeLa Hep2 cells (B) chemoresistant HeLa Hep2R cells. Values represent means ± SD of at least three experiments. *P<0.05 with one way-Anova test and Dunnett's post test for multiple comparisons. In HeLa Hep2 cells all docetaxels concentrations were significant in comparison to controls. In HeLa Hep2R cells all radiolabeled docetaxel concentrations (besides 500 and 1000 nM) were significant in comparison to controls.

4. DISCUSSION

In locally advanced or recurrent carcinoma of the uterine cervix, the established treatment strategies include radiation and/or chemotherapy. Still, the vast majority of such cervical cancers do not respond well to these individual treatment modalities and therefore new therapeutic strategies are sought to improve the survival rate and quality of life of thus affected patients [4].

Combining several treatment approaches in medical management of persistent or invasive cervical carcinoma may be advantageous due to several reasons. Firstly, combinations of factors with various cytostatic or cytotoxic mechanisms may suppress more efficiently cancer cell growth and induce cell demise. Furthermore, by acting on different targets and intracellular signaling pathways, such a combined strategy is more likely to avoid or bypass resistance of malignant cell populations regardless of its inherent or acquired nature. Secondly, active modulation of cell death promoting as well as suppressing signaling cascades may positively influence the total clinical response. Thirdly, mutually potentiating anti-tumor effects and overall higher cytotoxicity of combined modality treatments allow the significant reduction of dosing, thereby reducing side effects and improving their tolerance .

Amongst combined strategies, post-surgical chemoradiation has received much clinical attention despite its relatively limited curative potential [12]. Generally, ever since the discovery of curative effects of radiation in the treatment of tumors, its position in the treatment of many tumors including cervical cancer is well established [4]. Ionizing radiation induces many changes in exposed cell populations including single and double DNA breaks [18], the cleavage of the membrane-bound sphingomyelin [19] or production of ceramide [20]. Following the exposure to radiation, cells arrest in G_1, S and G_2 phases of the cell cycle which keeps them from undergoing mitotic cell divisions. Depending on the dose, tumor cells are thus at least partially synchronized and their accumulation (in particular in G_2/M) makes them a good target for the second radiation dose with more efficacious proapoptic effect [21]. Radiation-induced cell death-apoptosis occurs mostly via modulation of p53 pathway but some other mechanisms such as dowregulation of Bcl-2 have been reported as well [20,22]. Radiosensitivity of tumor cells depends on several factors including cell cycle position, cell cycle progression as well as intact DNA-damage sensing and repair mechanisms along with accurately timed and executed death signalling pathways [21].

Considering radiation sensitivity, cells synchronized and arrested in G_1 and G_2/M phases of the cell cycle represent an ideal target for radiation therapy. Therefore, the use of chemicals which induce cell cycle arrest in the above-mentioned phases might have a positive effect on the overall therapeutic response. One potent group of so called radiosensitisers are taxanes [16].

Docetaxel is a potent microtubule depolymerization inhibitor which is used in the treatment of many solid tumors, either in a single or combined approach [13,23]. The cytotoxic and proapoptotic effect of docetaxel on cancer cells is very complex and involves a large number of genes, intracellular signals and pathways. Docetaxel has been reported to arrest cells in G_2/M phase and induce apoptosis via p53 cascade [24]. Also, the roles of Bcl-2 and Bax genes in this process have been recognized [25]. In addition, due to its synchronization ability, docetaxel may be used as radiosensitizing agent too [26].

In our present work we wanted to examine cytotoxicity and cell death-inducing potential of ^{131}I-docetaxel and compare its effects with non-labeled docetaxel on chemosensitive and chemoresistant cervical cancer cell lines during 48 hours of treatment. Unlike an established concept of concurrent chemoradiotherapy where drugs are given prior or after radioation doses to enhance the efficacy of the treatment in terms of elimination of as many malignant cell cells as possible and preventing the clonogenic expansion of surviving ones, we present here a chemical which shows both radiation as well as antimicrotubular activity simultaneously. We found that in comparison to non-labeled docetaxel, ^{131}I-docetaxel - induced cytotoxicity was much more significant at both 24 hours and 48 hours treatment intervals. Furthermore, ^{131}I-docetaxel potently inbited the growth and proliferation of both employed cell lines which was not the case of non-labeled docetaxel whose effects on chemoresistant HeLa Hep2R cells were retarded and showed at the highest concentrations (500 and 100 nM) at 48 hours of treatment only (Fig. 2). These initial results are well in line with other reports showing potentiation of cytotoxicity in concurrent chemoradiation involving docetaxel [26,27,28]. However, since in our experimental model radiation and chemical inhibition of microtubules were meant to act simultaneously and not sequentially, we wanted to explore their potential interactions more deeply.

Therefore, to investigate molecular events and signals preceding and underlying observed cytotoxicity of both chemicals, first we folowed the morphology of treated cell populations. The photodocumentation (dynamic and sequential) revealed that non-labeled and radiolabeled docetaxel-treated chemosensitive cells displayed the typical features of apoptosis, i.e. cell rounding, formation of blebs and final shrinkage followed by secondary necrosis [29]. The spatial and temporal course of cell death were heterogeneous in individual cells and depended on the employed treatment concentration. In chemoresistant cells, docetaxel induced only a minor morphological changes during 48 hours of treatment. On the other hand, radiolabeled docetaxel-induced changes in chemoresistant cells comprised cell vacuolization, random cell shrinkage and a rather chaotic cell fragmentation with the absence of blebbing – the hallmarks of necrosis or necrosis-like cell death. The observed asynchronous behaviour of cells after the treatment with both chemicals in two cell lines might be explainable by a varying distribution of the cell cycle phases in individual cells and is supported by a fact that even synchronized tumor cell populations tend to display kinetic heterogeneity [30]. Converesely, docetaxel and radiation were reported to arrest cells in the particular cell cycle phases, thereby potentiating their cytotoxic activities [18,27,31]. In our experimental model of chemosensitive cells, both non-labeled and radiolabeled docetaxel induced time- and dose-dependent accumulation of cells in G_2/M phase which reached maximum at 36 hours of treatment (Fig. 4), with docetaxel being more potent (68% of cells compared to 48% after radiolabeled docetaxel). The situation was reversed in chemoresistant cells where the synchronization inceased in cells treated with radiolabeled docetaxel while oscillating (11 – 22%) in case of non-labeled docetaxel. Together, our results show that in sensitive cervical cancer cell line HeLa Hep2 antimicrotubular chemical (docetaxel) with intrinsic radioactivity is less capable of arresting cell in G_2/M phase than docetaxel while in chemoresistant cell line HeLa Hep2R radiation combined with antimicrotubular activity works better than antimicrotubular agent alone. We propose here that when administered simultaneously, combined DNA-damaging and antimicrotubular activity would achieve much more extensive alterations in exposed cells, thereby preventing them from entry into the cell cycle arrest and inducing them into cell death signalling instead. On the other hand, when one of the employed inhibiting effects does not work (chemoresistance or potentially radioresistance), arresting in the particular phase becomes more likely.

Ionizing radiation-specific effects on DNA in exposed cells are mostly responsible for cell cycle arrest and later cell death [18]. In order to determine the extent of DNA breaks in our experimental model, we estimated DNA damage by means single cell electrophoresis-comet assay. We found a dose-dependent increase in DNA strand breaks in both ^{131}I-docetaxel treated cell lines. The extent of DNA damage was significantly higher than in non-labeled docetaxel treated cells and in ionizing radiation only treated cells (data no shown). Thus indirectly, these results seem to point at mutually synergistic DNA-damaging effects of radiation and docetaxel. In suport of this notion, in non-labeled docetaxel treated chemosensitive cells an increase in numbers of cells with DNA breaks was noted at higher employed doses. Furthermore, in chemoresistant HeLa Hep2R cells where non-labeled docetaxel had only a little DNA-damaging effect, the percentage of cells with DNA breaks was lower after exposure to ^{131}I-docetaxel in comparison to radiation (unpublished observations). There have been reports about docetaxel-induced DNA strand breaks (single and double) in some experimental systems although no definite explanation for this phenomenon has been suggested [28]. Nevertheless, so far, no information is available regarding docetaxel associated modulation of DNA damage promoted by ionizing radiation when administered simultaneously. One may speculate that the simultaneous delivery of radiation and particular chemical insult is synergistically efective only if in tumor cells a certain damage threshold is reached. Indeed, it is a problem given the fact that combined treatment is often indicated in chemoresistant or radioresistant cell populations where this threshold is invariably increased. On the other hand, it is also possible that the suppressing effect of docetaxel on radiation incurred DNA damage was false because newly generated DNA lesions were concomitantly repaired. We cannot totally reject this possibility as (1) we did not carry out a detailed kinetic analysis of DNA damage and (2) we did not check the rate of DNA synthesis which might have informed us about putative DNA repir processes. It would also be interesting to see whether similar effects would occur in other cervical carcinoma cell lines, and in particular in radioresistant ones.

The ultimate goal of any antineoplastic therapy is a fast and efficient elimination of malignant cell populations. The most preferred way of eliminating these cells occurs by apoptosis; however some other types of cell death may be involved too [32]. Proapoptic effects of ionizing radiation are nowadays well established; there is ample evidence from various in vitro as well as in vivo studies that DNA strand breaks activate intracellular death signalling mainly via p53 pathway [22]. In addition, this pathway apparently integrates other proapoptotic signals too as was manifested in numerous models including, among others, those examining apoptosis induced by microtubule-inhibiting taxanes [33]. Considering the importance of p53 in cellular response to radiation and/or docetaxel, we detected the active protein p53 in HeLa Hep2 cervical cancer cell lines exposed to non-labeled and ^{131}I-docetaxel. As anticipated, both docetaxels induced p53 phosphorylation in chemosensitive cancer cells detectable at 12h of treatment albeit in a different manner. While non-labeled docetaxel acted mostly dose-dependently, ^{131}I-docetaxel produced the maximum effect at 100 nM concentration, with a severe decline in cells positive for phosphorylated p53 at higher concentrations. Based on these observations we may assume that the combination of antimicrotubular effect and DNA-damaging activity of radiolabeled docetaxel significantly activates p53 pathway in exposed cervical cancer cells. Furtheremore, beyond threshold concentrations of ^{131}I-docetaxel (in this case >100 nM) induce changes in signalling involving p53 which are either (1) much faster and occur very early, i.e. at first hours of treatment or (2) the extent of cellular damage is too large and proapoptic cascades are suppressed in favour of non-scheduled cell death such as necrosis. In chemoresistant cell line, docetaxel had a less significant effect on p53 than ^{131}I-docetaxel which induced significant p53 phosphorylation (maximum - 28% of cells at 100 nM concentration) but in a much more limited way.

In order to verify the type of cell death induced by docetaxels in both cell lines, we detected the presence of active caspase-3, an important apoptosis-execution enzyme. In docetaxel treated cells, activation of caspase-3 was dose dependent and occurred in both chemosensitive and chemoresistant cell lines although in chemoresistant cells the highest treatment concentrations were necessary to activate this enzyme in a significant number of cells. In the cell lines exposed to ^{131}I-docetaxel, activation of caspase-3 was maximal at 100 nM (chemosensitive cells) and 10 nM (chemoresistant cells), respectively. Still, in chemoresistant cells, only 30% of cells exhibited the presence of active caspase-3 while in chemosensitive cells almost 100% positivity was recorded. These results suggest that apoptosis is a mode of cell death induced by docetaxels in cervical carcinoma cell lines HeLa Hep2 and HeLa Hep2R. Still, ^{131}I-docetaxel likely induced some other type of cell death too as at higher treatment concentrations caspase-3 positivity was significantly lower and morphology of cells was different from lower concentrations treated cell populations.

Several studies have indicated that besides apoptosis docetaxel induces other cell death types too [15,34]. This appears to be a case here; however, our observed weak activation of caspase-3 after higher concentrations of ^{131}I-docetaxel may not be a definite proof of other type of cell death because of at least two reasons. Firstly, there are reports showing caspase-independent apoptosis in a variety of experimental models [35,36]. Secondly, kinetics of activation of caspase-3 might show a specific time profile, with its peak activity and decline occurring in a tight time frame. We do believe that both the stated arguments may hold true but, on the other hand, our morphological analysis as well as specific changes in mitochondria (not published results) in exposed cells argue for the presence of non-classical apoptosis in the treated cells. Considering thus presented evidence, we are planning to carry out further studies to elucidate the nature of this type of cell death in near future.

5. CONCLUSION

In conclusion, we found that that ^{131}I-docetaxel cytotoxicity and proapoptic activity towards chemosensitive and chemoresistant cervical cancer cell lines HeLa Hep2 is more significant that of docetaxel during 48h of treatment. ^{131}I-docetaxel therefore represents a unique combination of antineoplastic agent with radio and chemical activity which may be worth of further investigation both in vitro as well as in vivo.

6. ACKNOWLEDGMENT

This work was supported by Ministry of Education Research Project MSM 0021620820.

7. REFERENCES

[1]   Castellsague, X, Diaz, M, de Sanjose, S, Munoz, N, Herrero, R, Franceschi, S, Peeling, RW, Ashley, R, Smith, JS, Snijders, PJ, Meijer, CJ, Bosch, FX. Worldwide human papillomavirus etiology of cervical adenocarcinoma and its cofactors: implications for screening and prevention. *J Natl Cancer Inst*, 2006 98, 303-315.

[2]   Katz, IT, Wright, AA. Preventing cervical cancer in the developing world. *N Engl J Med*, 2006 354, 1110.

[3]   Sundar, S, Horne, A, Kehoe, S. Cervical cancer. *Clin Evid*, 2005 2285-2292.

[4]   Tambaro, R, Scambia, G, Di Maio, M, Pisano, C, Barletta, E, Iaffaioli, VR, Pignata, S. The role of chemotherapy in locally advanced, metastatic and recurrent cervical cancer. *Crit Rev Oncol Hematol*, 2004 52, 33-44.

[5]   Dreyer, G, Snyman, LC, Mouton, A, Lindeque, BG. Management of recurrent cervical cancer. *Best Pract Res Clin Obstet Gynaecol*, 2005 19, 631-644.

[6]   Rojas-Espaillat, LA, Rose, PG. Management of locally advanced cervical cancer. *Curr Opin Oncol*, 2005 17, 485-492.

[7]   Kuzuya, K. Chemoradiotherapy for uterine cancer: current status and perspectives. *Int J Clin Oncol*, 2004 9, 458-470.

[8]   Green, J, Kirwan, J, Tierney, J, Vale, C, Symonds, P, Fresco, L, Williams, C, Collingwood, M. Concomitant chemotherapy and radiation therapy for cancer of the uterine cervix. *Cochrane Database Syst Rev*, 2005 CD002225.

[9]   Peters, WA, 3rd, Liu, PY, Barrett, RJ, 2nd, Stock, RJ, Monk, BJ, Berek, JS, Souhami, L, Grigsby, P, Gordon, W, Jr., Alberts, DS. Concurrent chemotherapy and pelvic radiation therapy compared with pelvic radiation therapy alone as adjuvant therapy after radical surgery in high-risk early-stage cancer of the cervix. *J Clin Oncol*, 2000 18, 1606-1613.

[10] Green, JA, Kirwan, JM, Tierney, JF, Symonds, P, Fresco, L, Collingwood, M, Williams, CJ. Survival and recurrence after concomitant chemotherapy and radiotherapy for cancer of the uterine cervix: a systematic review and meta-analysis. *Lancet*, 2001 358, 781-786.

[11] Chauvergne, J, Lhomme, C, Rohart, J, Heron, JF, Ayme, Y, Goupil, A, Fargeot, P, David, M. Neoadjuvant chemotherapy of stage IIb or III cancers of the uterine cervix. Long-term results of a multicenter randomized trial of 151 patients. *Bull Cancer*, 1993 80, 1069-1079.

[12] Serkies, K, Jassem, J. Chemotherapy in the primary treatment of cervical carcinoma. *Crit Rev Oncol Hematol*, 2005 54, 197-208.

[13] Crown, J, O'Leary M. The taxanes: an update. *Lancet*, 2000 355, 1176-1178.

[14] Jordan, MA, Wilson, L. Microtubules and actin filaments: dynamictargets for cancer chemotherapy. *Curr Opin Cell Biol*, 1998 10, 123-130.

[15] Morse, DL, Gray, H, Payne, CM, Gillies, RJ. Docetaxel induces cell death through mitotic catastrophe in human breast cancer cells. *Mol Cancer Ther*, 2005 4, 1495-1504.

[16] Wenz, F, Greiner, S, Germa, F, Mayer, K, Latz, D, Weber, KJ. Radiochemotherapy with paclitaxel: synchronization effects and the role of p53. *Strahlenther Onkol*, 1999 175 Suppl 3, 2-6.

[17] Lawrence, TS, Blackstock, AW,McGinn, C. The mechanism of action of radiosensitization of conventional chemotherapeutic agents. *Semin Radiat Oncol*, 2003 13, 13-21.

[18] Warters, RL. Radiation-induced apoptosis in a murine T-cell hybridoma. *Cancer Res*, 1992 52, 883-890.

[19] Kolesnick, RN, Haimovitz-Friedman, A, Fuks, Z. The sphingomyelin signal transduction pathway mediates apoptosis for tumor necrosis factor, Fas, and ionizing radiation. *Biochem Cell Biol*, 1994 72, 471-474.

[20] Chen, M, Quintans, J, Fuks, Z, Thompson, C, Kufe, DW, Weichselbaum, RR. Suppression of Bcl-2 messenger RNA production may mediate apoptosis after ionizing radiation, tumor necrosis factor alpha, and ceramide. *Cancer Res*, 1995 55, 991-994.

[21] Pawlik, TM, Keyomarsi, K. Role of cell cycle in mediating sensitivity to radiotherapy. *Int J Radiat Oncol Biol Phys*, 2004 59, 928-942.

[22] Fei, P, El-Deiry, WS. P53 and radiation responses. *Oncogene*, 2003 22, 5774-5783.

[23] Roth, AD, Ajani, J. Docetaxel-based chemotherapy in the treatment of gastric cancer. *Ann Oncol*, 2003 14 Suppl 2, 41-44.

[24] Chang, JT, Chang, GC, Ko, JL, Liao, HY, Liu, HJ, Chen, CC, Su, JM, Lee, H, Sheu, GT. Induction of tubulin by docetaxel is associated with p53 status in human non small cell lung cancer cell lines. *Int J Cancer*, 2006 118, 317-325.

[25] Wang, LG, Liu, XM, Kreis, W, Budman, DR. The effect of antimicrotubule agents on signal transduction pathways of apoptosis: a review. *Cancer Chemother Pharmacol*, 1999 44, 355-361.

[26] Amorino, GP, Hamilton, VM, Choy, H. Enhancement of radiation effects by combined docetaxel and carboplatin treatment in vitro. *Radiat Oncol Investig*, 1999 7, 343-352.

[27] Creane, M, Seymour, CB, Colucci, S, Mothersill, C. Radiobiological effects of docetaxel (Taxotere): a potential radiation sensitizer. *Int J Radiat Biol*, 1999 75, 731-737.

[28] Araki, S, Miyagi, Y, Kawanishi, K, Yamamoto, J, Hongo, A, Kodama, J, Yoshinouchi, M, Kudo, T. Neoadjuvant treatment with docetaxel and the effects of irradiation for human ovarian adenocarcinoma and cervical squamous cell carcinoma in vitro. *Acta Med Okayama*, 2002 56, 13-18.

[29] Rudolf, E, Cervinka, M. Membrane blebbing in cancer cells treated with various apoptotic inducers. *Acta Medica (Hradec Kralove)*, 2005 48, 29-34.

[30] Tannock, I. Cell kinetics and chemotherapy: a critical review. *Cancer Treat Rep*, 1978 62, 1117-1133.

[31] Gallo, D, Ferlini, C, Distefano, M, Cantelmo, F, Gaggini, C, Fattorossi, A, Riva, A, Bombardelli, E,Proietti, E, Mancuso, S, Scambia, G. Anti-tumour activity of a panel of taxanes toward a cellular model of human cervical cancer. *Cancer Chemother Pharmacol*, 2000 45, 127-132.

[32] Blagosklonny, MV. Cell death beyond apoptosis. *Leukemia*, 2000 14, 1502-1508.

[33] Mollinedo, F, Gajate, C. Microtubules, microtubule-interfering agents and apoptosis. *Apoptosis*, 2003 8, 413-450.

[34] Oktem, G, Karabulut, B, Selvi, N, Sezgin, C, Sanli, UA, Uslu, R, Yurtseven, ME, Omay, SB. Differential effects of doxorubicin and docetaxel on nitric oxide production and inducible nitric oxide synthase expression in MCF-7 human breast cancer cells. *Oncol Res*, 2004 14, 381-386.

[35] Ahn, HJ, Kim, YS, Kim, JU, Han, SM, Shin, JW, Yang, HO. Mechanism of taxol-induced apoptosis in human SKOV3 ovarian carcinoma cells. *J Cell Biochem*, 2004 91, 1043-1052.

[36] Kim, R, Emi, M, Tanabe, K, Uchida, Y, Arihiro, K. The role of apoptotic or nonapoptotic cell death in determining cellular response to anticancer treatment. *Eur J Surg Oncol*, 2006 32, 269-277.

INDEX

H

I

J

K

L

M

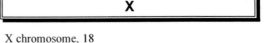

Z